BLUEPRINTS
OBSTETRICS &
GYNECOLOGY

Third Edition

BLUEPRINTS
OBSTETRICS &
GYNECOLOGY

Third Edition

Tamara L. Callahan, MD, MPP
Clinical Instructor in Obstetrics, Gynecology, and Reproductive Biology
Harvard Medical School
Attending Obstetrician/Gynecologist
Department of Obstetrics and Gynecology
Brigham and Women's Hospital
Boston, Massachusetts

Aaron B. Caughey, MD, MPP, MPH
Clinical Instructor in Maternal-Fetal Medicine
Department of Obstetrics and Gynecology
University of California, San Francisco
San Francisco, California
Doctoral Candidate, Health Services and Policy Analysis
University of California, Berkeley
Berkeley, California

Linda J. Heffner, MD, PhD
Associate Professor of Obstetrics, Gynecology, and Reproductive Biology
Harvard Medical School
Chief, Maternal-Fetal Medicine
Department of Obstetrics and Gynecology
Brigham and Women's Hospital
Boston, Massachusetts

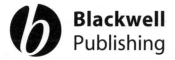

Blackwell
Publishing

© 2004 by Blackwell Publishing

Blackwell Publishing, Inc., 350 Main Street, Malden, Massachusetts 02148-5018, USA
Blackwell Publishing Ltd, 9600 Garsington Road, Oxford OX4 2DQ, UK
Blackwell Science Asia Pty Ltd, 550 Swanston Street, Carlton South, Victoria 3053, Australia
Blackwell Verlag GmbH, Kurfürstendamm 57, 10707 Berlin, Germany

03 04 05 06 5 4 3 2 1

ISBN: 1-4051-0331-0

Library of Congress Cataloging-in-Publication Data

Callahan, Tamara L.
    Blueprints obstetrics & gynecology / Tamara L. Callahan, Aaron B. Caughey ; faculty
advisor, Linda J. Heffner. — 3rd ed.
        p. ; cm. — (Blueprints)
    Rev. ed. of: Blueprints in obstetrics and gynecology / Tamara L. Callahan, Aaron B. Caughey.
2nd ed. c2001.
    Includes bibliographical references and index.
    ISBN 1-4051-0331-0 (pbk.)
    1. Obstetrics—Outlines, syllabi, etc.   2. Gynecology—Outlines, syllabi, etc.
    [DNLM: 1. Pregnancy Complications—Outlines.   2. Genital Diseases, Female—
Outlines. WQ 18.2 C156b 2003]   I. Title: Blueprints obstetrics and gynecology.   II. Title:
Obstetrics & gynecology.   III. Caughey, Aaron B.   IV. Callahan, Tamara L. Blueprints in
obstetrics and gynecology.   V. Title.   VI. Series.
    RG112.C35 2003
    618–dc21
                                                                                        2003006972

A catalogue record for this title is available from the British Library

Acquisitions: Nancy Anastasi Duffy
Development: Julia Casson
Production: Jennifer Kowalewski
Cover design: Hannus Design
Interior design: Mary McKeon
Typesetter: SNP Best-set Typesetter Ltd., Hong Kong
Printed and bound by Capital City Press in Vermont

For further information on Blackwell Publishing, visit our website:
www.blackwellpublishing.com

Notice: The indications and dosages of all drugs in this book have been recommended in the medical litera-
ture and conform to the practices of the general community. The medications described do not necessarily have
specific approval by the Food and Drug Administration for use in the diseases and dosages for which they are
recommended. The package insert for each drug should be consulted for use and dosage as approved by the
FDA. Because standards for usage change, it is advisable to keep abreast of revised recommendations, particularly those concerning new drugs.

Table of Contents

Contributing Authors

Sara Newmann, MD, MPH
Clinical Fellow in Obstetrics, Gynecology, and Reproductive Biology
Brigham and Women's Hospital
Massachusetts General Hospital
Boston, Massachusetts

Susan H. Tran, MD
Resident Physician
Kaiser San Francisco Hospital
San Francisco, California

Contributing Editors

Annette Chen, MD
Assistant Professor of Obstetrics and Gynecology
University of Massachusetts Medical School
Attending Physician in Gynecologic Oncology
University of Massachusetts Medical Center
Worcester, Massachusetts

Bruce B. Feinberg, MD
Assistant Professor of Obstetrics, Gynecology, and Reproductive Biology
Harvard Medical School
Attending Physician in Maternal-Fetal Medicine
Department of Obstetrics and Gynecology
Brigham and Women's Hospital
Boston, Massachusetts

Jing Wang, MD
Fellow, Gynecologic Oncology
Department of Obstetrics and Gynecology
University of California, Los Angeles
Los Angeles, California

Reviewers

Mila Felder, MD
Resident, Department of Emergency Medicine
Christ Hospital
Oak Lawn, Illinois

John Su, MD, MPH
Resident, Department of Family Medicine
Kaiser Permanente Los Angeles
Los Angeles, California

Raj Singh Rathee
Resident, Department of Obstetrics and Gynecology
Saginaw Cooperative Hospitals Inc
Saginaw, Michigan

Preface

In 1997, the first five books in the *Blueprints* series were published as board review for medical students, interns, and residents who wanted high-yield, accurate clinical content for USMLE Steps 2 & 3. Six years later, we are proud to report that the original books and the entire *Blueprints* brand of review materials have far exceeded our expectations.

The feedback we've received from our readers has been tremendously helpful and pivotal in deciding what direction the third edition of the core books will take. The student-to-student approach was highly acclaimed by our readers, so resident contributors have been recruited to ensure that the third edition of the series continues to provide content and an approach that made the original *Blueprints* a success. It was suggested that the review questions should reflect the current format of the Boards, so new board-format questions have been included in this edition with full explanations provided in the answers. Our readers asked for an enhanced art program, so a second color has been added to this edition to increase the usefulness of the figures and tables.

What we've also learned from our readers is that *Blueprints* is more than just Board review for USMLE, Steps 2 & 3. Students use the books during their clerkship rotations and subinternships. Residents studying for USMLE Step 3 often use the books for reviewing areas that were not their specialty. Students in physician assistant, nurse practitioner, and osteopath programs use *Blueprints* either as a companion or in lieu of review materials written specifically for their areas.

However you use *Blueprints*, we hope that you find the books in the series informative and useful. Your feedback and suggestions are essential to our continued success. Please send any comments you may have about this book or any book in the *Blueprints* series to *blue@blackwellpub.com*.

The Publisher
Blackwell Publishing

Acknowledgments

I would like to express my sincere and deep appreciation to Drs. Caughey, Newmann, Feinberg, Chen, Heffner, and Tran who gave liberally of their time and expertise to make this a book something of which we can all be proud. Without the extraordinary talent and commitment of these physicians, this project would not have been possible. This accomplishment is also credited in no small part to Michael, Mom, Dad, Jai, Tonya, Oneeka, and E—the incredible core of family and friends who lovingly and selflessly shepherded me through one of the most joyous and one of the darkest periods in my life. Their support was paramount to the success of this project and to my very survival. Lastly, I would like to acknowledge my mentors, Dr. William F. Crowley, Jr., and Dr. Nancy E. Oriol, and the many medical students and residents who have shared their input and enthusiasm with us along this exciting journey. It has been a privilege to be a small part of their never-ending learning experience.

Tamara L. Callahan, MD, MPP

I would like to acknowledge and extend my thanks to everyone involved in the third edition of our book, most important my coauthors and editors, Drs. Callahan, Newmann, and Tran as well as those involved in the first two editions, Drs. Chen, Feinberg, Wang, and Heffner and the staff at Blackwell Publishing. I would also like to thank my colleagues and friends for the supportive environment in which I work including the residents, faculty in the departments of Obstetrics and Gynecology at UCSF, and the Brigham and Women's Hospital, particularly Drs. Washington, Norton, Kuppermann, Ames-Castro, Repke, Blatman, Norwitz, Robinson, Parer, Thiet, and Sandberg as well as the students, staff, and faculty at UC Berkeley's Health Services and Policy Analysis program and the Department of Economics, particularly Matthew Rabin and Jeff Holman. Finally, to my family, Bill, Carol, Ethan, Samara, Big & Mugsy, Nicole, and of course, Susan, whose continued patience and support during all of my projects keeps me on task and productive.

Aaron B. Caughey, MD, MPP, MPH

Abbreviations

3β-HSD	3β-hydroxysteroid dehydrogenase
5-FU	5-fluorouracil
17-OHP	17α-hydroxyprogesterone
ABG	arterial blood gas
ACTH	adrenocorticotropic hormone
AD	autosomal dominant
ADH	antidiuretic hormone
AED	antiepileptic drug
AFE	amniotic fluid embolus
AFI	amniotic fluid index
AFLP	acute fatty liver of pregnancy
AFP	α-fetoprotein
AGUS	atypical glandular cells of undetermined significance
AIDS	aquired immunodeficiency syndrome
ALT	alanine transaminase
AMA	advanced maternal age
APA	antiphospholipid antibody
AR	autosomal recessive
ARDS	adult respiratory distress syndrome
AROM	artificial rupture of membranes
ART	assisted reproductive technology
ASC	atypical squamous cells
ASC-H	atypical squamous cells cannot exclude high-grade squamous intraepithelial lesion
ASC-US	artypical squamous cells of undetermined significance
AST	aspartate transaminase
AV	arteriovenous
AZT	zidovudine
β-hCG	beta human chorionic gonadotropin
BID	twice a day
BP	blood pressure
BPP	biophysical profile
BUN	blood urea nitrogen
BV	bacterial vaginosis
CAH	congenital adrenal hyperplasia
CBC	complete blood count
CF	cystic fibrosis
CHF	congestive heart failure
CIN	cervical intraepithelial neoplasia
CKC	cold knife cone (biopsy)
CMV	cytomegalovirus
CNS	central nervous system
CPD	cephalopelvic disproportion
CPK	creatine phosphokinase
CRS	congenital rubella syndrome
CSF	cerebrospinal fluid
CT	computed tomography (cat scan)
CVA	cerebrovascular accident
CVAT	costovertebral angle tenderness
CVD	collagen vascular disorders
CVS	chorionic villus sampling
CXR	chest x-ray
DA	developmental age
D&C	dilation and curettage
D&E	dilation and evacuation
DCIS	ductal carcinoma in situ
DES	diethylstilbestrol
DEXA	dual-energy x-ray absorptiometry
DHEA	dehydroepiandrosterone
DHEAS	dehydroepiandrosterone sulfate
DHT	dihydrotestosterone
DIC	disseminated intravascular coagulation
DTRs	deep tendon reflexes
DUB	dysfunctional uterine bleeding
DVT	deep venous thrombosis
ECG	electrocardiogram
EDC	estimated date of confinement
EDD	estimated date of delivery
EFW	estimated fetal weight
EIF	echogenic intracardiac focus
ELISA	enzyme-linked immunosorbent assay
EMB	endometrial biopsy
EMG	electromyography
ESR	erythrocyte sedimentation rate
FAS	fetal alcohol syndrome
FH	fetal heart
FHR	fetal heart rate
FIGO	International Federation of Gynecology and Obstetrics
FIRS	fetal immune response syndrome
FISH	fluorescent in situ hybridization

FNA	fine-needle aspiration	IUI	intrauterine insemination
FSE	fetal scalp electrode	IUP	intrauterine pregnancy
FSH	follicle-stimulating hormone	IUPC	intrauterine pressure catheter
FTAABS	fluorescent treponemal antibody absorption	IUT	intrauterine transfusion
FTP	failure to progress	IVC	inferior vena cava
G	gravidity	IVF	in vitro fertilization
GA	gestational age	IVP	intravenous pyelography
GBS	group B streptococcus	JVP	jugular venous pressure
GDM	gestational diabetes mellitus	KB	Kleihauer-Betke test
GFR	glomerular filtration rate	KOH	potassium hydroxide
GH	gestational hypertension	KUB	kidneys/ureter/bladder (x-ray)
GI	gastrointestinal	LBW	low birth weight
GIFT	gamete intrafallopian transfer	LCHAD	long-chain hydroxyacyl-CoA dehydrogenase
GLT	glucose loading test	LCIS	lobular carcinoma in situ
GnRH	gonadotropin-releasing hormone	LDH	lactate dehydrogenase
GSI	genuine stress incontinence	LDL	low-density lipoprotein
GTD	gestational trophoblastic disease	LEEP	loop electrosurgical excision procedure
GTT	glucose tolerance test	LFT	liver function test
GU	genitourinary	LGA	large for gestational age
HAART	highly active antiretroviral therapy	LGV	lymphogranuloma venereum
Hb	hemoglobin	LIQ	lower inner quadrant
HbH	hemoglobin H disease	LH	luteinizing hormone
hCG	human chorionic gonadotropin	Lletz	large loop excision of the transformation zone
hCS	human chorionic somatomammotropin	LMP	last menstrual period
Hct	hematocrit	LOQ	lower outer quadrant
HDL	high-density lipoprotein	LOT	left occiput transverse
HELLP	hemolysis, elevated liver enzymes, low platelets	LSIL	low-grade squamous intraepithelial lesion
HIV	human immunodeficiency virus	LTL	laparoscopic tubal ligation
HLA	human leukocyte antigen	Lytes	electrolytes
hMG	human menopausal gonadotropin	MAO	monoamine oxidase
HPI	history of present illness	MESA	microsurgical epididymal sperm aspiration
HPL	human placental lactogen		
HPV	human papillomavirus	MHATP	microhemagglutination assay for antibodies to *T. pallidum*
HR	heart rate		
HRT	hormone replacement therapy	MI	myocardial infarction
HSG	hysterosalpingography	MIF	müllerian inhibiting factor
HSIL	high-grade squamous intraepithelial lesion	MLK	myosin light-chain kinase
		MRI	magnetic resonance imaging
HSV	herpes simplex virus	MRKH	Mayer-Rokitansky-Kuster-Hauser (syndrome)
I&D	incision and drainage		
ICSI	intracytoplasmic sperm injection	MSAFP	maternal serum α-fetoprotein
ID/CC	identification and chief complaint	MTHFR	methyl tetrahydrofolate reductase
Ig	immunoglobulin	NPO	nil per os (nothing by mouth)
IM	intramuscular	NPV	negative predictive value
INH	isoniazid	NRFT	nonreassuring fetal testing
INR	International Normalized Ratio	NSAID	nonsteroidal anti-inflammatory drug
IUD	intrauterine device	NST	nonstress test
IUFD	intrauterine fetal demise or death	NSVD	normal spontaneous vaginal delivery
IUGR	intrauterine growth restricted	NT	nuchal translucency

NTD	neural tube defect	SERM	selective estrogen receptor modulators
OA	occiput anterior	SGA	small for gestational age
OCP	oral contraceptive pill	SHBG	sex hormone binding globulin
OCT	oxytocin challenge test	SIDS	sudden infant death syndrome
OI	ovulation induction	SLE	systemic lupus erythematosus
OP	occiput posterior	SPT	septic pelvic thrombophlebitis
OT	occiput transverse	SROM	spontaneous rupture of membranes
OTC	over-the-counter	SSRIs	selective seratonin reuptake inhibitors
P	parity	STD	sexually transmitted disease
PBS	peripheral blood smear	SUI	stress urinary incontinence
PCOD	polycystic ovarian disease	SVT	superficial vein thrombophlebitis
PCOS	polycystic ovarian syndrome	SVT	supraventricular tachycardia
PCR	polymerase chain reaction	TAB	therapeutic abortion
PDA	patent ductus arteriosus	TAC	transabdominal cerclage
PE	physical exam	TAHBSO	total abdominal hysterectomy and bilateral salpingo-oophorectomy
PE	pulmonary embolus		
PET	preeclampsia/toxemia	TBG	thyroid binding globulin
PFTs	pulmonary function tests	TENS	transcutaneous electrical nerve stimulation
PID	pelvic inflammatory disease		
PIH	pregnancy induced hypertension	TFTs	thyroid function tests
PMN	polymorphonuclear leukocyte	TIBC	total iron-binding capacity
PMOF	premature ovarian failure	TLC	total lung capacity
PMS	premenstrual syndrome	TNM	tumor/node/metastasis
PMTs	premenstrual tension syndrome	TOA	tubo-ovarian abscess
PO	per os (by mouth)	TOLAC	trial of labor after cesarean
POC	products of conception	TOV	transposition of the vessels
POF	premature ovarian failure	tPA	tissue plasminogen activator
PPCM	peripartum cardiomyopathy	TPAL	term, preterm, aborted, living
PPD	purified protein derivative	TRH	thyrotropin-releasing hormone
PPROM	preterm premature rupture of membranes	TSE	testicular sperm extraction
		TSH	thyroid-stimulating hormone
PPS	postpartum sterilization	TSI	thyroid-stimulating immunoglobulins
PPV	positive predictive value	TSS	toxic shock syndrome
PROM	premature rupture of membranes	TSST	toxic shock syndrome toxin
PSTT	placental site trophoblastic tumor	TTTS	twin-to-twin transfusion syndrome
PT	prothrombin time	UA	urinalysis
PTL	preterm labor	UAE	uterine artery embolization
PTT	partial thromboplastin time	UG	urogenital
PTU	propylthiouracil	UIQ	upper inner quadrant
PUBS	percutaneous umbilical blood sampling	UOQ	upper outer quadrant
		UPI	uteroplacental insufficiency
PUS	pelvic ultrasound	US	ultrasound
QD	each day	UTI	urinary tract infection
QID	four times a day	V/Q	ventilation/perfusion ratio
RBC	red blood cell	VAIN	vaginal intraepithelial neoplasia
RDS	respiratory distress syndrome	VBAC	vaginal birth after cesarean
ROM	rupture of membranes	V_D	volume of distribution
ROT	right occiput transverse	VDRL	Venereal Disease Research Laboratory
RPR	rapid plasma reagin	VIN	vulvar intraepithelial neoplasia
RR	respiratory rate	VLDL	very low density lipoprotein
SAB	spontaneous abortion	VS	vital signs
SCC	squamous cell carcinoma		

VSD	ventricular septal defect	XAFP	expanded maternal serum alpha fetoprotein (test)
VZIG	varicella zoster immune globulin		
VZV	varicella zoster virus	XR	x-ray
WBC	white blood cell	ZIFT	zygote intrafallopian tube transfer

Pregnancy and Prenatal Care

■ PREGNANCY

Pregnancy is the state of having products of conception implanted normally or abnormally in the uterus or occasionally elsewhere. Pregnancy is terminated by spontaneous or elective abortion or delivery. A myriad of physiologic changes occur in a pregnant woman, which affect every organ system.

Diagnosis

In a patient who has regular menstrual cycles and is sexually active, a period delayed by more than a few days to a week is suggestive of pregnancy. Even at this early stage, patients may exhibit signs and symptoms of pregnancy. The classic finding of "morning sickness" can begin this early and often continues through 12 to 16 weeks of gestation. On physical examination, a variety of findings indicate pregnancy (Table 1-1).

Many over-the-counter (OTC) urine pregnancy tests have a high sensitivity and will be positive around the time of the missed menstrual cycle. These urine tests and the hospital laboratory serum assays test for the beta subunit of human chorionic gonadotropin (β-hCG). This hormone produced by the placenta will rise to a peak of 100,000 mIU/mL by 10 weeks of gestation, decrease throughout the second trimester, and then level off at approximately 20,000 to 30,000 mIU/mL in the third trimester.

A viable pregnancy can be confirmed by ultrasound, which may show the gestational sac as early as 5 weeks, or at a β-hCG of 1500 to 2000 mIU/mL, and the fetal heart as soon as 6 weeks, or a β-hCG of 5000 to 6000 mIU/mL.

Terms and Definitions

From the time of fertilization until the pregnancy is 8 weeks along (10 weeks gestational age [GA]), the conceptus is called an embryo. After 8 weeks until the time of birth, it is designated a fetus. The term infant is used for the period between delivery and 1 year of age. Pregnancy is divided into trimesters. The first trimester lasts until 12 weeks but is also defined as up to 14 weeks GA, the second trimester from 12 to 14 until 24 to 28 weeks GA, and the third trimester from 24 to 28 weeks until delivery. An infant delivered prior to 24 weeks is considered to be previable, from 24 to 37 weeks is considered preterm, and from 37 to 42 weeks is considered term. A pregnancy carried beyond 42 weeks is considered postdate or postterm.

Gravidity (G) refers to the number of times a woman has been pregnant, and parity (P) refers to the number of pregnancies that led to a birth beyond 20 weeks GA or of an infant weighing more than 500 g. A more specific designation of pregnancy outcomes divides them into term and preterm deliveries, number of abortuses, and number of living children. This is known as the TPAL designation. A woman who has given birth to one set of preterm twins, one term infant, and with two miscarriages would be a G4 P1-1-2-3. A multiple gestation is just one delivery but obviously may change the number of living children by more than one. In this designation, abortuses includes both therapeutic and spontaneous abortions.

Dating of Pregnancy

The GA of a fetus is the age in weeks and days measured from the last menstrual period (LMP).

■ TABLE 1-1

Signs and Symptoms of Pregnancy

Signs

Bluish discoloration of vagina and cervix (Chadwick's sign)

Softening and cyanosis of the cervix at or after 4 weeks (Goodell's sign)

Softening of the uterus after 6 weeks (Ladin's sign)

Breast swelling and tenderness

Development of the linea nigra from umbilicus to pubis

Telangiectasias

Palmar erythema

Symptoms

Amenorrhea

Nausea and vomiting

Breast pain

Quickening—fetal movement

Developmental age (DA) is the number of weeks and days since fertilization. Because fertilization usually occurs about 14 days after the first day of the prior menstrual period, the GA is 2 weeks more than the DA.

Classically, **Nägele's rule** for calculating the **estimated date of confinement** (EDC), or estimated date of delivery (EDD), is to subtract 3 months from the LMP and add 7 days. Thus, a pregnancy with an LMP of 4/13/02 would have an EDC of 1/20/03. Exact dating uses an EDC calculated as 280 days after a certain LMP. If the date of ovulation is known, as in assisted reproductive technology (ART), the EDC can be calculated by adding 266 days. This dating can be confirmed and should be consistent with the examination of the uterine size at the first prenatal appointment.

With an uncertain LMP, ultrasound is often used to determine the EDC. Ultrasound has a level of uncertainty that increases during the pregnancy but it is rarely off by more than 7% to 8% at any GA. A safe rule of thumb is that the ultrasound should not differ from LMP dating by more than 1 week in the first trimester, 2 weeks in the second trimester, and 3 weeks in the third trimester. The dating done with crown-rump length in the first half of the first trimester is probably even more accurate, to within 3 to 5 days.

Other measures used to estimate gestational age include pregnancy landmarks such as auscultation of the fetal heart (FH) at 20 weeks by nonelectronic fetoscopy or at 10 weeks by Doppler ultrasound, as well as maternal awareness of fetal movement or "quickening," which occurs between 16 and 20 weeks.

Physiology of Pregnancy

Cardiovascular

During pregnancy, **cardiac output** increases by 30% to 50%. Most increases occur during the first trimester, with the maximum being reached between 20 and 24 weeks gestation and maintained until delivery. **Systemic vascular resistance** decreases during pregnancy, resulting in a fall in arterial blood pressure. This decrease is most likely due to the elevated progesterone leading to smooth muscle relaxation. There is a decrease in systolic blood pressure of 5–10 mm Hg and in diastolic blood pressure of 10–15 mm Hg that nadirs at week 24. Between 24 weeks gestation and term, blood pressure slowly returns to prepregnancy levels but should never exceed them.

Pulmonary

There is an increase of 30% to 40% in tidal volume (V_T) during pregnancy (Figure 1-1) despite the fact that the total lung capacity is decreased by 5% due to the elevation of the diaphragm. This increase in V_T decreases the expiratory reserve volume by about 20%. The increase in V_T with a constant respiratory rate leads to an increase in minute ventilation of 30% to 40%, which in turn leads to an increase in alveolar (PAo_2) and arterial (Pao_2) Po_2 levels and a decrease in $PAco_2$ and $Paco_2$ levels.

$Paco_2$ decreases to approximately 30 mm Hg by 20 weeks gestation from 40 mm Hg prepregnancy. This change leads to an increased CO_2 gradient between mother and fetus and is likely caused by elevated progesterone levels that either increase the respiratory system's responsiveness to CO_2 or act as a primary stimulant. Dyspnea of pregnancy occurs in 60% to 70% of patients. This is possibly secondary to decreased $Paco_2$ levels, increased V_T, or decreased total lung capacity (TLC).

Gastrointestinal

Nausea and vomiting occur in more than 70% of pregnancies. This has been termed **"morning sickness"** even though it can occur anytime throughout the day. These symptoms have been attributed to the

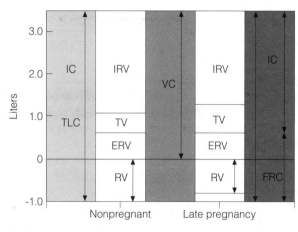

TLC–total lung capacity
VC–vital capacity
IC–inspiratory capacity
FRC–functional residual capacity
IRV–inspiratory reserve volume
TV–tidal volume
ERV–expiratory reserve
RV– residual volume

Figure 1-1 • Lung volumes in nonpregnant and pregnant women.

elevation in estrogen, progesterone, and hCG. The nausea and vomiting should routinely resolve by 14 to 16 weeks gestation. During pregnancy, the stomach has prolonged gastric emptying times, and the gastroesophageal sphincter has decreased tone. Together, these changes lead to reflux and possibly combine with decreased esophageal tone to cause ptyalism, or spitting, during pregnancy. The large bowel also has decreased motility, which leads to increased water absorption and constipation.

Renal

The kidneys actually increase in size and the ureters dilate during pregnancy, which may lead to increased rates of pyelonephritis. The glomerular filtration rate (GFR) increases by 50% early in pregnancy and is maintained until delivery. As a result of increased GFR, blood urea nitrogen and creatinine decrease by about 25%. An increase in the renin-angiotensin system leads to increased levels of aldosterone. This ultimately results in increased sodium resorption. However, plasma levels of sodium do not increase because of the simultaneous increase in GFR.

Hematology

Although the plasma volume increases by 50% in pregnancy, the red blood cell volume increases by only 20% to 30%, which leads to a decrease in the hematocrit. The white blood cell (WBC) count increases during pregnancy to a mean of 10.5 million/mL with a range of 6 to 16. During labor, stress may cause the WBC count to rise to over 20 million/mL. There is a slight decrease in the concentration of platelets, probably secondary to increased plasma volume and an increase in peripheral destruc-

tion. Although 7% to 8% of patients' platelets may be between 100 and 150 million/mL, a drop in the platelet count below 100 million/mL or over a short time period is not normal and should be investigated promptly.

Pregnancy is considered to be a hypercoagulable state, and the number of thromboembolic events increases. There are elevations in the levels of fibrinogen and factors VII–X. However, the actual clotting and bleeding times do not change. The increased rate of thromboembolic events in pregnancy may be secondary to an increase in venous stasis and vessel endothelial damage.

Endocrine

Pregnancy is a hyperestrogenic state. The increased estrogen is produced primarily by the placenta, with the ovaries contributing to a lesser degree. Unlike estrogen production in the ovaries, where estrogen precursors are produced in ovarian theca cells and transferred to the ovarian granulosa cells, estrogen in the placenta is derived from circulating plasma-borne precursors produced by the maternal adrenal glands. Fetal well-being has been correlated with maternal serum estrogen levels with low estrogen levels being associated with conditions such as fetal death and anencephaly.

The hormone hCG is composed of two dissimilar alpha and beta subunits. The alpha subunit of hCG is identical to the alpha subunits of luteinizing hormone (LH), follicle-stimulating hormone (FSH), and thyroid-stimulating hormone (TSH), whereas the beta subunits differ. The placenta produces hCG, which acts to maintain progesterone production by the corpus luteum. Levels of hCG double approximately every 48 hours during early pregnancy, reaching a peak at approximately 10 to 12 weeks, and thereafter declining to reach a steady state after week 15.

Human placental lactogen (hPL) is produced in the placenta and is important for ensuring a constant nutrient supply to the fetus. hPL, also known as human chorionic somatomammotropin (hCS), causes lipolysis with a concomitant increase in circulating free fatty acids. hPL also acts as an insulin antagonist, along with various other placental hormones, thereby having a diabetogenic effect. This leads to increased levels of insulin and protein synthesis.

Progesterone is produced by the corpus luteum during early pregnancy, after which time biosynthesis occurs primarily in the placenta. Progesterone precursors are derived from low-density-lipoprotein cholesterol and progesterone levels increase over the course of pregnancy. Progesterone causes relaxation of smooth muscle, which has multiple effects on the gastrointestinal, cardiovascular, and genitourinary systems.

High estrogen levels cause an increase in thyroid binding globulin (TBG). Placental hormones such as hCG may also have thyroid-stimulating properties that lead to an elevation in total T3 and T4. Together, these changes lead to a relatively euthyroid state, although free T3 and T4 levels may decrease slightly during pregnancy. Levels of prolactin are markedly increased during pregnancy. These levels paradoxically decrease after delivery but later increase in response to suckling.

Musculoskeletal and Dermatologic

The obvious change in the center of gravity during pregnancy can lead to a shift in posture and lower back strain. Numerous changes in the skin occur during pregnancy, including spider angiomata and palmar erythema secondary to increased estrogen levels and hyperpigmentation of the nipples, umbilicus, abdominal midline (the **linea nigra**), perineum, and face (**melasma or chloasma**) secondary to increased levels of α-melanocyte-stimulating hormone and the steroid hormones.

Nutrition

Nutritional requirements increase during pregnancy and breastfeeding. The average woman requires 2000 to 2500 kcal/day. The caloric requirement is increased by 300 kcal/day during pregnancy and by 500 kcal/day when breast-feeding. Most patients should gain between 20 and 30 pounds during pregnancy. Obese women are advised to gain less, between 15 and 20 pounds; thin women are advised to gain slightly more, 25 to 35 pounds.

In addition to the increased caloric requirements, there are increased nutritional requirements for protein, iron, folate, calcium, and other vitamins and minerals. The protein requirement increases from 60 g/day to 70 or 75 g/day. Recommended calcium intake is 1.5 g/day. Many patients develop iron deficiency anemia because of the increased demand on hematopoiesis both by the mother and the fetus. Folate requirements increase from 0.4 to 0.8 mg/day and are important in preventing neural tube defects.

All patients are advised to take prenatal vitamins during pregnancy. These are designed to compensate for the increased nutritional demands of pregnancy. Furthermore, any patient whose hematocrit falls during pregnancy is advised to increase iron intake with oral supplementation (Table 1-2).

KEY POINTS

1. A urine pregnancy test will often be positive at the time of the missed menstrual cycle.
2. Physiologic changes during pregnancy, mediated by the placental hormones, affect every organ system.
3. Cardiovascular changes include a decrease in systemic vascular resistance and blood pressure and a 50% rise in total blood volume.
4. Elevation in serum progesterone levels is responsible for smooth muscle relaxation in the vascular system, GI tract, and genitourinary system, leading to many of the concomitant physiologic changes.

◼ PRENATAL CARE

Prenatal visits are designed to screen for various complications of pregnancy and to educate the patient. They include a series of outpatient office visits that involve routine physical examinations and various screening tests that occur at different points in the prenatal care. Important issues of prenatal care include initial patient evaluation, routine patient evaluation, nutrition, disease states during the pregnancy, and preparing for the delivery.

■ TABLE 1-2

Recommended Daily Dietary Allowances for Nonpregnant, Pregnant, and Lactating Women

	Nonpregnant Women by Age					Pregnant Women	Lactating Women
	11–14	15–18	19–22	23–50	51+		
Energy (kcal)	2400	2100	2100	2000	1800	+300	+500
Protein (g)	44	48	46	46	46	+30	+20
Fat-soluble vitamins							
Vitamin A activity (RE)	800	800	800	800	800	1000	1200
(IU)	4000	4000	4000	4000	4000	5000	6000
Vitamin D (IU)	400	400	400	—	—	400	400
Vitamin E activity (IU)	12	12	12	12	12	15	15
Water-soluble vitamins							
Ascorbic acid (mg)	45	45	45	45	45	60	80
Folacin (µg)	400	400	400	400	400	800	600
Niacin (mg)	16	14	14	13	12	+2	+4
Riboflavin (mg)	1.3	1.4	1.4	1.2	1.1	+0.3	+0.5
Thiamin (mg)	1.2	1.1	1.1	1	1	+0.3	+0.3
Vitamin B_6 (mg)	1.6	2	2	2	2	2.5	2.5
Vitamin B_{12} (µg)	3	3	3	3	3	4	4
Minerals							
Calcium (mg)	1200	1200	800	800	800	1200	1200
Iodine (µg)	115	115	100	100	80	125	150
Iron (mg)	18	18	18	18	10	+18	18
Magnesium (mg)	300	300	300	300	300	450	450
Phosphorus (mg)	1200	1200	800	800	800	1200	1200
Zinc (mg)	15	15	15	15	15	20	25

Source: From Gabbe SG, Niebyl JR, and Simpsen JL, Obstetrics: Normal and Problem Pregnancies. 4th ed. New York: Churchill Livingstone, 2002:196.
Note: IU = International Unit.

Initial Visit

This is often the longest of the prenatal visits because it involves obtaining a complete history and doing a physical as well as a battery of initial laboratory tests. It should occur early in the first trimester, between 6 and 10 weeks, although occasionally patients will not present for their initial prenatal visit until later in their pregnancy.

History

The patient's history includes the present pregnancy, the last menstrual period, and symptoms during the pregnancy. After this, an obstetric history of prior pregnancies including date, outcome (e.g., SAB [spontaneous abortion], TAB [therapeutic abortion], term delivery), mode of delivery, length of time in labor and second stage, birth weight, and any complications. Finally, a complete medical, surgical, family, and social history should be obtained.

Physical Examination

A complete physical examination is performed, paying particular attention to the patient's prior medical and surgical history. The pelvic examination includes a Pap smear, unless one has been done in the past 6 months, and cultures for gonorrhea and chlamydia. On bimanual examination, the size of the uterus should be consistent with the gestational age from the LMP.

Diagnostic Evaluation

The panel of tests in the first trimester includes a complete blood count, primarily for hematocrit, blood type, antibody screen, rapid plasma reagin

(syphilis)

(RPR), rubella antibody screen, hepatitis B surface antigen, urinalysis, and urine culture. If a patient has no history of chickenpox, a titer for varicella zoster virus (VZV) antibodies is sent. A purified protein derivative (PPD) is usually placed during the first or second trimester. A urine pregnancy test should be sent if the patient is not entirely certain she is pregnant. If there has been any bleeding or cramping, a β-hCG level should be obtained. While there is some debate over the use of routine toxoplasma titers, they are often ordered as well. All patients are counseled about human immunodeficiency virus (HIV) and testing should be offered routinely (Table 1-3). In addition to this battery of tests, there are a variety of other screens offered to high-risk patients (Table 1-4).

Routine Prenatal Visits

On each follow-up prenatal care visit blood pressure, weight, urine dipstick, measurement of the uterus, and auscultation of the fetal heart are performed and assessed. Maternal blood pressure decreases during the first and second trimester and slowly returns to baseline during the third trimester; elevation may be a sign of preeclampsia. Maternal weight is followed serially throughout the pregnancy as a proxy for adequate nutrition. Also, large weight gains toward the end of pregnancy can be a sign of fluid retention and preeclampsia. Measurement of the uterine fundal height in centimeters corresponds roughly to the weeks of gestation. If the fundal height is progressively decreasing or is 3 cm less than gestational age,

an ultrasound is done to more accurately assess fetal growth. After 10 to 14 weeks, Doppler ultrasound is used to auscultate the fetal heart rate. Urine is routinely dipped for protein, glucose, blood, and leukocyte esterase. Protein may be indicative of preeclampsia, glucose of diabetes, and leukocyte esterase of urinary tract infection.

At each visit, the patient is asked about symptoms that indicate complications of pregnancy. These symptoms include vaginal bleeding, vaginal discharge or leaking of fluid, and urinary symptoms. In addition, after 20 weeks, patients are asked about contractions and fetal movement. Vaginal bleeding is a sign of miscarriage or ectopic pregnancy in the first trimester, and of placental abruption or previa as the pregnancy advances. Vaginal discharge may be a sign of infection or cervical change, whereas leaking fluid can indicate ruptured fetal membranes. While irregular (Braxton-Hicks) contractions are common throughout the third trimester, regular contractions more frequent than five or six per hour may be a sign of preterm labor and should be assessed. Changes in or absence of fetal movement should be evaluated by auscultation of the fetal heart in the previable fetus and with further testing such as a nonstress test or biophysical profile in the viable fetus.

First-Trimester Visits

During the first trimester—patients, particularly nulliparous women—need to be familiarized with pregnancy. The symptoms of pregnancy and what will occur at each prenatal visit should be reviewed. At the second prenatal visit, all of the initial labs should

TABLE 1-3		
Routine Tests in Prenatal Care		
Initial Visit and First Trimester	**Second Trimester**	**Third Trimester**
Hematocrit	MSAFP/triple screen	Hematocrit
Blood type and screen	Ultrasound	RPR
RPR	Amniocentesis in	GLT
Rubella antibody screen	AMA patients	Repeat gonorrhea
Hepatitis B surface antigen		and chlamydia
Gonorrhea culture		Chest x-ray if PPD + IP Group B
Chlamydia culture		strep culture
PPD		
Pap smear		
Urinalysis and culture		
VZV titer in patients with no history of exposure		
HIV offered		

(handwritten annotation above Second Trimester header: "α feto protein"; and below AMA patients: "advanced maternal age")

■ TABLE 1-4

Initial Screens in Specific High-Risk Groups

High-Risk Group	Specific Test
African American	Sickle-cell prep/Hgb electrophoresis
Age 35 or older at time of EDC	Prenatal genetics referral
Prior gestational diabetic, family history of diabetes, Hispanic, Native American, Southeast Asian	Glucose loading test
Pregestational diabetic, unsure dates, recurrent miscarriages	Dating sonogram
Hypertension, renal disease, pregestational diabetic, prior preeclampsia, renal transplant, SLE	24 hour urine collection for protein and creatinine clearance
Pregestational diabetic, prior cardiac disease, hypertension	Electrocardiogram (ECG)
Pregestational diabetic	Hgb A1C, ophthalmology for eye exam
Graves' disease	Thyroid-stimulating immunoglobulins
All thyroid disease	TSH, possibly free T4
Systemic lupus erythematosus (SLE)	Anti-Rho, anti-La antibodies

be reviewed with the patient. Patients with poor weight gain or decreased caloric intake secondary to nausea and vomiting may be referred to a nutritionist. Patients treated for infections noted at the initial prenatal visit should be cultured for test of cure.

Second-Trimester Visits

During the second trimester, much of the screening for genetic and congenital abnormalities is done. This allows a patient to obtain an elective termination if there are abnormalities. Screening for **maternal serum alpha fetoprotein** (MSAFP) is usually performed between 15 and 18 weeks. An elevation in MSAFP is correlated with an increased risk of neural tube defects and a decrease is seen in some aneuploidies including Down syndrome. The sensitivity of aneuploidy screening is augmented using β-hCG and estriol along with MSAFP called the **triple screen**. Between 18 and 20 weeks gestation, most patients are offered a screening ultrasound. This provides the opportunity to do a thorough fetal anatomic survey. Also noted are the amniotic fluid volume, placental location, and gestational age.

The fetal heart is usually first heard during the second trimester and the first fetal movement, or "quickening," is felt late in the second trimester. Most patients have resolution of their nausea and vomiting by the second trimester, although some continue with these symptoms throughout their pregnancy. Because the risk of spontaneous abortions decreases after 12 weeks of gestation, childbirth classes and tours of the labor floor are usually offered in the second and third trimesters.

Third-Trimester Visits

During the third trimester, the fetus is viable. Patients will begin to have occasional Braxton Hicks contractions and, if these contractions become regular, the cervix is examined to rule out preterm labor. Prenatal visits increase to every 2 to 3 weeks from 28 to 36 weeks and then to every week after 36 weeks. In addition, patients who are Rh negative should receive RhoGAM at 28 weeks. Beyond 32 to 34 weeks Leopold's maneuvers (Figure 3-1) are performed to determine fetal presentation. Beyond 37 weeks, which is considered term, the cervix is usually examined at each visit.

Third-Trimester Labs

At 27 to 29 weeks, the third-trimester labs are ordered. These consist of the hematocrit, RPR, and **glucose loading test** (GLT). At this time, the hematocrit is getting close to its nadir. Patients with a hematocrit below 32% to 33% (hemoglobin less than 11 mg/dL) are usually started on iron supplementation. Because this will cause further constipation, stool softeners are given in conjunction. The GLT is a screening test for gestational diabetes. It consists of giving a 50-g oral glucose loading dose and checking a serum glucose 1 hour later. If this value is greater than or equal to 140 mg/dL, a **glucose tolerance test** (GTT) is administered.

The GTT consists of a fasting serum glucose measurement and then administration of a 100-g oral glucose loading dose. The serum glucose is then measured at 1, 2, and 3 hours after the oral dose is given. This test is indicative of gestational diabetes if the fasting glucose is over 105 mg/dL or if any two of three values are over 190, 165, or 145 mg/dL, respectively.

In high-risk populations, vaginal cultures for gonorrhea and chlamydia are repeated late in the third trimester. These infections are transmitted vertically during birth and should be treated if cultures or DNA tests return positive. At 36 weeks, many institutions perform screening for group B streptococcus. Patients who have a positive culture should be treated with intravenous penicillin when they present in labor.

KEY POINTS

1. The initial prenatal visit is used to screen for many of the problems that can occur in pregnancy and to verify dating of the pregnancy.
2. Much of the screening for genetic and congenital abnormalities is performed in the second trimester.
3. Blood pressure, weight gain, fundal height, fetal heart rate, and symptoms including contractions, vaginal bleeding, or discharge are assessed at each prenatal visit.

◼ ROUTINE PROBLEMS OF PREGNANCY

Back Pain

Low back pain in pregnancy is quite common, particularly in the third trimester when the patient's center of gravity has shifted and there is increased strain on the lower back. Mild exercise—particularly stretching—may release endorphins and reduce the amount of back pain. Gentle massage, heating pads, and Tylenol can be used for mild pain. For patients with severe back pain, muscle relaxants or occasionally narcotics can be used.

Constipation

The decreased bowel motility secondary to elevated progesterone levels leads to increased transit time in the large bowel. In turn, there is greater absorption of water from the gastrointestinal tract. This can result in constipation. Increased PO fluids, particularly water, should be recommended. In addition, stool softeners or bulking agents may help. Laxatives can be used, but are usually avoided in the third trimester because of the theoretical risk of preterm labor.

Contractions

Occasional irregular contractions are considered Braxton Hicks contractions and will occur several times per day. Patients should be warned about these and assured that they are perfectly normal. Dehydration may cause increased contractions, and patients should be advised to drink many (10 to 14) glasses of water and juice per day. Regular contractions, as often as every 10 to 15 minutes, should be considered a sign of preterm labor and should be assessed by cervical examination. If a patient has had several days of contractions and no documented cervical change, this is reassuring to both the obstetrician and the patient that delivery is not imminent.

Dehydration

Because of the expanded intravascular space and increased third spacing of fluid, patients have a difficult time maintaining their intravascular volume status. Dietary recommendations should include increased fluids. As mentioned above, dehydration may lead to uterine contractions, possibly secondary to cross-reaction of vasopressin with oxytocin receptors.

Edema

Compression of the inferior vena cava (IVC) and pelvic veins by the uterus can lead to increased hydrostatic pressure in the lower extremities and eventually to edema in the feet and ankles. Elevation of the lower extremities above the heart can ease this. Also, patients should be advised to sleep on their sides to decrease compression. Severe edema of the face and hands may be indicative of preeclampsia and merits further evaluation.

Gastroesophageal Reflux Disease

Relaxation of the lower esophageal sphincter and increased transit time in the stomach can lead to reflux and nausea. Patients with reflux should be started on antacids, advised to eat multiple small meals per day, and avoid lying down within an hour of eating. For patients with continued symptoms, H_2 blockers or proton pump inhibitors can be given.

Hemorrhoids

Patients will have increased venous stasis and IVC compression, leading to congestion in the venous system. Congestion of the pelvic vessels combined with increased abdominal pressure with bowel movements secondary to constipation can lead to hemorrhoids. Hemorrhoids are treated symptomatically with topical anesthetics and steroids for pain and swelling. Prevention of constipation with increased fluids, increased fiber in the diet, and stool softeners may prevent or decrease the exacerbation of hemorrhoids.

Pica

Rarely, a patient will have cravings for nonedible items such as dirt or clay. As long as these substances are nontoxic, the patient is advised to maintain adequate nutrition and encouraged to stop ingesting the inedible items. However, if patients have been consuming toxic substances, immediate cessation along with a toxicology consult is advised.

Round Ligament Pain

Usually late in the second trimester or early in the third trimester, there may be some pain in the adnexa or lower abdomen. This pain is likely secondary to the rapid expansion of the uterus and stretching of the ligamentous attachments, such as the round ligaments. This is often self-limited but may be relieved with Tylenol.

Urinary Frequency

Increased intravascular volumes and elevated glomerular filtration rate (GFR) can lead to increased urine production during pregnancy. However, the most likely cause of urinary frequency during pregnancy is that as the uterus grows, it increasingly compresses the bladder. A urinary tract infection may also be present with isolated urinary frequency but is often accompanied by dysuria. A urinalysis and culture should therefore be ordered to rule out infection. If no infection is present, patients can be assured  that the increasing voiding is normal. Patients should be advised to keep up PO hydration despite urinary frequency.

Varicose Veins

The lower extremities or the vulva may develop varicosities during pregnancy. The relaxation of the venous smooth muscle and increased intravascular pressure probably both contribute to the pathogenesis. Elevation of the lower extremities or the use of pressure stockings may help reduce existing varicosities and prevent more from developing. If the problem does not resolve by 6 months postpartum, patients may be referred for surgical therapy.

KEY POINTS

1. Many of the routine problems of pregnancy are related to hormonal effects of the placenta.
2. It is important to discuss the side effects of pregnancy in order to best prepare the patient.
3. While pregnancy is often the cause of many somatic complaints, other causes should still be ruled out as in the nonpregnant patient.

■ PRENATAL ASSESSMENT OF THE FETUS

Throughout pregnancy, the fetus is screened and diagnosed by a variety of modalities. Parents can be screened for common diseases such as cystic fibrosis, Tay-Sachs, sickle-cell disease, and thalassemia. If both parents are carriers, the fetus is then diagnosed. Fetal karyotype can be obtained via amniocentesis or chorionic villus sampling (CVS). The fetus can be imaged and many of the congenital anomalies diagnosed via second trimester ultrasound. First and second trimester genetic screening and prenatal diagnosis is discussed further in Chapter 3. Other fetal testing includes fetal blood sampling, fetal lung maturity testing, and assessment of fetal well-being.

Fetal Blood Sampling

Percutaneous umbilical blood sampling (PUBS) is performed by placing a needle transabdominally into the uterus and phlebotomizing the umbilical cord. This procedure may be used when the fetal hematocrit needs to be obtained, particularly in the setting of Rh isoimmunization, other causes for fetal anemia, and hydrops. PUBS is also used for rapid karyotype analysis and to assess fetal platelet count in alloimmune thrombocytopenia.

Fetal Lung Maturity

There are many tests for fetal lung maturity. Classically, the lecithin to sphingomyelin (L/S) ratio has been used as a predictor of fetal lung maturity. Type II pneumocytes secrete a surfactant that uses phospholipids in its synthesis. Commonly, lecithin increases as the lungs mature, whereas sphingomyelin decreases beyond about 32 weeks. The L/S ratio should therefore increase as the pregnancy progresses. Repetitive studies have shown that a L/S ratio of greater than 2 is associated with only rare cases of respiratory distress syndrome (RDS). With a L/S ratio below 1.5, the risk of RDS is 70%. Examples of other fetal lung maturity tests include measuring the levels of phosphatidylglycerol, saturated phosphatidyl choline (SPC), the presence of lamellar bodies, and surfactant to albumin ratio (S/A).

Ultrasound

Ultrasound can be used to date a pregnancy with an unknown or uncertain LMP, and is most accurate in the first trimester. In the setting of prenatal diagnosis of fetal malformations, most patients undergo a routine screening ultrasound at 18 to 20 weeks. Routinely, an attempt is made to identify placental location, amniotic fluid volume, gestational age, and any obvious malformations. In high-risk patients, careful attention is paid to commonly associated anomalies such as cardiac anomalies in pregestational diabetics. Fetal echocardiography and, rarely, MRI are used to augment assessment of the fetal heart and brain, respectively.

In the third trimester, ultrasound can be used to monitor high-risk pregnancies by obtaining biophysical profiles (BPP), fetal growth, and fetal Doppler studies. The BPP looks at five categories and gives a score of either 0 or 2 for each: amniotic fluid volume, fetal tone, fetal activity, fetal breathing movements, and the nonstress test (NST), which is a test of the fetal heart rate. A BPP of 8 to 10 or better is reassuring. Ultrasound can also be used to assess the blood flow velocity in the umbilical cord. A decrease, absence, or reversal of diastolic flow in the umbilical artery is progressively more worrisome.

Antenatal Testing of Fetal Well-being

Formal antenatal testing includes the NST, the oxytocin challenge test (OCT), and the BPP. The NST is considered formally reactive if there are two accelerations of the fetal heart rate in 20 minutes that are at least 15 beats above the baseline heart rate and last for at least 15 seconds. An OCT or contraction stress test (CST) is obtained by getting at least three contractions in 10 minutes and analyzing the fetal heart rate (FHR) tracing during that time. The reactivity criteria are the same as for the NST. In addition, late decelerations with at least half of the contractions constitute a positive test and is worrisome. Commonly, most antenatal testing units use the NST beginning at 32 to 34 weeks of gestation in high-risk pregnancies and at 40.5 to 41 weeks for undelivered patients. If the NST is nonreactive, the fetus is assessed via ultrasound. If the fetal heart tracing has any worrisome decelerations or the BPP is not reassuring, an OCT is performed.

KEY POINTS

1. Common screening tests for fetal abnormalities include MSAFP and the triple screen.
2. The fetus may be diagnosed with abnormalities using amniocentesis, CVS, and ultrasound.
3. Fetal status can be assessed antepartum with ultrasound, NST, BPP, and OCT.

Early Pregnancy Complications

■ ECTOPIC PREGNANCY

An **ectopic pregnancy** is one that implants outside the uterine cavity. Implantation occurs in the fallopian tube in up to 99% of the cases (Figure 2-1). Implantation may also occur on the ovary, the cervix, the outside of the fallopian tube, the abdominal wall, or the bowel. The incidence of ectopic pregnancies has been increasing over the past 10 years, and now occurs in more than 1:100 pregnancies. This is thought to be secondary to the increase in assisted fertility, sexually transmitted disease (STD), and pelvic inflammatory disease (PID). Patients who present with vaginal bleeding and/or abdominal pain should always be evaluated for ectopic pregnancy because a ruptured ectopic pregnancy is a true emergency. It can result in rapid hemorrhage, leading to shock and eventually death.

Risk Factors

Several risk factors predispose patients to extrauterine implantation (Table 2-1). Many affect the fallopian tubes, causing either tubal scarring or decreased peristalsis of the tube. Use of an intrauterine device (IUD) for birth control leads to an increased rate of ectopic pregnancy in those women who become pregnant because the IUD has prevented normal intrauterine implantation.

Diagnosis

The diagnosis of ectopic pregnancy is made by history, physical examination, laboratory tests, and ultrasound. On history, patients often complain of unilateral pelvic or lower abdominal pain and vaginal bleeding. Physical examination may reveal an adnexal mass that is often tender, a uterus that is small for gestational age, and bleeding from the cervix. Patients with ruptured ectopic pregnancies may be hypotensive, unresponsive, or show signs of peritoneal irritation secondary to hemoperitoneum.

On laboratory studies, the classic finding is a beta human chorionic gonadotropin (β-hCG) level that is low for gestational age and does not increase at the expected rate. In patients with a normal **intrauterine pregnancy** (IUP), the trophoblastic tissue secretes β-hCG in a predictable manner that should lead to doubling of the total β-hCG level approximately every 48 hours. An ectopic pregnancy has a poorly implanted placenta; thus the level of β-hCG does not double every 48 hours. The hematocrit may be low or may drop in patients with ruptured ectopic pregnancies.

Ultrasound may show an adnexal mass or an extrauterine pregnancy. A gestational sac with a yolk sac seen in the uterus on ultrasound indicates an intrauterine pregnancy. However, there is always a small risk of **heterotopic pregnancy**, a multiple gestation with at least one IUP and at least one ectopic pregnancy. At early gestations, neither an IUP nor an adnexal mass can be seen on ultrasound.

Patients who cannot be diagnosed with ectopic pregnancy because they do not have an adnexal mass on physical examination or ultrasound and are seemingly stable may be followed with serial β-hCG levels every 48 hours to assess the possibility of ectopic pregnancy. β-hCG levels that do not double every 48 hours are suspicious for ectopic pregnancy. As a guideline, an IUP should be seen on transvaginal ultrasonography with a β-hCG between 1500 and 2000 mIU/mL. A fetal heartbeat should be seen with β-hCG >5000 mIU/mL.

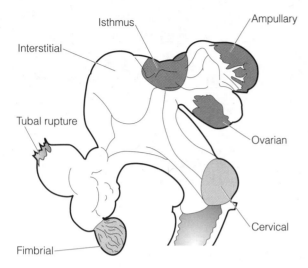

Figure 2-1 • Sites of ectopic pregnancies.

TABLE 2-1

Risk Factors for Ectopic Pregnancy

History of STDs or PID

Prior ectopic pregnancy

Previous tubal surgery

Prior pelvic or abdominal surgery resulting in adhesions

Endometriosis

Current use of exogenous hormones including progesterone or estrogen

In vitro fertilization and other assisted reproduction

DES-exposed patients with congenital abnormalities

Congenital abnormalities of the fallopian tubes

Use of an IUD for birth control

Treatment

If a patient presents with a ruptured ectopic pregnancy and is unstable, the first priority is to stabilize with intravenous fluids, blood products, and pressors if necessary. The patient should then be taken to the operating room where exploratory laparotomy can be performed to stop the bleeding and remove the ectopic pregnancy. If the patient is stable with a likely ruptured ectopic pregnancy, the procedure of choice at many institutions is an exploratory laparoscopy that can be performed to evacuate the hemoperitoneum, coagulate any ongoing bleeding, and resect the ectopic pregnancy.

Patients who present with an unruptured ectopic pregnancy should be monitored for signs of rupture—increased abdominal pain, bleeding, or signs of shock. These patients are often treated surgically with laparoscopic resection of the ectopic pregnancy. **Methotrexate** therapy for treatment of the ectopic pregnancy is used at most institutions for uncomplicated, nonthreatening, ectopic pregnancies.

KEY POINTS

1. Ectopic pregnancy is implantation of the pregnancy outside the uterine cavity.
2. Approximately 1% of pregnancies are ectopic.
3. Patients present with bleeding and unilateral pelvic pain, and diagnosis is made with palpation of an adnexal mass or visualization of an extrauterine pregnancy on ultrasound.
4. Treatment is often surgical and includes stabilizing the patient and removing the pregnancy. Stable, unruptured ectopics can be managed medically with methotrexate therapy.

■ SPONTANEOUS ABORTION (SAB)

A **spontaneous abortion**, or miscarriage, is a pregnancy that ends before 20 weeks gestation. SABs are estimated to occur in 15% to 25% of all pregnancies. This number may be even higher because losses that occur at 4 to 6 weeks gestational age are often confused with late menses. The type of SAB is defined by whether any or all of the **products of conception** (POC) have passed and whether or not the cervix is dilated. Definitions are as follows:

- **Abortus**—fetus lost before 20 weeks gestation, less than 500 g, or less than 25 cm.
- **Complete abortion**—complete expulsion of all POC before 20 weeks gestation (Figure 2-2).
- **Incomplete abortion**—partial expulsion of some but not all POC before 20 weeks gestation.
- **Inevitable abortion**—no expulsion of products, but bleeding and dilation of the cervix such that a viable pregnancy is unlikely.
- **Threatened abortion**—any intrauterine bleeding before 20 weeks, without dilation of the cervix or expulsion of any POC.
- **Missed abortion**—death of the embryo or fetus before 20 weeks with complete retention of POC;

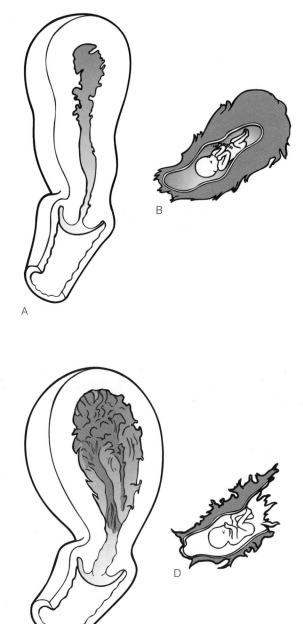

Figure 2-2 • A: Complete abortion. B: Product of complete abortion. C: Incomplete abortion. D: Product of incomplete abortion.

these often proceed to complete abortions in 1 to 3 weeks but are occasionally retained much longer.

First-Trimester Abortions

It is estimated that 60% to 80% of all SABs in the first trimester (early abortions are at <12 weeks gestational age) are associated with abnormal chromosomes. This percentage may be higher because many abortions likely occur before implantation. Other factors associated with SABs include infections, maternal anatomic defects, immunologic factors, and endocrine factors. A large number of first-trimester abortions have no obvious cause.

Diagnosis

Most patients present with bleeding from the vagina (Table 2-2). Other findings include cramping, abdominal pain, and decreased symptoms of pregnancy. The physical examination should include vital signs to rule out shock and febrile illness. A pelvic examination can be performed to look for sources of bleeding other than uterine and for changes in the cervix suggestive of an inevitable abortion. The laboratory tests ordered include a quantitative level of β-hCG, complete blood count, blood type, and antibody screen. An ultrasound can assess fetal viability and placentation.

Because patients with ectopic pregnancy also present with vaginal bleeding, it needs to be ruled out of the differential diagnosis. An ultrasound showing fetal cardiac activity or serial β-hCG levels doubling every 48 hours in early pregnancy are consistent with a viable IUP.

Treatment

The treatment plan is based on specific diagnosis and on the decisions made by the patient and her caregivers. Initially, all pregnant and bleeding patients need to be stabilized if hypotensive. A complete abortion can be followed for recurrent bleeding and signs of infection such as elevated temperature. Any tissue that the patient may have passed at home and at the hospital should be sent to pathology, both to

TABLE 2-2

Differential Diagnosis of First-Trimester Bleeding

Spontaneous abortion

Postcoital bleeding

Ectopic pregnancy

Vaginal or cervical lesions or lacerations

Extrusion of molar pregnancy

Nonpregnancy causes of bleeding

assess that POC have passed and for chromosome analysis if applicable.

An incomplete abortion can be allowed to finish on its own if the patient prefers expectant management, but can also be taken to completion with either a dilation and curettage (D&C) or administration of prostaglandins (e.g., misoprostol) to induce cervical dilatation and uterine contractions. Any tissue that has passed or been evacuated needs to be sent to pathology. Inevitable abortions and missed abortions are similarly managed.

A patient with a threatened abortion should be followed for continued bleeding and placed on pelvic rest with nothing per vagina. Often, the bleeding will resolve. However, these patients are at increased risk for preterm labor (PTL) and preterm premature rupture of membranes (PPROM). Finally, all Rh-negative pregnant women who experience vaginal bleeding during pregnancy should receive RhoGAM.

KEY POINTS

1. The most common cause of first trimester abortions is fetal chromosomal abnormalities.
2. It is important to rule out ectopic pregnancy with history, physical examination, laboratory studies, and ultrasound.
3. First trimester incomplete, inevitable, and missed abortions are usually completed with a D&C or medical management with prostaglandins, although expectant management is also used.
4. RhoGAM should be given to all Rh-negative patients with bleeding.

Second-Trimester Abortions

Second-trimester abortions (12 to 20 weeks gestational age) have multiple etiologies. Infection, maternal uterine or cervical anatomic defects, maternal systemic disease, exposure to fetotoxic agents, and trauma are all associated with late abortions. Abnormal chromosomes are not a frequent cause of late abortions. Late second-trimester abortions and periviable deliveries are also seen with PTL and incompetent cervix.

Diagnosis

Patients commonly present with bleeding from the vagina. Other findings include cramping, abdominal pain, and decreased symptoms of pregnancy. Occasionally, patients will note a lack of fetal movement in a previously active fetus. The physical examination, laboratory studies, and ultrasound are similar to those for a first-trimester abortion.

Treatment

As in first-trimester abortions, once the diagnosis of ectopic pregnancy has been eliminated, the treatment plan is based on the specific clinical scenario. All hemodynamically unstable patients need to be stabilized. Similar to first-trimester abortions, complete abortions can be followed for recurrence of bleeding and signs of infection. If there is any concern for retained POC, a dilation and evacuation (D&E) can be done to ensure completion of the abortion. The distinction between a D&C and D&E depends on gestational age at the time of procedure (i.e., first or second trimester). The fetus is larger in the second trimester making the procedure more difficult.

Incomplete and missed abortions can be allowed to finish on their own but are often taken to completion with a D&E. Commonly, between 16 and 24 weeks, either a D&E may be performed or labor may be induced with high doses of oxytocin or prostaglandins. The advantages of a D&E is that the procedure is self-limited and performed faster than an induction of labor. However, aggressive dilation prior to the procedure with laminaria is necessary, and there is a significant risk of uterine perforation and cervical lacerations. An induction of labor can take longer, but allows completion of the abortion without the inherent risks of instrumentation. With either method, great care should be taken to ensure the complete evacuation of all POC.

In the second trimester, the diagnoses of PTL and incompetent cervix need to be ruled out. Particularly in the setting of inevitable abortions or threatened abortions, the etiology is likely to be related to the inability of the uterus to maintain the pregnancy. PTL begins with contractions leading to cervical change, whereas an incompetent cervix is characterized by painless dilation of the cervix. In the case of an incompetent cervix, an emergent cerclage may be offered. PTL can be managed with tocolysis.

KEY POINTS

1. Most second-trimester abortions are secondary to uterine or cervical abnormalities, trauma, systemic disease, or infection.
2. D&E, prostaglandins, or oxytocic agents can be used for the management of spontaneous abortions in the second trimester that need assistance to completion.
3. The risk of uterine perforation from D&E is greater in the second trimester than in the first.

■ INCOMPETENT CERVIX

Patients with an **incompetent cervix** present with painless dilation and effacement of the cervix, often in the second trimester of pregnancy. As the cervix dilates, the fetal membranes are exposed to vaginal flora and risk of increased trauma. Thus, infection, vaginal discharge, and rupture of the membranes are common findings in the setting of incompetent cervix. Patients may also present with short-term cramping or contracting, leading to advancing cervical dilation or pressure in the vagina with the chorionic and amniotic sacs bulging through the cervix. Cervical incompetence is estimated to cause approximately 15% of all second-trimester losses.

Risk Factors

Surgery or other cervical trauma is the most common cause of cervical incompetence (Table 2-3). The other possible cause is a congenital abnormality of the cervix that can sometimes be attributed to diethylstilbestrol (DES) exposure in utero. However, many patients who present with cervical incompetence have no known risk factors.

■ TABLE 2-3

Risk Factors for Cervical Incompetence

History of cervical surgery, such as a cone biopsy or dilation of the cervix

History of cervical lacerations with vaginal delivery

Uterine anomalies

History of DES exposure

Diagnosis

Patients with incompetent cervix often present with a dilated cervix noted on routine examination, ultrasound, or in the setting of bleeding, vaginal discharge, or rupture of membranes. Occasionally, patients experience mild cramping or pressure in the lower abdomen or vagina. On examination, the cervix is dilated more than expected with the level of contractions experienced. In this setting, it is difficult to differentiate between incompetent cervix and PTL. However, patients who present with mild cramping and have advancing cervical dilation on serial examinations and/or an amniotic sac bulging through the cervix are more likely to have an incompetent cervix, with the cramping being instigated by the dilated cervix and exposed membranes.

Treatment

Individual obstetric issues should be treated accordingly. If the fetus is previable (i.e., less than 24 weeks gestational age), expectant management and elective termination are options. Patients with viable pregnancies are treated with betamethasone to decrease the risk of prematurity and are managed expectantly with strict bed rest. If there is a component of preterm contractions or PTL, tocolysis may be used with viable pregnancies.

One alternative course of management for incompetent cervix in a previable pregnancy is the placement of an emergent cerclage. The cerclage is a suture placed vaginally around the cervix either at the cervical-vaginal junction (McDonald cerclage) or at the internal os (Shirodkar cerclage). The intent of a cerclage is to close the cervix. Complications include rupture of membranes, PTL, and infection.

If incompetent cervix was the suspected diagnosis in a previous pregnancy, a patient is usually offered an elective cerclage with subsequent pregnancies (Figure 2-3). Placement of the elective cerclage is similar to that of the emergent cerclage with either the McDonald or Shirodkar methods being used, usually at 12 to 14 weeks gestation. The cerclage is maintained until 36 to 38 weeks of gestation if possible. At that point it is removed and the patient is followed expectantly until labor ensues. In patients for whom one or both of the vaginal cerclages have failed, a transabdominal cerclage (TAC) is often the next management offered. This can be placed electively either prior to the pregnancy or at 12 to 14 weeks. Patients with a TAC need to be delivered via cesarean section.

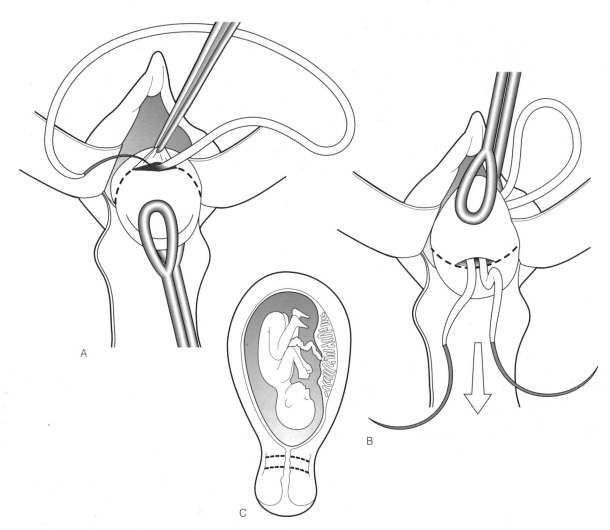

Figure 2-3 • Cerclage of the cervix (Shirodkar) with incompetent os in pregnant patient. A: Placement of the suture. B: Cinching the suture down to tie the knot posteriorly. C: The tightened cerclage almost at the internal os.

KEY POINTS

1. Incompetent cervix is painless dilation of the cervix. This dilation may lead to infection, PPROM, or PTL.
2. If the fetus is previable, incompetent cervix is treated with expectant management, elective termination, or emergent cerclage.
3. Patients with a history of incompetent cervix should be offered an elective, prophylactic cerclage at 12 to 14 weeks gestational age.

■ RECURRENT PREGNANCY LOSS

A recurrent or habitual aborter is a woman who has had three or more consecutive SABs. Less than 1% of the population is diagnosed with **recurrent pregnancy loss**. The risk of an SAB after one prior SAB is 20% to 25%; after two consecutive SABs, 25% to 30%; and after three consecutive SABs, 30% to 35%.

Pathogenesis

The etiologies of recurrent pregnancy loss are generally similar to those of SABs. These include chromosomal abnormalities, maternal systemic disease, maternal anatomic defects, and infection. Fifteen percent of patients with recurrent pregnancy loss have **antiphospholipid antibody (APA) syndrome**. Another group of patients are thought to have a **luteal phase defect** and lack an adequate level of progesterone to maintain the pregnancy.

Diagnosis

Patients who are habitual aborters should be evaluated for the etiology. Patients with only two consecutive SABs are occasionally assessed as well, particularly those with advancing maternal age or for whom continued fertility may be an issue. Patients are often screened in the following manner. First, a karyotype of both parents is obtained, as well as the karyotypes of the POC from each of the SABs. Second, maternal anatomy should be examined, initially with a hysterosalpingogram (HSG). If the HSG is abnormal or nondiagnostic, a hysteroscopic or laparoscopic exploration may be performed. Third, screening tests for hypothyroidism, diabetes mellitus, APA syndrome, hypercoagulability and systemic lupus erythematosus (SLE) should be performed. These tests should include lupus anticoagulant, factor V Leiden deficiency, and ANA. Additionally, anticardiolipin antibody and tests for protein S and protein C are also considered. Fourth, a level of serum progesterone should be obtained in the luteal phase of the menstrual cycle. Finally, cultures of the cervix, vagina, and endometrium can be taken to rule out infection. An endometrial biopsy can be done during the luteal phase as well to look for proliferative endometrium.

Treatment

Treatment of patients with recurrent pregnancy loss depends on the etiology of the SABs. For many (approximately 30% to 50%), no etiology is ever found. For others, the etiology itself needs to be diagnosed as described above and can often be treated on an individual basis. For patients with chromosomal abnormalities such as balanced translocations, in vitro fertilization can be performed using donor sperm or ova. Anatomic abnormalities may or may not be correctable. If incompetent cervix is suspected, a cerclage may be placed. If a luteal phase defect is suspected, progesterone may be given. Patients with APA syndrome are treated with low-dose aspirin. Maternal diseases should be treated with the appropriate therapy (e.g., hypothyroidism with thyroid hormone, infection with antibiotics). However, with some systemic diseases, treatment may not decrease the risk of SAB. Because even patients with three prior consecutive SABs will have a subsequent normal pregnancy two-thirds of the time, it is difficult to estimate whether certain treatments of recurrent abortions are effective.

KEY POINTS

1. Recurrent pregnancy loss is defined as three or more consecutive SABs.
2. Despite extensive evaluation to diagnose the etiology of SABs, the cause of recurrent SABs is undiagnosed in greater than one-third of all cases.
3. Treatment is specific to the etiology, but efficacy is difficult to measure because two-thirds of subsequent pregnancies will be normal without therapy.

3

Prenatal Screening, Diagnosis, and Treatment

Prenatal screening, diagnosis, and treatment represents a relatively new field within obstetrics. It has been particularly tied to the advent of real-time ultrasound imaging over the past two decades. Prenatal genetic diagnoses are and will be increasingly available as the association of genes and their phenotypes are discovered. The distinction between screening and diagnosis should be further defined. **Screening** allows high-risk individuals to be selected out of a population at low risk for a given complication. The sensitivity and specificity and resulting false-positive rates of screening tests are highly important both because of the number of patients that may be missed by a screen as well as the number of patients who are falsely concerned. **Prenatal diagnosis** is usually far more specific than screening, but in the case of amniocentesis and chorionic villus sampling (CVS), it also bears greater risk of complications.

■ SCREENING PATIENTS FOR GENETIC DISEASES

Many diseases are passed genetically from parents to their offspring. This is best understood using the principles of Mendelian genetics. **Autosomal dominant** (AD) syndromes are passed from one parent with the disease by way of a single gene defect. Risk of disease is 50%. **Autosomal recessive** (AR) diseases require two affected alleles. Thus assuming both parents are carriers, the risk to the child is 25%. **X-linked recessive** syndromes (e.g., hemophilia) are usually carried by the mother and passed on only to their sons. The sons have the disease 50% of the time and the daughters are carriers 50% of the time. Rare **X-linked dominant** syndromes can be passed from either parent to

either child similar to that of autosomal dominant syndromes. Phenotypes may vary, however, because of mixed penetrance, X-chromosome lyonization, and genomic imprinting. The first step in determining fetal risk is to screen the mother for the disease, which is usually done in higher risk groups.

Cystic Fibrosis

Cystic fibrosis (CF) is an autosomal recessive disorder that results from a mutation in the gene responsible for chloride channels. Almost all CF patients have chronic lung disease due to recurrent infections, leading eventually to irreversible lung damage and strain on the right ventricle (cor pulmonale). Eighty-five percent of CF patients have pancreatic insufficiency manifested by chronic malabsorption and failure to thrive. Chronic lung disease and its sequelae are the life-limiting factor for most CF patients. Median survival is currently 30 years for CF patients in the United States with high patient to patient variation.

CF requires that the mutant allele is present in a double dose (homozygosity) although, for the majority of AR disorders, affected individuals have two different allelic mutations at the same locus (compound heterozygote). For example, ΔF508/G542X, are two of the most common mutations in CF. These mutations can be screened for in asymptomatic carrier patients. If the mother has a positive screen, her partner can be screened as well. If he is also positive, then the risk of the fetus being affected is 25%. Amniocentesis or CVS can then be performed to diagnose the fetus. The CF mutations are more common in Caucasians (1 : 28 is a carrier); but one problem in this screening program is that not all mutations have been identified. Therefore, even with a negative screen, there remains a small probability that a child could be affected.

Sickle-Cell Disease

Sickle-cell disease is an autosomal recessive disease caused by a single point mutation in the gene for the beta chain in hemoglobin. The resulting hemoglobin (Hb S) forms polymers when deoxygenated that cause the cells to lose their biconcave shape and take on a "sickle" appearance. Patients have a hemolytic anemia, shortened life expectancy, and frequent pain crises secondary to vaso-occlusion by dysmorphic erythrocytes. Because this disease is more common among African Americans, all persons of African descent should be screened in pregnancy. It is likely that the increased carrier status in African Americans was selected because of their **heterozygote advantage**. This was seen because the resistance to malaria in individuals heterozygous for sickle-cell anemia was greater than those without the gene defect. Red blood cells in these individuals function in normal conditions but are inhospitable to *Plasmodium vivax*, the parasitic protozoan responsible for malaria.

The maternal screen is usually accomplished with a hemoglobin electrophoresis. This will distinguish Hb S from the normal Hb A. If the patient is positive, then her partner can be screened. If he is also positive, then the fetus carries a 25% chance of being affected, and the couple can choose to undergo fetal diagnosis.

Tay-Sachs Disease

Tay-Sachs is an AR disease that is most commonly seen in Eastern European Jews and French Canadians. Approximately 1 in 27 Ashkenazi Jews is a carrier for the Tay-Sachs allele, making the incidence of the disease in this population approximately 100 times greater than in other populations. It is thought that this is due to a **founder effect**, where the high frequency of a mutant gene in a population is founded by a small ancestral group when one or more founders is a carrier for the mutation.

Infants with Tay-Sachs develop symptoms 3 to 10 months after birth. These symptoms include a loss of alertness and an excessive reaction to noise (hyperacusis). There is a progressive neurologic degeneration with developmental delay in intellectual and neurologic function. Myoclonic and akinetic seizures can present 1 to 3 months later. One physical exam finding is the cherry-red spots seen on the fundoscopic eye exam where the prominent red macular fovea centralis is contrasted by the pale macula. These children eventually suffer from paralysis, blindness, and dementia, and die by age 4.

The disease is due to the deficiency of hexosaminidase A (hex A), the enzyme responsible for the degradation of G_{M2} gangliosides. Hex A is a multimeric protein composed of three parts: alpha and beta subunits that comprise the enzyme and an activator protein. The activator protein must associate with both the enzyme and the substrate before the enzyme can cleave the ganglioside between the N-acetyl-α-galactosamine and galactose residues. Gangliosides are continually degraded in lysosomes where multiple degradative enzymes function to sequentially remove the terminal sugars from the gangliosides. The impact of Tay-Sachs is mainly in the brain where gangliosides are found in the highest concentration, particularly in the gray matter. The deficiency of hex A results in the accumulation of gangliosides in the lysosomes resulting in enlarged neurons containing lipid-filled lysosomes, cellular dysfunction, and ultimately neuronal death.

Similar to other AR syndromes, Tay-Sachs is screened for particularly among high-risk patients and in their partners if they are positive. Fetal diagnosis can then be performed if both partners are carriers.

Thalassemia

The **thalassemias** are a set of hereditary hemolytic anemias that are caused by mutations that result in the reduction in the synthesis of either the α or β chains that make up the hemoglobin molecule. The reduction of a particular chain leads to the imbalance of globin chain synthesis and subsequently a distortion in the $\alpha:\beta$ ratio. As a result, unpaired globin chains produce insoluble tetramers that precipitate in the cell and cause damage to membranes. The red cells are susceptible to premature red cell destruction by the reticuloendothelial system in the bone marrow, liver, and spleen.

Beta Thalassemia

In β-**thalassemia**, there is an impairment of β-globin production that leads to an excess of alpha chains. These disorders are typically diagnosed several months after birth because the presence of β-globin is only important postnatally when it would normally replace the α-globin as the major non-α chain. There are multiple types of mutations that can lead to β-thalassemia. Almost any point mutation that causes a decrease in synthesis of mRNA or protein can cause this disease. β-thalassemia is essentially an AR disorder seen more commonly among patients of Mediterranean descent, as well as Asians and Africans. Because the heterozygotes will have a mild hemolytic anemia and low MCV, they can be screened by getting a CBC. Confirmation can then be made by hemoglobin electrophoresis, which will show an increase in α:β ratio.

Alpha Thalassemia

The alpha chain is encoded by four alleles. Additionally, two out of four mutations can occur cis or trans, with cis being on the same chromosome and trans being on two different chromosomes. Cis mutations are seen more commonly among Asians, whereas trans mutations are seen more commonly among Africans. With α-thalassemia, deletions or alterations of one, two, three, or four genes causes an increasingly severe phenotype. The most severe form of α-thalassemia causes fetal hydrops and is incompatible with life. The infants are pale, premature, hydropic, severely anemic, and have splenomegaly. A hemoglobin electrophoresis would reveal no HbF, no HbA, and approximately 90% to 100% Hbα4 also referred to as **Hb Bart**. **Hemoglobin H disease** (HbH) is due to the deletion of three alpha globin genes resulting in the accumulation of excess beta chains in the red cell. Beta tetramers form which are unstable and undergo oxidation. Membrane damage results and these red cells are susceptible to early clearance and destruction. These infants are born with anemia and the initial hemoglobin electrophoresis shows some Hb Bart and some HbH. Within the following few months, Hb Bart disappears and the hemoglobins detected are HbH and HbA. **Alpha thalassemia trait** (two deletions) carries a milder phenotype with mainly a microcytic anemia and a normal hemoglobin electrophoresis. Patients with only one gene deletion are silent carriers. In that case, diagnosis is confirmed by gene-mapping techniques.

Like beta-thalassemia, alpha-thalassemia is also screened for with a CBC in high-risk groups. Patients can then undergo hemoglobin electrophoresis if they have a microcytic anemia. Sorting out whether patients are cis or trans is particularly important. When both partners have a cis mutation, their child has a 25% chance of getting the most severe variant

that usually results in fetal death. If they both have the trans mutation, the child will end up with the trans mutation as well, and primarily remain an asymptomatic carrier.

KEY POINTS

1. Mothers can be asymptomatic carriers of autosomal recessive diseases, and can often be screened for carrier status.
2. If a mother is a carrier, the father of the baby can be screened as well to determine his carrier status. If the father is negative, there is no risk to the baby; if he is positive, there is a 25% chance of the disease in the fetus.
3. Two common ways that AR disorders are introduced and maintained in a population is by the founder effect (Tay-Sachs) and heterozygote advantage (sickle-cell disease).

■ CHROMOSOMAL ABNORMALITIES

In addition to genetic disorders caused by single gene mutations, another family of disorders in the fetus is caused by chromosomal abnormalities. Aneuploidy—that is, extra or missing chromosome(s)—is generally the cause of these syndromes. These chromosomal abnormalities are usually accompanied by obvious phenotypic differences and congenital anomalies. However, these may not always be appreciated on prenatal ultrasound. Thus, fetal karyotype remains the best way to diagnose them. Screening tests exist for some syndromes, including the expanded maternal serum alpha fetoprotein (XAFP) test, which includes MSAFP, estriol and beta-hCG. While trisomy and monosomy of any of the chromosomes exists, most result in early miscarriage. In addition, triploidy (i.e., three sets of chromosomes) also occurs and usually results in miscarriage or gestational trophoblastic disease. Despite the high rate of miscarriages, an infant is occasionally born with a triploidy and can survive for up to 1 year.

Down Syndrome

Trisomy 21, or an extra chromosome 21, is the most common cause of **Down syndrome**. This karyotype results in a higher rate of miscarriages and stillbirths. However, there are several thousand Down syndrome infants born each year. Because chromosomal abnormalities increase with maternal age, the baseline average risk per patient is increasing. The typical phenotype of Down syndrome is that of a short stature, classic facies, developmental delay and mental retardation with IQs ranging from 40 to as high as 90. Associated anomalies include cardiac defects, duodenal atresia or stenosis, and short limbs. Some of these anomalies can be seen by ultrasound, but up to 50% of Down syndrome fetuses will not have diagnosable anomalies by ultrasound, making this a poor screening tool. Currently, Down syndrome is screened for using the XAFP test between 15 and 19 weeks gestation.

Trisomy 18

Trisomy 18 (**Edward's syndrome**) is another common trisomy that can also be screened for using the XAFP test. It is not compatible with life beyond age 2, and commonly results in fetal or neonatal death. This syndrome is associated with multiple congenital anomalies seen on ultrasound, making this modality a reasonable screening tool. Edward's syndrome is classically associated with clenched fists, overlapping digits, and rocker bottom feet. Cardiac defects including ventricular septal defect (VSD) and tetralogy of Fallot, omphalocele, congenital diaphragmatic hernia, neural tube defects, and choroid plexus cysts have also been associated with trisomy 18 (Figure 3-1).

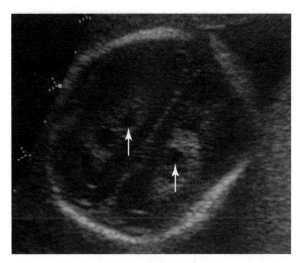

Figure 3-1 • Choroid plexus (CP) cysts located in the lateral ventricles of the brain.
(Image provided by Departments of Radiology and Obstetrics & Gynecology, University of California, San Francisco.)

Trisomy 13

Trisomy 13 (**Patau's syndrome**) has many findings similar to trisomy 18. Eighty-five percent of these newborns will not live past age 1. Commonly associated anomalies include holoprosencephaly; cleft lip and palate; cystic hygroma; single nostril or absent nose; omphalocele; cardiac anomalies including hypoplastic left heart; and limb anomalies including club foot and hand, polydactyly, and overlapping fingers. Unfortunately, the serum analytes of the XAFP are variable in these pregnancies making this a poor screening test. However, it is very rare that trisomy 13 fetuses would not have anomalies visible on ultrasound, and thus will be commonly diagnosed by routine ultrasound exam.

Sex Chromosomal Abnormalities

45,XO (**Turner's syndrome**, or monosomy X) and 47,XXY (**Klinefelter's syndrome**) are the most common sex chromosome anomalies. This may be because 47,XXX and 47,XYY karyotypes exhibit little variation from standard phenotypes, and are not identified as often. Individuals affected by Turner's syndrome are phenotypically female and of short stature. They experience primary amenorrhea, sexual infantilism, webbed neck, low-set ears, low posterior hairline, epicanthal folds, wide carrying angle of the arms, shield-like chest, wide-set nipples, short fourth metacarpal, renal anomalies, lymphedema of the extremities at birth, and cardiovascular anomalies—especially coarctation of the aorta. The only anomaly in Turner's syndrome commonly seen on ultrasound is cystic hygroma. Unfortunately, no screening test for Turner's syndrome exists as yet.

No screening test for Klinefelter's syndrome is available, however, both it and other sex chromosome abnormalities are diagnosed by karyotype when patients undergo amniocentesis or CVS. Testicular development is initially normal in these individuals. However, the presence of at least two X chromosomes causes the germ cells to die off when they enter meiosis, eventually resulting in small, firm testes and hyalinization of the seminiferous tubules. Other classic findings in Klinefelter's syndrome include infertility, gynecomastia, mental retardation, and elevated gonadotropin levels due to the decreased levels of circulating androgens.

■ FETAL CONGENITAL ANOMALIES

Congenital anomalies can occur in any organ system. The affected organ system often depends on which time during gestation a teratogenic insult is received by the fetus. These teratogens can include medications ingested by the mother, infections, particularly viral that the mother contracts and transmits transplacentally, and rarely chemotherapy or radiation. In order to better understand how these anomalies occur, a review of organogenesis is useful.

Early Embryogenesis and Organogenesis

After fertilization of the ovum by the sperm, the resulting zygote undergoes a series of cell divisions reaching the 16-cell morula stage by day 4 (Figure 3-2). After the morula enters the uterine cavity, an influx of fluid separates the morula into the inner and outer cell masses, which forms the blastocyst. This gives rise to the embryo and the trophoblast, respectively. The blastocyst implants into the endometrium by the end of the week 1. By the start of week 2, the trophoblast begins to differentiate into the inner cytotrophoblast and the outer syncytiotrophoblast, and together they eventually give rise to the placenta. Meanwhile, the inner cell mass divides into the bilaminar germ disc composed of the epiblast and the hypoblast.

During week 3 of development, the embryo is primarily preoccupied with the process of gastrulation. This is characterized by the formation of the primitive streak on the epiblast followed by the invagination of epiblast cells to form the three germ layers of the embryo: the inner endoderm, the middle mesoderm, and the outer ectoderm. The endodermal layer eventually gives rise to the gastrointestinal and respiratory systems. The mesoderm forms the cardiovascular, musculoskeletal, and genitourinary systems. The ectoderm layer will differentiate into the nervous system, skin, and many sensory organs (e.g., hair, eyes, nose, and ears). The period of organogenesis primarily lasts from week 3 to week 8 after conception (i.e., week 5–10 gestational age) and is the time when most of the major organ systems are formed.

Neural Tube Defects (NTDs)

The formation of the neural tube begins on days 22 to 23 after conception (week 4) in the region of the fourth and sixth somites. Fusion of the neural folds

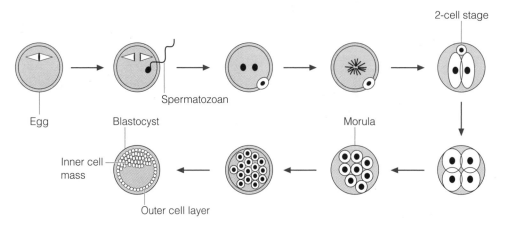

Figure 3-2 • Progression of the ova through fertilization to the blastula phase.

occurs in cranial and caudal directions. The anterior neuropore (future brain) closes by day 25 and the posterior pore (future spinal cord) closes by day 27. Closure of the neural tube coincides with establishment of its vascular supply. The majority of **neural tube defects** (NTDs) develop as a result of defective closure by week 4 of development (week 6 GA/LMP).

NTDs, including spina bifida and anencephaly, are a classic example of multifactorial inheritance, emphasizing the interactions between environmental and genetic factors. Geographic and ethnic variations may reflect environmental and genetic influences on the incidence of NTDs. Decreased levels of maternal folic acid are associated with the development of NTDs. Supplementation with periconceptional folic acid effectively reduces the incidence as well as recurrence of NTDs. The risk of NTDs is doubled in cases of homozygosity for a common mutation in the gene for methyl tetrahydrofolate reductase (MTHFR), the C677T allelic variant that encodes an enzyme with reduced activity. However, even if the association were causal, this MTHFR variant would account for only a small fraction of NTDs prevented by folic acid. The risk of NTDs seen with certain genotypes may vary depending on maternal factors, such as the blood levels of vitamin B_{12} or folate.

Fetuses with **spina bifida** can be identified on ultrasound, which is accomplished not by visualization of the opening of the spinal canal (Figure 3-3), but by the associated findings. Spina bifida leads to classic ultrasound findings of the "lemon" sign (concave frontal bones), and the "banana" sign (a cerebellum that is pulled caudally and flattened) (Figure 3-4). Ventriculomegaly and club feet are also seen. Prior to the existence of real-time ultrasound, one of the first prenatal screening programs was created using MSAFP to screen for neural tube defects. An open neural tube leads to elevated amniotic fluid α-fetoprotein (AFP) that crosses into the maternal serum.

Function of the infant and child with spina bifida is entirely dependent upon the level of the spinal lesion. If the lesion is quite low in the sacral area, bowel and bladder function may be normal, and ambulation can be achieved with crutches. However, in higher lesions, there may be complete disuse of the lower extremities, as well as lack of bowel or bladder control. Currently, there is a trial underway to see if in utero surgical repair can help those who are severely affected.

Cardiac Defects

Whereas the heart is merely a four-chamber pump, there are a number of ways to change the structure that can lead to some interesting pathophysiology. Cardiac development begins during week 3 after conception when an angiogenic cell cluster forms at the anterior central portion of the embryo. As the embryo folds cephalocaudally, the cardiogenic area also folds into a heart tube. Even at this early stage, the embryonic heart tube is already receiving venous flow from its caudal end and pumping blood through the first aortic arch and into the dorsal aorta. Simul-

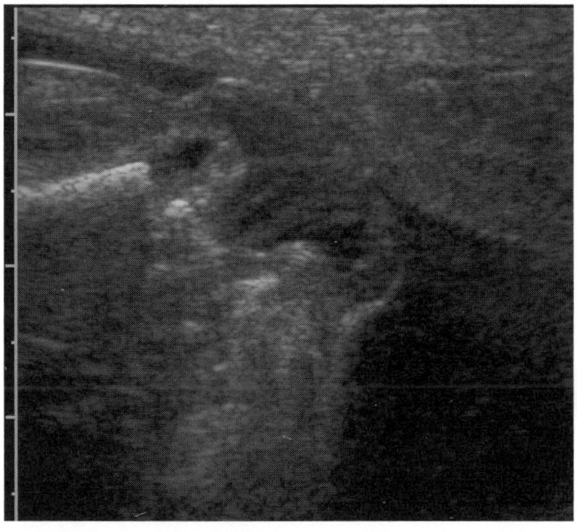

Figure 3-3 • Meningomyelocele—nonclosure of the neural tube at the lower aspect of the spine.
(Image provided by Departments of Radiology and Obstetrics & Gynecology, University of California, San Francisco.)

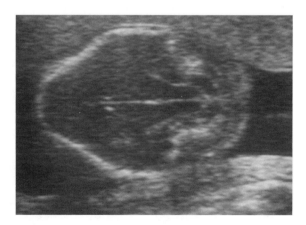

Figure 3-4 • Cerebral findings of the "lemon" and "banana" signs in spina bifida.
(Image provided by Departments of Radiology and Obstetrics & Gynecology, University of California, San Francisco.)

taneously, mesoderm around the endocardial tube form the three layers of the heart wall composed of an outer epicardium, a muscular wall of myocardium, and the endocardium that is the internal endothelial lining. Between days 23 and 28, the heart tube elongates and bends to create the cardiac loop with a common atrium and a narrow atrioventricular junction connecting it to the primitive ventricle. The bulbus cordis is the caudal section of the heart tube and will eventually form three structures: the proximal third will form the trabeculated part of the right ventricle, the midportion (conus cordis) will form the outflow tracts of the ventricles, and the distal segment (truncus arteriosus) will eventually give rise to the proximal portions of the aorta and pulmonary artery (Figure 3-5).

Between days 27 and 37, the heart continues to develop through the formation of the major septa. Septum formation is achieved via the formation of tissue, called endocardial cushions, which subdivide the lumen into two cavities. The right and left atria are created by the formation of the septum primum and septum secundum that subdivides the primitive atrium while allowing for an interatrial opening (foramen ovale) to continue the right-to-left shunting of blood. At the end of week 4, endocardial cushions also appear in the atrioventricular canal to form the right and left canals as well as the mitral and tricuspid valves. During this time, the medial walls of the ventricles gradually fuse together to form the muscular interventricular septum. The conus cordis comprises the middle third of the bulbis cordis and,

during week 5 of development, cushions subdivide the conus to form the outflow tract of the right and left ventricle as well as the membranous portion of the interventricular septum. Cushions also appear in the truncus arteriosus (distal third of bulbus cordis) and grow in a spiral pattern to form the aorticopulmonary septum and divide the truncus into the aortic and pulmonary tracts.

Any of these points of development can go awry leading to disastrous complications. For example, if the ventricular walls fail to fuse, there is a VSD that, if not repaired, can lead to Eisenmenger's physiology; that is, right ventricular hypertrophy, pulmonary hypertension, and a right-to-left shunt. A commonly seen constellation of cardiac findings is tetralogy of Fallot. This is a VSD with an overriding aorta, pulmonary stenosis (or atresia) and right ventricular hypertrophy. Just as the chambers and valves can be anomalous, so can the great vessels as seen in transposition of the vessels (TOV), where the pulmonary artery and the aorta are connected to the wrong ventricles. Other common anomalies of vessels are coarctation of the aorta, an atretic portion prior to the insertion of the ductus arteriosus; and a patent ductus arteriosus (PDA), which can also lead to Eisenmenger's physiology.

Diagnosis of these anomalies varies widely and depends on the lesion and the quality of the ultrasonographer imaging the fetal heart. Some of the more common lesions will be identified by the standard four-chamber view of the heart, but many—including coarctation of the aorta, VSD, and

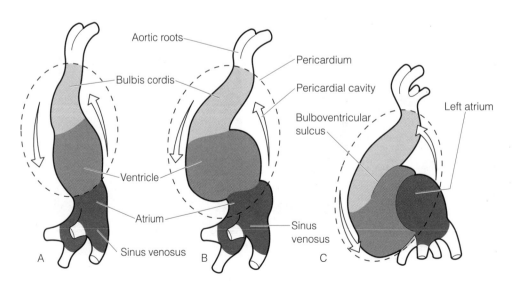

Figure 3-5 • A–C: Folding of the heart tube into the four-chamber heart.

ASD—often will not. Outcomes of these congenital anomalies are quite variable. Most of these may be surgically repaired, although hypoplastic left heart, in particular, can have high mortality at a young age.

Potter's Syndrome

Potter's syndrome results from renal failure leading to anhydramnios, which in turn causes pulmonary hypoplasia and contractures in the fetus. Potter's disease is bilateral renal agenesis. However, a fetus can also develop renal failure if there is distal obstruction of the urinary system as with posterior urethral valves. To better understand the etiology of this system, we should consider its embryology.

The kidneys are formed from intermediate mesoderm. Kidney development begins in week 4 with the formation of the first of three kidney scaffolds that arise and regress sequentially before the permanent kidney develops. This first scaffold is the pronephros, which is nonfunctional. In week 5 the *meso*nephros develops and functions briefly, creating the *meso*nephric duct (wolffian duct). The ureteric bud is an offshoot of the mesonephric duct that dilates and subdivides to form the urinary collecting system (collecting tubules, calyces, renal pelvis, and ureter) in both males and females. In the presence of testosterone, the mesonephric duct in males also forms the vas deferens, epididymis, ejaculatory duct, and seminal vesicles. In females, it degenerates entirely except for the vestigial Gartner's duct that can form a benign cyst along the broad ligament. The third scaffold—the *meta*nephros—also appears in week 5 of gestation and becomes the functioning kidney by week 9 of gestation. The ureteric bud from the *meso*nephric duct contacts the *meta*nephros and induces it to form nephrons. If this contact does not occur, renal agenesis results. The adjacent dorsal aorta also sends out collaterals into the *meta*nephros that ultimately develop into glomerular tufts.

Before week 7, the cloaca (the proximal portion of the allantois distally connected to the yolk sac) is divided into the urogenital (UG) sinus and the anorectal canal. During this process, the caudal-most portion of the mesonephric duct is absorbed. Thus, the ureteric bud no longer buds off of the mesonephric duct but enters the UG sinus directly. As such, the UG sinus forms the bladder and the ureteric buds form the ureters. The UG sinus forms the bladder and is continuous with the urethra caudally and the allantois cranially. The urachus is the fibrotic cord that remains when the allantois is obliterated and becomes the median umbilical ligament in the adult.

There are many renal anomalies (e.g., horseshoe kidney, ectopic kidney, double ureter) that go undiagnosed and are without much consequence. Renal agenesis, however, is not one of these. Without kidneys, the fetus can still excrete waste via placental exchange, however it essentially has anhydramnios. Without amniotic fluid, the fetal lungs do not have constant pressure on them causing them to expand and grow. This leads to pulmonary hypoplasia. Without amniotic fluid, the fetus cannot move much, so develops dramatic contractures of the limbs. There have been attempts to put amniotic fluid into the amniotic cavity via amniocentesis. However, this has been unsuccessful because the fluid is resorbed rapidly. An indwelling catheter has also been considered, but the infectious risks are quite high. At this point in time, there is minimal treatment available for Potter's disease. However, in Potter's syndrome secondary to bladder outlet obstruction, there have been attempts to place catheters into the bladder or to perform in utero laser ablation of the obstruction. In theory, as long as the fetal kidneys have not been damaged, this idea should work. However, the results thus far are mixed.

KEY POINTS

1. Fetal congenital anomalies primarily arise during embryogenesis. However, they can progress (as seen in Potter's syndrome) as development continues.
2. NTDs are associated with folate deficiency and can be screened for by noting an elevated MSAFP.
3. Cardiac anomalies that are surgically repaired can often result in minimal impairment, although this is highly lesion dependent.
4. Organ systems are often interconnected during development, as in the case of the lungs and kidneys in Potter's syndrome.

■ PRENATAL SCREENING

Screening for fetal chromosomal and congenital anomalies is dependent upon finding screens that are both sensitive and specific for the condition being screened. Before we move on to discuss these modalities, we should quickly review the terms used with screening tests.

Epidemiology

The classic two-by-two table in epidemiology is divided into cases and controls versus exposed and unexposed. In screening tests, the two dimensions are affected/not affected versus screen positive/screen negative (Table 3-1).

As can be seen in Table 3-1, the sensitivity is the proportion of those who are affected and test positive. On the other hand, the specificity is that proportion of individuals who are unaffected and test negative. Sometimes we are more interested in what it means to have a particular test result. In this setting, the positive predictive value (PPV) reports what percentage of patients with a positive screen are affected. The negative predictive value (NPV) looks at the percentage of people with a negative screen who indeed are not affected. Another set of useful test characteristics are likelihood ratios. The positive likelihood ratio (LR+) tells how much to multiply the prior odds to get the posterior odds; that is, if one knows the odds of some event occurring is 1:100, and runs a test with a LR+ of 5, then the odds after getting a positive result is 5:100. Similarly, the negative likelihood ratio (LR–) does the same for a negative result.

First-Trimester Screening

First trimester was traditionally the time for the first prenatal visit, and to check labs. However, there has recently been an interest in first-trimester serum and ultrasound screening for two theoretical benefits. One is to find screening tests that are more sensitive than the current second-trimester tests. The other is that by making the diagnosis sooner, the option

of termination is safer. **Nuchal translucency** (NT) appears to be an excellent way to screen for aneuploidy and Down syndrome in particular. NT involves a measurement of the posterior fetal neck taken in profile view. Its sensitivity for Down syndrome has been reported to be between 60% to 90%, and is generally assumed to be about 70% or greater.

Several maternal serum analytes have been studied to generate a first-trimester serum screen. Currently, a combination of free b-hCG and PAPP-A (pregnancy-associated plasma protein A) are being studied alone and in combination with NT. Using a 5% false positive rate, they appear to have a sensitivity of approximately 60% used alone and, when combined, the two appear to give an approximate sensitivity of 80%. Commonly, thresholds for these tests are established at a 5% false positive rate, or where the posterior probability of disease is somewhere between 1:190 to 1:300.

Second-Trimester Screening

The initial second-trimester serum screen was the MSAFP. This was designed to screen for fetuses with NTD. When the data from studies was being analyzed it was noted that the cases of Down syndrome had low MSAFP. This has been combined with low serum estriol and high β-hCG as the expanded AFP (XAFP), or triple screen (Table 3-2). Overall, the current XAFP has only a 60% sensitivity for Down syndrome with a 5% false positive rate. Maternal age is essentially another screening tool because it has been found that the risk of aneuploidy increases exponentially beyond age 35 (Figure 3-6). At age 35, the overall risk is about 1:190 of aneuploidy. The XAFP is combined with maternal age to generate an overall risk profile of both Down syndrome and trisomy 18. Among women over 35, the XAFP has a sensitivity of 80%, whereas in women under age 35, the sensitivity drops to about 50%.

Another finding from studies of MSAFP has been in patients whose MSAFP was elevated, but did not have NTD. Common reasons for this include inaccurate dating (MSAFP increases with gestation), abdominal wall defects, multiple gestations, and fetal demise. Patients whose MSAFP is elevated without an elevated amniotic fluid AFP or these other etiologies have been found to be at greater risk of pregnancy complications associated with the placenta: placental abruption, preeclampsia, IUGR, and possibly IUFD. These problems have been associated with elevated β-hCG as well.

■ TABLE 3-1

	Screen Positive (Pos)	Screen Negative (Neg)
Affected	a	b
Not affected	c	d

Notes: Sensitivity (sens) = a / (a + b).
Specificity (spec) = d / (c + d).
False negative = b / (a + b).
False positive = c / (c + d).
Positive predictive value (PPV) = a / (a + c).
Negative predictive value (NPV) = d / (b + d).
Positive likelihood ratio (LR+) = sens / (1 − spec) = [a/(a + b)]/[c/(c + d)].
Negative likelihood ratio (LR−) = (1 − sens) / spec = [b/(a + b)]/[d/(c + d)].

■ TABLE 3-2

Triple Screen Table			
	Trisomy 21	Trisomy 18	Trisomy 13
MSAFP	Decreased	Decreased	Depends on defects
Estriol	Decreased	Decreased	Depends on defects
β-hCG	Elevated	Decreased	Depends on defects

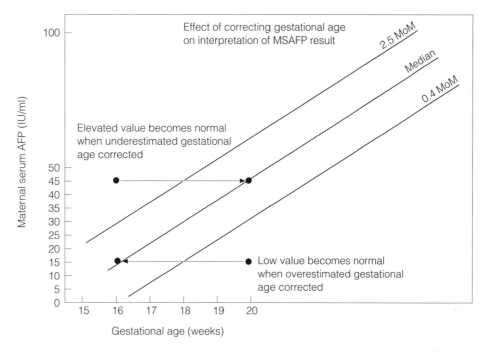

Figure 3-6 • Median maternal serum α-fetoprotein levels throughout gestation. Increasing values with increasing gestational age require accurate dating to interpret low or high MSAFP.

Real-time ultrasound is used to document a singleton, viable gestation and a rudimentary anatomy scan in more than 90% of pregnancies in the United States. The level-I obstetric ultrasound scan is a fair screening tool, but its sensitivity varies between providers. One study showed that there was a two- to threefold difference in the number of anomalies identified between primary and tertiary medical centers. The level-I ultrasound is not designed to be all encompassing and does not look at fetal limbs, identify sex, the face or provide extensive views of the heart. These are generally all done in a level-II or targeted ultrasound. A level-II ultrasound is utilized in patients who are at risk for congenital anomalies or who have had an abnormal level-I scan. These tests are generally performed by specially trained perinatologists or radiologists.

There are a number of "soft" findings on obstetrical ultrasound that have been associated with aneuploidies. Trisomy 18 has been associated with the finding of a choroid plexus cyst, and Down syndrome has been associated with many ultrasound findings, most notably the **echogenic intracardiac focus** (EIF). Pathologically, the EIF (Figure 3-7) is a calcification of the papillary muscle without any particular pathophysiology. It is seen in 5% of pregnancies, and is more common in the fetuses of Asian women. Unfortunately, the LR+ for this test is 1.5:2.0, so it at most doubles the pretest odds. For example, a young, 25-year-old woman whose Down syndrome risk is 1:1000 prior to finding the EIF will therefore have an "increased" risk of 1:500 after finding the EIF. Thus, these tests end up needlessly worrying many patients only to identify a few abnormal fetuses.

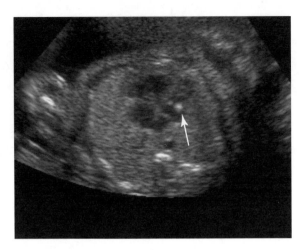

Figure 3-7 • Echogenic intracardiac focus (EIF).
(Image provided by Departments of Radiology and Obstetrics & Gynecology, University of California, San Francisco.)

KEY POINTS

1. The sensitivity of a screening test is that percentage of patients who would be identified by the test.
2. Common screening tests for fetal abnormalities include the XAFP and level-I ultrasound.
3. One component of the XAFP—the MSAFP—is used to screen for NTDs.
4. The overall sensitivity of the XAFP for Down syndrome is 60%.

■ PRENATAL DIAGNOSIS

In patients who are known carriers of a genetic disease, at high risk for aneuploidy based on age, or who have a positive screening test, the next step is to obtain prenatal diagnosis. This involves obtaining fetal cells in order to perform a karyotype and possibly DNA tests. There are currently three ways that fetal cells are obtained: amniocentesis, CVS, and percutaneous umbilical blood sampling (PUBS).

Amniocentesis

An amniocentesis may be performed beyond 15 weeks to obtain a fetal karyotype, once the chorion and amnion have fused. Amniocentesis is also offered to any patient of advanced maternal age (AMA). **Amniocentesis** involves placing a needle transabdominally through the uterus into the amniotic sac

and withdrawing some of the fluid. The fluid contains sloughed fetal cells that can be cultured. These cultured cells can then be karyotyped and also utilized in DNA tests.

The cultures take about 5 to 7 days to grow, but a newer technique—**fluorescent in-situ hybridization (FISH)**—can be used to look for aneuploidy and gets results in 24 to 48 hours. Generally, the risk of complications secondary to amniocentesis is considered to be about 1:200. The common risks are rupture of membranes, preterm labor and, rarely, fetal injury. This risk of 1:200 is one of the reasons why the threshold risk for offering patients fetal diagnosis is about 1:200, which is roughly equivalent to age 35. While it is true that the numbers are the same, the outcomes—Down syndrome and miscarriage—are quite different.

Chorionic Villous Sampling (CVS)

Chorionic villous sampling (CVS) can be used to obtain a fetal karyotype sooner than amniocentesis because it can be performed between week 9 to week 11. CVS involves placing a catheter into the intrauterine cavity, either transabdominally or transvaginally, and aspirating a small quantity of chorionic villi from the placenta. The risk of complications from CVS is likely higher than the amniocentesis rate of 1:200. Because a greater amount of cells are obtained, CVS results are often faster than those of amniocentesis. However, the cells are from the placenta; therefore, in rare cases of confined placental mosaicism, the cells may be misleading. Complications include preterm labor, premature rupture of membranes, previable delivery, and fetal injury. When performed earlier than week 9, CVS has been associated with limb anomalies, which is assumed to be secondary to vascular interruption.

Fetal Blood Sampling

PUBS is performed by placing a needle transabdominally into the uterus and phlebotomizing the umbilical cord. This procedure may be used when a fetal hematocrit needs to be obtained, particularly in the setting of Rh alloimmunization, other causes of fetal anemia, and hydrops. PUBS is also used for rapid karyotype analysis. Because the amount of fetal cells in a PUBS is so high, there is no need to culture the cells prior to analysis. The PUBS needle can then be used to transfuse the fetus in cases of fetal anemia. Intrauterine transfusion (IUT) was performed before the advent of real-time ultrasound by placing needles into the fetal peritoneal cavity and performing intraperitoneal transfusions, but transumbilical transfusions are more effective.

Fetal Imaging

Currently, ultrasound is used most commonly to image a fetus prenatally. As described above, a level-I ultrasound is commonly performed between weeks 18 and 22. The fetal anatomy can be difficult to visualize well prior to week 18, and if an anomaly is seen, the further work-up can take more than a week, giving the patient just a few days prior to week 24 to decide about termination of the pregnancy in the setting of congenital anomalies. A targeted, level-II ultrasound can identify cleft lip, polydactyly, club foot (Figure 3-8), fetal sex, NTDs, abdominal wall defects, and renal anomalies. It can usually identify cardiac and brain anomalies as well, but may not be able to make the specific diagnosis. It is poor at identifying esophageal atresia and tracheo-esophageal fistula, in which sometimes the only sign may be a small or nonvisualized stomach in the setting of polyhydramnios.

Fetal echocardiogram is usually used to make specific diagnoses of fetal cardiac anomalies detected on ultrasound. Doppler ultrasound can characterize the blood flow through the chambers of the heart as well as the vessels entering and leaving the heart. Fetal echo is used in some institutions as the first line diagnostic modality in patients at high risk for cardiac anomalies, in particular, pregestational diabetic patients.

Fetal MRI is one of the newest modalities to image a fetus. It is particularly useful in examining the fetal brain, and recognizes hypoxic damage sooner than ultrasound. It is also superior in measuring volumes. Another new modality that may be better in mea-

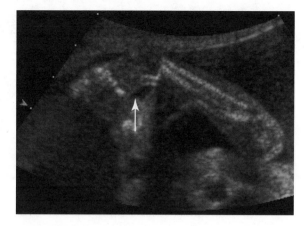

Figure 3-8 • Club foot—The fibula and tibia can be seen with the foot at almost a right angle to them.
(Image provided by Departments of Radiology and Obstetrics & Gynecology, University of California, San Francisco.)

suring volumes is three-dimensional (3-D) ultrasound. While the image provided certainly looks more like an actual fetus than the more common 2-D images, it is unclear whether 3-D ultrasound offers increased diagnostic capabilities.

KEY POINTS

1. Karyotype and DNA tests require fetal or trophoblastic cells for analysis.
2. Fetal diagnosis in the first trimester is by CVS, which obtains trophoblastic cells.
3. In the second trimester, amniocentesis is used to obtain fetal cells in the amniotic fluid.
4. Prenatal diagnosis can also be made by imaging studies, most commonly 2-D ultrasound. Fetal echocardiogram, MRI, and 3-D ultrasound are also used.

Normal Labor and Delivery

■ LABOR AND DELIVERY

When a patient first presents to the labor floor, a quick initial assessment is made using the history of present pregnancy, obstetric history, and the standard medical and social history. Routinely, patients are queried regarding contractions, vaginal bleeding, leakage of fluid, and fetal movement. Beyond the standard physical examination, the obstetric examination includes maternal abdominal examination for contractions and the fetus (**Leopold maneuvers**), cervical examination, fetal heart tones, and a sterile speculum examination if rupture of membranes is suspected.

Obstetric Examination

The physical examination includes determination of fetal lie and presentation and a cervical examination. **Fetal lie**, that is, whether the infant is longitudinal or transverse within the uterus, is relatively easy to determine with Leopold maneuvers (Figure 4-1). The maneuvers involve palpating first at the fundus of the uterus in the maternal upper abdominal quadrants, then on either side of the uterus (maternal left and right), and finally, palpation of the presenting part just above the pubic symphysis. Determination of **fetal presentation**, either breech or vertex (cephalic), can be more difficult, and even the most experienced examiner may require ultrasound to confirm presentation.

Rupture of Membranes

In 10% of pregnancies, the membranes surrounding the fetus rupture at least 1 hour prior to the onset of labor; this is called premature rupture of membranes (PROM). When PROM occurs more than 18 hours before labor, it is considered prolonged PROM and puts both mother and fetus at increased risk for infection. PROM is often confused with PPROM, which is preterm, premature rupture of membranes, with preterm being before week 37 gestational age.

Diagnosis

Diagnosis of rupture of membranes (ROM) is suspected with a history of a gush or leaking of fluid from the vagina, although sometimes it is difficult to differentiate between stress incontinence and small leaks of amniotic fluid. Diagnosis can be confirmed by the **pool**, **nitrazine**, and **fern** tests.

Using a sterile speculum to examine the vaginal vault, the pool test is positive if there is a collection of fluid in the vagina. This can be augmented by asking the patient to cough or bear down, potentially allowing one to observe fluid escaping from the cervix. Vaginal secretions are normally acidic, whereas amniotic fluid is alkaline. Thus, when the fluid is placed on nitrazine paper, the paper should immediately turn blue. The estrogens in the amniotic fluid cause crystallization of the salts in the amniotic fluid when it dries. Under low microscopic power, the crystals resemble the blades of a fern, giving the test its name. Caution should be exercised to sample fluid that is not directly from the cervix because cervical mucus also ferns and may result in a false positive reading. If these tests are equivocal, an ultrasound examination can determine the quantity of fluid around the infant. If fluid volume was previously normal and there is no other reason to suspect low fluid, **oligohydramnios** is indicative of ROM. In situations when an accurate diagnosis is necessary (e.g., PPROM where antibiotic prophylaxis would be

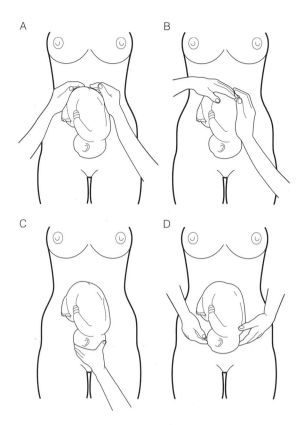

A   B

C   D

Figure 4-1 • A–D: Leopold's maneuvers used to determine fetal presentation, position, and engagement.

indicated), amniocentesis may be used to inject dilute indigo carmine dye into the amniotic sac to look for leakage of fluid from the cervix onto a tampon.

Cervical Examination

The cervical examination allows the obstetrician to determine whether a patient is in labor, the phase of labor, and how labor is progressing. The five components of the cervical examination are dilation, effacement, station, cervical position, and consistency of the cervix. These five aspects of the examination make up the **Bishop score** (Table 4-1). A Bishop score greater than 8 is consistent with a cervix favorable for both spontaneous and, as it is more commonly used, induced labor.

Dilation is assessed by using either one or two fingers of the examining hand to determine how open the cervix is at the level of the **internal os**. The measurements are in centimeters and range from closed, or 0 cm, to fully dilated, or 10 cm. On average, 10-cm dilation is necessary to accommodate the term infant's biparietal diameter.

Effacement is also a subjective measurement made by the examiner. It determines how much length is left of the cervix how effaced (i.e., thinned out) it is (Figure 4-2). The typical cervix is 3–5 cm in length; thus, if the cervix feels like it is about 2 cm from external to internal os, it is 50% effaced. Complete or 100% effacement occurs when the cervix is as thin as the adjoining lower uterine segment.

The relation of the fetal head to the ischial spines of the female pelvis is known as **station** (Figure 4-3). When the most descended aspect of the presenting part is at the level of the ischial spines, it is designated 0 station. Station is negative when the presenting part is above the ischial spines and positive when it is below. There are two systems of measuring the distance of the presenting part in relation to the ischial spines. One divides the distance to the pelvic inlet into thirds and thus station is −3 to 0 and then 0 to +3, which is at the level of the introitus. The other system uses centimeters, which gives stations of −5 to +5. Either system is effective and both are widely used among different institutions,

■ TABLE 4-1

The Bishop Score

	Score			
	0	1	2	3
Cervical dilation (cm)	Closed	1–2	3–4	<5
Cervical effacement (%)	0–30	40–50	60–70	<80
Station	−3	−2	−1, 0	<+1
Cervical consistency	Firm	Medium	Soft	
Cervical position	Posterior	Mid	Anterior	

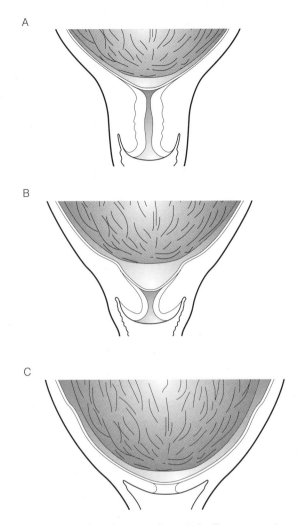

A

B

C

Figure 4-2 • A: The absence of cervical effacement prior to labor. B: The cervix is approximately 50% effaced. C: The cervix is as thin as the adjoining lower uterine segment, 100% effaced.

however, the American College of Obstetricians and Gynecologists (ACOG) recommends the usage of the (+5) system in its clinical guidelines.

Cervical **consistency** is self-explanatory. Whether the cervix feels firm, soft or somewhere in between should be noted. Cervical **position** ranges from posterior to mid to anterior. A posterior cervix is high in the pelvis, located behind the fetal head and often quite difficult to reach, let alone examine. The anterior cervix can usually be felt easily on examination and is often lower down in the vagina. During early labor, the cervix often changes its consistency to soft and advances its position from posterior to mid to anterior.

Fetal Presentation and Position

The fetal presentation can be **vertex** (head down), **breech** (buttocks down), or **transverse** (neither down). Although presentation may already be known from the Leopold maneuvers, it can be confirmed by examination of the presenting part during cervical examination. Assuming that the cervix is somewhat dilated, the fetal presenting part may be palpated as well during this examination. In the early stages of labor when the cervix is not very dilated, digital exam of the presenting part can be difficult, leading to inaccurate determination of presentation. However, palpation of hair or sutures on the fetal vertex or the gluteal cleft or anus on the breech usually leaves little doubt. A fetus presenting head-first should actually be designated cephalic rather than vertex, unless the head is flexed and the vertex is truly presenting. If the fetus is cephalic with an extended head, it may be presenting with either the face or brow.

Fetal **position** in the vertex presentation is usually based on the relationship of the fetal occiput to the maternal pelvis. Position is determined by palpation of the sutures and fontanelles. The vault, or roof, of the fetal skull is composed of five bones: two frontal, two parietal, and one occipital. The **anterior fontanelle** is the junction between the two frontal bones and two parietal bones and is larger and diamond-shaped. The **posterior fontanelle** is the junction between the two parietal bones and the occipital bone and is smaller and more triangular-shaped. In the setting of extensive molding of the fetal skull or asynclitism, where the sagittal suture is not midline within the maternal pelvis, palpation of the fetal ear can be used to determine position. With face presentations, the chin or mentum is the fetal reference point, while with breech presentations the reference is the fetal sacrum (Figure 4-4). If fetal presentation cannot be determined by physical examination, ultrasound can confirm presentation. Ultrasound is also useful in determining whether a breech presentation is frank, complete, or footling. Breech presentations are discussed further in Chapter 6.

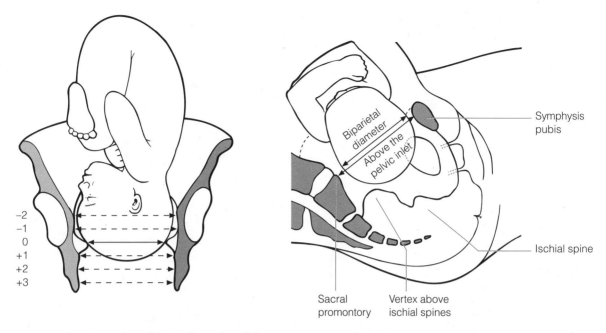

Figure 4-3 • The relationship of the leading edge of the presenting part of the ischial spine determines the station. Station +1 is depicted in the frontal view on the left; station −2 to −1 is depicted in the lateral view on the right.

KEY POINTS

1. The physical exam of a pregnant woman on labor and delivery often includes Leopold maneuvers, a sterile speculum exam, and a cervical exam.
2. It is important to determine both the presentation of the fetus and status of the cervix. The cervical exam includes dilation, effacement, station, consistency, and position.

■ NORMAL LABOR

Labor is defined as contractions that cause cervical change in either effacement or dilation. **Prodromal labor** or "false labor" is common in the differential diagnosis of labor. These patients usually present with irregular contractions that vary in duration, intensity, and intervals and yield little or no cervical change.

The diagnosis of labor strictly defined is regular uterine contractions that cause cervical change. However, clinicians use many other signs of labor, including patient discomfort, bloody show, nausea and vomiting, and palpability of contractions. These signs and symptoms vary from patient to patient; although they can add to the assessment, clinicians should rely on an objective definition.

■ INDUCTION AND AUGMENTATION OF LABOR

Induction of labor is the attempt to begin labor in a nonlaboring patient, whereas **augmentation of labor** is intervening to increase the already present contractions. Labor is induced with **prostaglandins**, **oxytocic agents**, mechanical dilation of the cervix, and/or **artificial rupture of membranes**. The indications for induction are based on either maternal, fetal, or fetoplacental reasons. Common indications for induction of labor include postterm pregnancy, preeclampsia, premature ROM, nonreassuring fetal testing, and intrauterine growth restriction. The patient's desire to end the pregnancy is *not* an indication for induction of labor.

Preparing for Induction

When proper indications for induction exist, the situation should be discussed with the patient and a plan for induction formed. When the indication is more pressing, induction should be started without significant delay. The success of an induction (defined as achieving vaginal delivery) is often correlated with favorable cervical status as defined by the **Bishop score**. A Bishop score of 5 or less leads to a failed

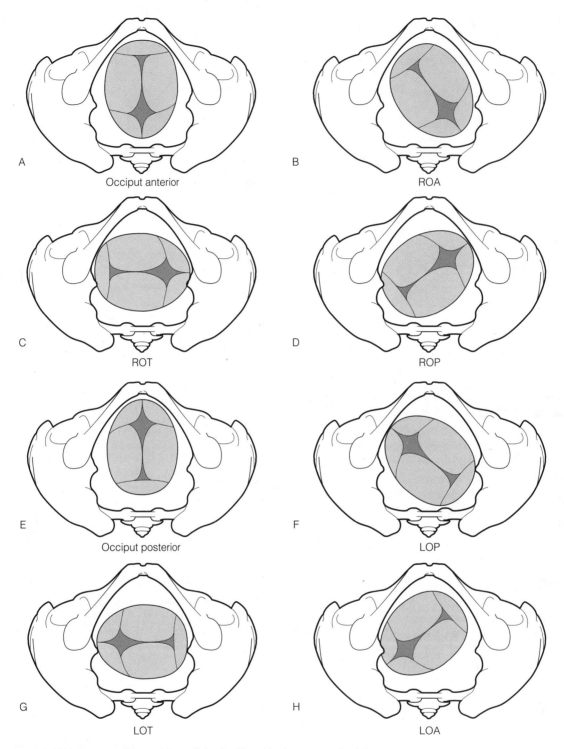

Figure 4-4 • A–H: Various possible positions of the fetal head in the maternal pelvis.

induction as often as 50% of the time. In these patients, prostaglandin E_2 (PGE_2) gel, PGE_2 pessary (cervidil), or PGE_1M (misoprostol) are often used to "ripen" the cervix.

There are both maternal and obstetric contraindications for the use of prostaglandins. Maternal reasons include asthma and glaucoma. Obstetric reasons include having had more than one prior cesarean section and nonreassuring fetal testing. Because PGE_2 gel cannot be turned off with the ease of Pitocin, there is a risk of uterine hyperstimulation and tetanic contractions. In this setting, a mechanical dilator such as laminaria or a 30 cc foley bulb can be used. The laminaria tents are placed inside the cervical canal and, over the course of 6 to 12 hours, dilate the cervix as they absorb water and expand. The foley is placed inside the cervix adjacent to the amniotic sac, inflated, and placed on gentle traction. It usually dilates the cervix within 4 to 6 hours.

Induction

Labor may begin with the ripening and dilation of the cervix performed with prostaglandins or mechanical means. However, induction is usually begun pharmacologically with pitocin. This is a synthesized, but identical, version of the octapeptide oxytocin normally released from the posterior pituitary that causes uterine contractions. Pitocin is given continuously via IV since it is rapidly metabolized.

Labor may also be induced by **amniotomy**. Amniotomy is performed with an amnio hook that is used to tear the amniotic sac around the fetus and release some of the amniotic fluid. After the amniotomy is performed, a careful examination should be performed to ensure that prolapse of the umbilical cord has not occurred. When performing amniotomy, it is important not to elevate the fetal head from the pelvis to release more of the amniotic fluid because this may lead to prolapse of the umbilical cord beyond the fetal head.

Augmentation

Pitocin and amniotomy are also used to augment labor. The indications for augmentation of labor include those for induction in addition to inadequate contractions or a prolonged phase of labor. The adequacy of contractions is indirectly assessed by the progress of cervical change. It may also be measured directly using an **intrauterine pressure catheter** (IUPC) that determines the absolute change in pressure during a contraction and thus estimates the strength of contractions.

■ MONITORING OF THE FETUS IN LABOR

It is easy to monitor the mother in labor with vital signs and laboratory studies. Monitoring the infant is indirect and thus more difficult than maternal assessment. Determination of the baseline rate and assessment of fetal heart rate variations with contractions can be done by auscultation. The normal range for the fetal heart rate is between 110 and 160 beats per minute. With baselines above 160, fetal distress secondary to infection, hypoxia, or anemia is of concern. Any bradycardia of greater than 2 minutes duration with a heart rate less than 90 is of concern and requires immediate action.

External Electronic Monitors

Since the advent of electronic fetal monitoring, auscultation is rarely used. Continuous fetal heart monitors are standard in most hospitals in the United States because they afford several advantages over auscultation. The information gathered is more subtle and includes variations in heart rate. Probably the greatest advantage is that the information is easier to gather and record, thus allowing more time for analyzing the data.

The external tocometer has a pressure transducer that is placed against the patient's abdomen, usually near the fundus of the uterus. During uterine contractions, the abdomen becomes firmer, and this pressure is transmitted through the transducer to a tocometer that records the contraction. The relative heights of the tracings on different patients or at different locations on the same patient cannot be used to compare strength of contractions. External tocometers are most useful for measuring the frequency of contractions and comparing to the fetal heart rate tracing to determine the type of decelerations occurring.

A fetal heart rate tracing is examined for several characteristics that are considered reassuring. First, the baseline is determined and should be in the normal range (110 to 160 beats per minute). Then the variations from the baseline should be examined. A flat tracing is not reassuring. The tracing should be jagged from the beat-to-beat variability of the heart rate. There should also be at least three to five cycles per minute of the heart rate around the baseline. Finally, a tracing can be considered formally reactive (Figure 4-5) if there are at least two accelerations of at least 15 beats per minute over the baseline that last for at least 15 seconds within 20 minutes.

Decelerations of the Fetal Heart Rate

The fetal heart rate tracing should also be used to examine decelerations (decels) and can be used along with the tocometer to determine the type and severity. There are three types of decelerations: early, variable, and late. **Early decelerations** begin and end approximately at the same time as contractions (Figure 4-6A). They are a result of increased vagal tone secondary to head compression during a contraction. **Variable decelerations** can occur at any time and tend to drop more precipitously than either early or late decels (Figure 4-6C). They are a result of umbilical cord compression. Repetitive variables with contractions can be seen when the cord is

entrapped either under a fetal shoulder or around the neck and is compressed with each contraction. **Late decelerations** begin at the peak of a contraction and slowly return to baseline after the contraction has finished (Figure 4-6B). These decels are a result of uteroplacental insufficiency and are the most worrisome type. They may degrade into bradycardias as labor progresses, particularly with stronger contractions.

Fetal Scalp Electrode

In the case of repetitive decels or in fetuses who are difficult to trace externally with Doppler, a **fetal scalp electrode** (FSE) is often used. A small electrode is attached to the fetal scalp that senses the potential differences created by the depolarization of the fetal heart. The information obtained from the scalp electrode is more sensitive in terms of the beat-to-beat variability and is in no danger of being lost during contractions as the fetal position changes.

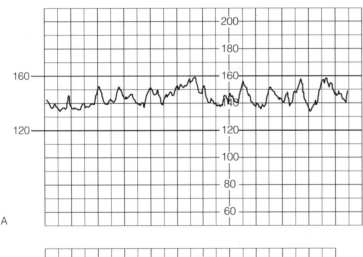

A

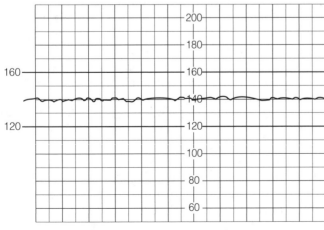

B

Figure 4-5 • A: Normal short- and long-term beat-to-beat variability. **B:** Reduced variability. This may occur during fetal sleep, following maternal intake of drugs, or with reduced fetal CNS function, as in asphyxia.

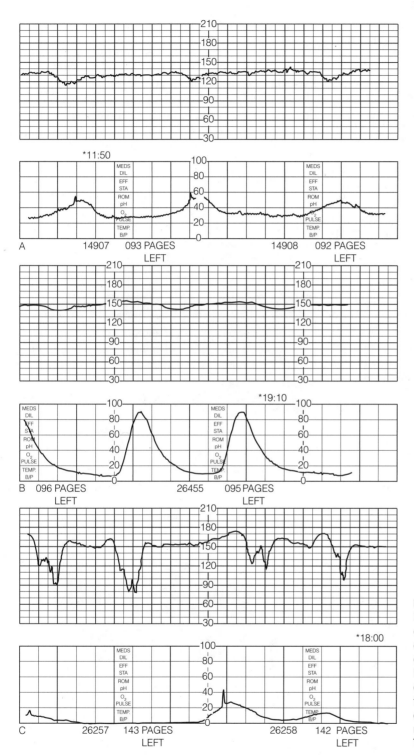

Figure 4-6 • A: An early deceleration pattern is depicted in this FHR tracing. Note that each deceleration returns to baseline before the completion of the contraction. The remainder of the FHR tracing is reassuring. **B:** Repetitive late decelerations in conjunction with decreased variability. **C:** Variable decelerations are the most common periodic change of the FHR during labor. Repetitive mild to moderate variable decelerations are present. The baseline is normal.

Contraindications include a history of maternal hepatitis or human immunodeficiency virus (HIV) or fetal thrombocytopenia.

Intrauterine Pressure Catheter

The external tocometer records the onset and end of contractions. The absolute values of the readings mean little and are entirely position dependent. Further, on some patients—particularly those who are obese—the tocometer does not show much in the way of fluctuation from the baseline. If it is particularly important to determine the timing or strength of contractions, an IUPC may be used (Figure 4-7). This catheter is threaded past the fetal presenting part into the uterine cavity to measure the pressure changes during contractions. The baseline intrauterine pressure is usually between 10 and 15 mm Hg. Contractions during labor will increase by 20–30 mm Hg in early labor and by 40–60 mm Hg as labor progresses. The most commonly used measurement of uterine contractions is the **Montevideo unit**, which is an average of the variation of the intrauterine pressure from the baseline multiplied by the number of contractions in a 10-minute period. Some institutions use the Alexandria unit, which multiplies the Montevideo units by the length of each contraction as well.

Fetal Scalp pH

If a fetal heart rate tracing is nonreassuring, the fetal scalp pH may be obtained to directly assess fetal hypoxia and acidemia (Figure 4-8). Fetal blood is obtained by making a small nick in the fetal scalp and drawing up a small amount of fetal blood into capillary tubes. The results are reassuring when the scalp pH is greater than 7.25, indeterminant between 7.20 and 7.25, and nonreassuring when less than 7.20. Care must be taken to avoid contamination of the blood sample with amniotic fluid, which is basic and will elevate the results falsely. Although this tool is used less frequently now that technology has improved fetal monitoring, it can still provide additional information on fetal well being.

KEY POINTS

1. Labor can be induced or augmented with prostaglandins, pitocin, laminaria, foley bulb, and artificial rupture of membranes.
2. The fetus can be monitored in labor with external fetal monitoring, fetal scalp electrode, ultrasound, and fetal scalp pH.

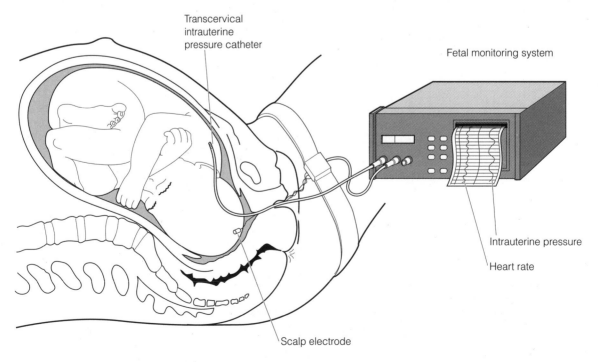

Transcervical intrauterine pressure catheter

Fetal monitoring system

Intrauterine pressure

Heart rate

Scalp electrode

Figure 4-7 • Technique for continuous electronic monitoring of FHR and uterine contractions.

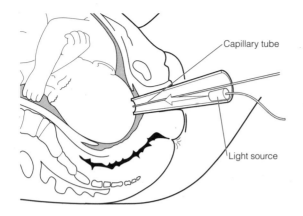

Figure 4-8 • Technique for fetal scalp blood sampling via an amnioscope. After making a small stab incision in the fetal scalp, the blood is drawn off through a capillary tube.

The Progression of Labor

Labor is assessed by the progress of cervical effacement, cervical dilation, and descent of the fetal presenting part. To assess the progress of labor, it is important to understand the cardinal movements or mechanisms of labor.

Cardinal Movements of Labor

The cardinal movements are engagement, descent, flexion, internal rotation, extension, and external rotation (also called restitution or resolution) (Figure 4-9). When the fetal presenting part enters the pelvis, it is said to have undergone **engagement**. The head will then undergo **descent** into the pelvis, followed by **flexion**, which allows the smallest diameter to present to the pelvis. With descent into the midpelvis, the fetal vertex undergoes **internal rotation** from an occiput transverse (OT) position so that the sagittal suture is parallel to the anteroposterior diameter of the pelvis—either occiput anterior (OA) or occiput posterior (OP). As the vertex passes beneath and beyond the pubic symphysis, it will **extend** to deliver. Once the head delivers, **external rotation** occurs and the shoulders may be delivered.

Stages of Labor

Labor and delivery are divided into three stages. Each stage involves different concerns and considerations. Stage 1 begins with the onset of labor and lasts until dilation and effacement of the cervix are completed. Stage 2 is from the time of full dilation until delivery of the infant. Stage 3 begins after delivery of the infant and ends with delivery of the placenta.

Stage 1

The first stage of labor ranges from the onset of labor until complete dilation of the cervix has occurred. An average first stage of labor lasts approximately 10 to 12 hours in a nulliparous patient and 6 to 8 hours in a multiparous patient. The range of what is considered within normal limits is quite wide, from 6 hours up to 20 hours in a nulliparous patient and from 2 to 12 hours in a multiparous patient. The first stage is divided further into the latent and active phases (Figure 4-10).

The **latent phase** generally ranges from the onset of labor until 3 or 4 cm of dilation and is characterized by slow cervical change. The **active phase** follows the latent phase and extends until greater than 9 cm of dilation and is defined by the period of time when the slope of cervical change against time increases. A third phase is often delegated at this point called deceleration or transition phase as the cervix completes dilation. During the active phase, at least 1.0 cm/hr of dilation is expected in the nulliparous patient and 1.2 cm/hr in the multiparous patient. This minimal expectation is approximately the fifth percentile of women undergoing labor and the median rates of dilation range from 2.0 to 3.0 cm/hr during the active phase.

The three "Ps"—powers, passenger, and pelvis— can all affect the transit time during the active phase of labor. The "powers" are determined by the strength and frequency of uterine contractions. The size and position of the infant affect the duration of the active phase, as do the size and shape of the maternal pelvis. If the "passenger" is too large for the "pelvis" **cephalopelvic disproportion** (CPD) results. If the rate of change of cervical dilation falls below the fifth percentile (1.0 cm/hr), these three Ps should be assessed to determine whether a vaginal delivery can be expected. Strength of uterine contractions can be measured with an IUPC, and is considered adequate with greater than 200 Montevideo units. Signs of CPD include development of fetal caput and extensive molding of the fetal skull with palpable overlapping sutures.

Stage 2

When the cervix has completely dilated, stage 2 has begun. Stage 2 is completed with delivery of the infant. Stage 2 is considered prolonged if its duration is longer than 2 hours in a nulliparous patient,

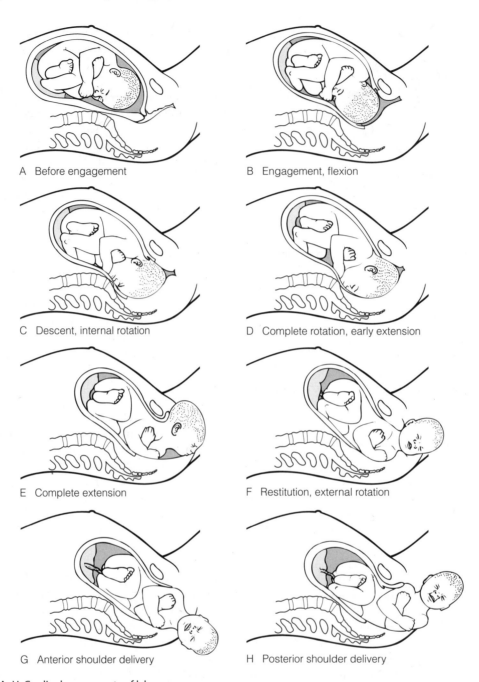

A Before engagement

B Engagement, flexion

C Descent, internal rotation

D Complete rotation, early extension

E Complete extension

F Restitution, external rotation

G Anterior shoulder delivery

H Posterior shoulder delivery

Figure 4-9 • A–H: Cardinal movements of labor.

although 3 hours are allowed in patients who have epidurals. In multiparous women, stage 2 is prolonged if its duration is longer than 1 hour without an epidural and 2 hours with an epidural. In multiparous women, it is rare for stage 2 to last longer than 30 minutes unless there is fetal macrosomia, persistent occiput posterior position, compound presentation, or asynclitism.

Monitoring

Repetitive early and variable decels are common during the second stage. The clinician can be reassured if these decels resolve quickly after each contraction and there is no loss of variability in the tracing. Repetitive late decels, bradycardias, and loss of variability are all signs of nonreassuring fetal status. With these tracings, the patient should be placed on

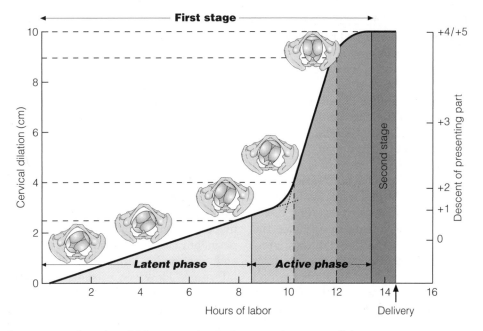

Figure 4-10 • The progress of rotation of OA presentation in the successive stages of labor.

face mask O_2, turned onto her left side to decrease inferior vena cava (IVC) compression and increase uterine perfusion; if it is being used, the pitocin should be immediately discontinued until the tracing resumes a reassuring pattern. If a bradycardia is felt to be the result of uterine **hypertonus** (a single contraction lasting 2 minutes or longer) or **tachysystole** (greater than five contractions in a 10-minute period), which can be diagnosed by palpation or examination of the tocometer, the patient can be given a dose of terbutaline to help relax the uterus. If a nonreassuring pattern does not resolve with these interventions, the fetal position and station should be assessed to determine whether an operative vaginal delivery can be performed. If fetal station is above +2 or the position cannot be determined, cesarean delivery is the mode of choice.

Vaginal Delivery

As the fetus begins crowning, the delivering clinician should be dressed with goggles, sterile gown, and sterile gloves (for self-protection as much as for prevention of maternal/fetal infection) and have two clamps, scissors, suction bulb, and—when meconium is suspected or confirmed—a DeLee suction trap. Various approaches can be taken to vaginal delivery, but most clinicians would agree that a smooth, controlled delivery leads to less perineal trauma. A modified Ritgen's maneuver (Figure 4-11) using the heel of the delivering hand to exert pressure on the peri-

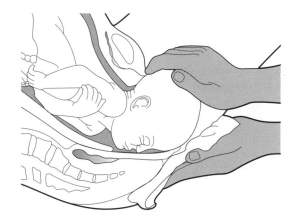

Figure 4-11 • Near completion of the delivery of the fetal head by the modified Ritgen maneuver. Moderate upward pressure is applied to the fetal chin by the posterior hand covered with a sterile towel while the suboccipital region of the fetal head is held against the symphysis.

neum and to extend the fetal head to hasten delivery and maintain station between contractions may be performed. Simultaneously, the opposite hand should be used to flex the head to keep it from extending too far and causing periurethral and labial lacerations. This hand can also be used to massage the labia over the head during delivery.

Once the head of the infant is delivered, the mouth and upper airway are bulb suctioned. If there is meconium in the amniotic fluid, the DeLee suction tube is passed down the infant's nares and mouth and vigorous suctioning is performed before delivery of the shoulders. After suctioning is complete, the infant's neck is checked for a wrapped umbilical cord. If a nuchal cord exists, an attempt is made to reduce the cord over the infant's head. If it is too tight, two options exist. If the clinician is extremely confident that delivery will be accomplished shortly, the cord is clamped and cut at this point. If a shoulder dystocia is suspected, an attempt is made to deliver the infant with the nuchal cord intact.

Delivery of the rest of the infant follows first with delivery of the anterior shoulder by exerting direct downward pressure on the infant's head. Once the anterior shoulder is visualized, a direct upward pressure is exerted to deliver the posterior shoulder (Figure 4-12). After this, exertion of gentle traction will deliver the torso and the rest of the infant. At this point, the cord is clamped and cut and the infant passed either to the labor nurse and mother or to the waiting pediatricians.

Episiotomy

An **episiotomy** is an incision made in the perineum to facilitate delivery. Indications for episiotomy include need to hasten delivery and impending or ongoing shoulder dystocia. A relative contraindication for episiotomy is the assessment that there will be a large perineal laceration. Once the episiotomy is cut, great care should be taken to support the peri-neum around the episiotomy to avoid extension into the rectal sphincter or rectum itself. In the past, episiotomies were used routinely in the setting of spontaneous and operative vaginal deliveries. However, evidence suggests that the rate of third- and fourth-degree lacerations increases with the use of routine midline episiotomy.

There are two common types of episiotomies: median (or midline) and mediolateral (Figure 4-13). The median episiotomy, the most common type used in the United States, uses a vertical midline incision from the posterior fourchette into the perineal body. The mediolateral episiotomy is an oblique incision made from either the 5 or 7 o'clock position on the perineum and cut laterally. It is used less frequently and reportedly causes more pain and wound infections. However, mediolateral episiotomies are thought to lead to fewer third- and fourth-degree extensions, particularly in patients with short peri-neums or with operative deliveries.

Operative Vaginal Delivery

In the case of a prolonged stage 2, maternal exhaustion, or the need to hasten delivery, an operative vaginal delivery may be indicated. The two possibilities are forceps delivery or vacuum-assisted delivery. Both are effective methods to facilitate vaginal delivery and have similar indications. The decision of which method to choose is based on clinician preference and experience.

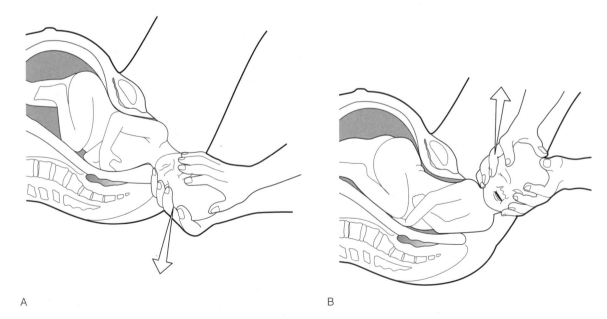

A   B

Figure 4-12 • A: Delivery of the anterior shoulder. B: Delivery of posterior shoulder.

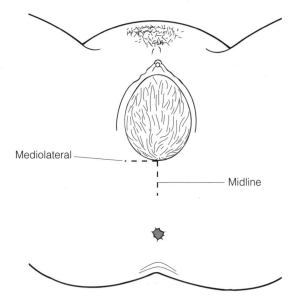

Figure 4-13 • Placement of mediolateral and midline episiotomy.

Forceps Delivery

Forceps (Figure 4-14) have blades that are placed around the infant's head and are shaped with a cephalic curve to accommodate the head. In addition, most have a pelvic curve that conforms to the maternal pelvis. The blade of each forcep is at the end of a shank that is connected to a handle. The two forceps are connected at the lock between the shank and the handle. Once the forceps are placed around the fetal head, the operator pulls on the handles to aid maternal expulsive efforts (Table 4-2).

The conditions necessary for safe application of forceps include full dilation of the cervix, ruptured membranes, engaged head and at least +2 station, absolute knowledge of the position, no evidence of cephalopelvic disproportion, adequate anesthesia, empty bladder, and—most important—an experienced operator. In some institutions mid-forceps applications (fetal station between 0 and +2) and rotational forceps (fetal head more than 45 degrees from either direct OA or OP position) are also used. An experienced operator is, again, the most important component of these deliveries. Use of high forceps with the fetal vertex above 0 station is no longer considered a safe obstetric procedure. Complications from forceps application include bruising on the face and head, lacerations to the fetal head and birth canal, facial nerve palsy, and, rarely, skull fracture and/or intracranial damage.

Vacuum Extraction

The **vacuum extractor** consists of a vacuum cup that is placed on the fetal scalp and a suction device that is connected to the cup to create the vacuum. Conditions for the safe use of the vacuum extractor are identical to that of forceps. Vacuum should never be chosen because position is unknown or the station is too high. Exertion on the cup and consequently on the fetal scalp is made parallel to the axis of the maternal pelvis concomitant with maternal bearing-down efforts and uterine contractions. The most common complications of use of the vacuum are scalp laceration and cephalohematoma. There is great debate between clinicians as to which of these forms of operative delivery are safer, but a large retrospective study shows no difference in fetal outcomes between forceps and vacuum deliveries.

Stage 3

Stage 3 begins once the infant has been delivered. It is completed with delivery of the placenta. Placental

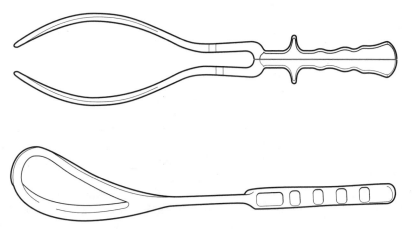

Figure 4-14 • Forceps.

■ TABLE 4-2

Classification of Forceps Delivery According to Station and Rotation

Type of Procedure	Classification
Outlet forceps	1. Scalp is visible at the introitus without separating the labia
	2. Fetal skull has reached pelvic floor
	3. Sagittal suture is in anteroposterior diameter or right or left occiput anterior or posterior position
	4. Fetal head is at or on perineum
	5. Rotation does not exceed 45 degrees
Low forceps	Leading point of fetal skull is at station 2 or greater, but not on the pelvic floor
	a. Rotation < 45 degrees (left or right occiput anterior to occiput anterior, or left or right occiput posterior to occiput posterior)
	b. Rotation > 45 degrees
Mid forceps	Station above +2 cm but head engaged
High forceps	Not included in classification

Source: From Cunningham FG, et al. Williams Obstetrics. 19th ed. Norwalk: Appleton & Lange, 1993: 557.

separation usually occurs within 5 to 10 minutes of delivery of the infant; however, up to 30 minutes is usually considered within normal limits. With the abrupt decrease in intrauterine cavity size after delivery of the fetus, the placenta is mechanically sheared from the uterine wall with contractions. Classically, the use of oxytocin was contraindicated during stage 3. However, this was established prior to the use of ultrasound out of concern for causing abruption in the case of an undiagnosed twin. If there is no doubt about completion of stage 2, oxytocin can be used during the stage 3 to strengthen uterine contractions to decrease both placental delivery time and blood loss.

The three signs of placental separation include cord lengthening, a gush of blood, and uterine fundal rebound as the placenta detaches from the uterine wall. No attempt to deliver the placenta should be made until all these signs are noted. The placenta is delivered by gentle traction on the cord. It is important not to use too much traction because the cord may avulse or uterine inversion may occur. When the patient begins bearing down for delivery of the placenta, it is imperative that one of the examiner's hands is applying suprapubic pressure to keep the uterus from inverting or prolapsing (Figure 4-15). When the placenta is evident at the introitus, the delivery should be controlled to avoid both further perineal trauma and tearing of any of the membranes that often trail the placenta at delivery.

Retained Placenta

The diagnosis of retained placenta is made when the placenta does not deliver within 30 minutes after the infant. Retained placenta is common in preterm deliveries, particularly previable deliveries. However, it is also a sign of placenta accreta, where the placenta has invaded into or beyond the endometrial stroma. The retained placenta may be removed by manual extraction. A hand is placed in the intrauterine cavity and the fingers used to shear the placenta from the surface of the uterus (Figure 4-16). If the placenta cannot be completely extracted manually, a curettage is performed to ensure no products of conception (POC) are retained.

Laceration Repair

Lacerations are repaired after placental delivery. A thorough examination of the perineum, labia, periurethral area, vagina, and cervix is performed to assess lacerations. The most common lacerations are perineal lacerations, which are described by the depth of tissues they involve (Figure 4-17). A first-degree laceration involves the mucosa or skin. Second-degree lacerations extend into the perineal body but do not involve the anal sphincter. Third-degree lacerations extend into or completely through the anal sphincter. A fourth-degree tear occurs if the anal mucosa itself is entered.

Repair of any superficial lacerations, including first-degree perineal tears, is usually accomplished

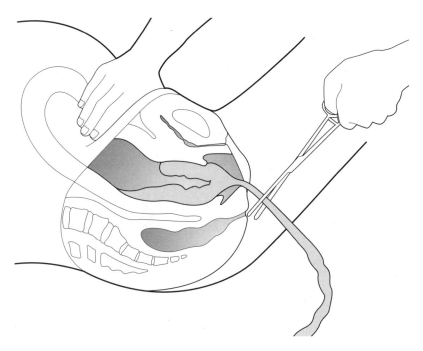

Figure 4-15 • Delivery of the placenta with traction on the cord and suprapubic pressure on the uterus to prevent uterine inversion.

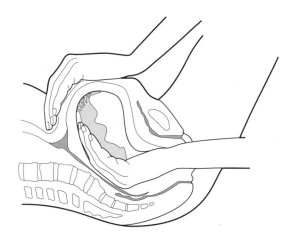

Figure 4-16 • Manual removal of placenta. The fingers are alternately abducted, adducted, and advanced until the placenta is completely detached.

with interrupted sutures. A second-degree laceration is repaired in layers. The apex of the laceration, which often lies beyond the hymenal ring, is located and a suture is anchored at the apex. This suture is then run down to the level of the hymenal ring, bringing together the vaginal tissue. This suture is then passed beyond the hymenal ring and used to bring together the perineal body. Sometimes a separate suture is used to place a "crown stitch" that brings together the perineal body. Finally, the skin of

the perineum is closed with a subcuticular closure (Figure 4-18).

Third-degree lacerations require repair of the anal sphincter with several interrupted sutures and then the rest of the repair is completed as in a second-degree repair. Fourth-degree repairs are begun with repair of the anal mucosa. Mucosal repair is performed meticulously to prevent fistula formation. Once the rectum is repaired, a fourth-degree laceration is completed just as a third-degree repair.

Cesarean Section

Cesarean section has been used effectively throughout the twentieth century and is one of the most common operations performed today. The current cesarean rate in the United States is approximately 23%. Although maternal mortality from cesarean section is low, approximately 0.01%, it is still higher than from vaginal delivery. Further, the morbidity from infections, thrombotic events, wound dehiscence, and recovery time is greater than that of vaginal delivery.

The most common indication for primary cesarean section is that of failure to progress in labor. Failure to progress can be caused by problems with any of the three Ps. If the pelvis is too small or the fetus too large (depending on the viewpoint taken), the diagnosis is CPD, which leads to failure to progress. If the uterus simply does not generate

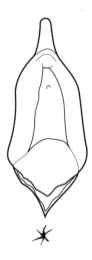
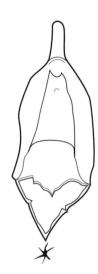
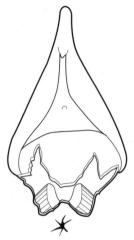
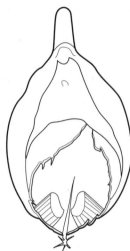

| First-degree tear (Superficial) | Second-degree tear (Into the body of the perineum) | Third-degree tear (Into the anal sphincter) | Fourth-degre tear (Into the rectum) |

Figure 4-17 • Perineal tears.

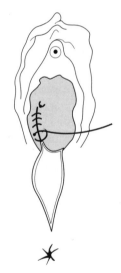

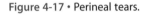
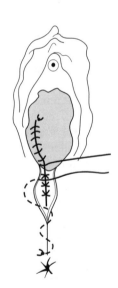
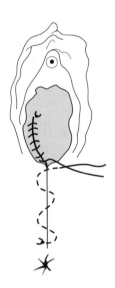

1   2   3

Figure 4-18 • A: Repair of a second-degree laceration. 1—The vaginal mucosa is repaired down to the level of the hymenal ring. 2—The subcutaneous tissue of the perineum is then brought together. 3—Finally, the skin of the perineum is reapproximated in a subcuticular fashion.

enough pressure during contractions, labor can stall and lead to failure to progress. If labor seems to be stalling, there are a number of measures that can be taken to augment it, such as pitocin or ROM.

Other common indications for primary cesarean section (Table 4-3) are breech presentation, shoulder or compound presentation, placenta previa, placental abruption, nonreassuring fetal status, cord prolapse, prolonged stage 2, failed operative vaginal delivery, or active herpes lesions. The most common indication for cesarean section is a previous cesarean section.

Vaginal Birth After Cesarean Section

Vaginal birth after cesarean section (VBAC) can be attempted if the proper setting exists. This includes knowledge of the prior hysterotomy, in-house obstetrician and anesthesiologist, and informed patient consent. The prior hysterotomy needs to be either a Kerr (low transverse incision) or Kronig (low vertical incision) without any extensions into the cervix or upper uterine segment. The greatest risk during a

TABLE 4-3

Indications for Cesarean Section

Type	Indication
Maternal/fetal	Cephalopelvic disproportion
	Failed induction of labor
Maternal	Maternal diseases
	Eclampsia/severe preeclampsia
	Active genital herpes
	Cervical cancer
	Prior uterine surgery
	Classic cesarean section
	Full-thickness myomectomy
	Prior uterine rupture
	Obstruction to the birth canal
	Fibroids
	Ovarian tumors
Fetal	Nonreassuring fetal testing
	Bradycardia
	Absence of FHR variability
	Scalp pH < 7.20
	Cord prolapse
	Fetal malpresentations
	Breech, transverse lie, brow
	Multiple gestations
	Nonvertex first twin
	Higher-order multiples
	Fetal anomalies
	Hydrocephalus
	Osteogenesis imperfecta
Placental	Placenta previa
	Abruptio placentae

trial of labor after cesarean (TOLAC) is that of rupture of the prior uterine scar, which occurs approximately 0.5% to 1.0% of the time. Prior classical hysterotomies, or vertical incisions through the thick upper segment of the uterine corpus, are at a higher risk for uterine rupture in labor and women who have had this type of cesarean are not usually allowed to attempt a trial of labor. Other factors associated with success or failure of a TOLAC and with uterine rupture are listed in Table 4-4. Common signs of rupture include abdominal pain, FHR decelerations or bradycardia, sudden decrease of pressure on an IUPC, and maternal sensation of a "pop." Therefore, the patient needs to be monitored closely in labor and delivered emergently if uterine rupture is suspected.

KEY POINTS

1. Labor is divided into stages: stage 1 extends until complete cervical dilation, stage 2 until delivery of the infant, and stage 3 until delivery of the placenta.
2. Forceps delivery and vacuum extraction are two forms of operative vaginal delivery that are used to expedite vaginal delivery.
3. Cesarean delivery has multiple indications and is the most common operation performed in the United States.

■ OBSTETRIC ANALGESIA AND ANESTHESIA

Natural Childbirth

Certainly a component of the discomfort during labor comes from the anticipation of pain and the apprehension that accompanies this event. The concept behind natural childbirth is to educate patients regarding the experiences of labor and delivery in order to prepare them for the event. In addition, a variety of relaxation techniques, showers, and massage are used to help patients cope with the pain from uterine contractions. These techniques have been formalized in the Lamaze method, which involves a series of classes for both the patient and a birthing coach that teach relaxation and breathing techniques.

Systemic Pharmacologic Intervention

Either narcotics or sedatives can be useful in the first stage of labor to relax patients and decrease pain. Because they cross the placenta, sedating medications should not be used close to the time of expected delivery because they may result in a depressed infant. Other complications of these medications are respiratory depression and increased risk of aspiration.

Pudendal Block

The pudendal nerve travels just posterior to the ischial spine at its juncture with the sacrospinous ligament. With the pudendal block, anesthetic is injected at that site, bilaterally, to give perineal anesthesia. A pudendal block is commonly used in the

■ **TABLE 4-4**

Risk Factors for Uterine Rupture and Success or Failure in a TOLAC

Increased Success of TOLAC	Increased Risk of Uterine Rupture
Prior vaginal birth	More than one prior cesarean delivery
Prior VBAC	Prior classical cesarean
Nonrecurring indication for prior C/S	Induction of labor
(herpes, previa, breech)	Use of prostaglandins
Presentation in labor at:	Use of high amounts of oxytocin
>3 cm dilated	Time from last cesarean < 18 months
>75% effaced	Uterine infection at time of last cesarean
Decreased Success of TOLAC	**Decreased Risk of Uterine Rupture**
Prior C/S for cephalopelvic disproportion	Prior vaginal birth
Induction of labor	

case of operative vaginal delivery with either forceps or vacuum. It may be combined with local infiltration of the perineum to ensure perineal anesthesia (Figure 4-19).

Local Anesthesia

In patients without anesthesia who are going to require an episiotomy, local infiltration with an anesthetic is used. Local anesthetic is also used before repair of vaginal, perineal, and periurethral lacerations.

Epidural and Spinal Anesthesia

Epidurals are commonly administered to patients who wish to have anesthesia throughout the active phase and delivery of the infant. Many patients worry about nerve damage and the pain of the epidural itself. An early consult with an anesthesiologist to help answer questions about the epidural can be reassuring. The epidural catheter is placed in the L3–L4 interspace when the patient requires analgesia, although usually not until labor is deemed to be in the active phase. Once the catheter is placed, an

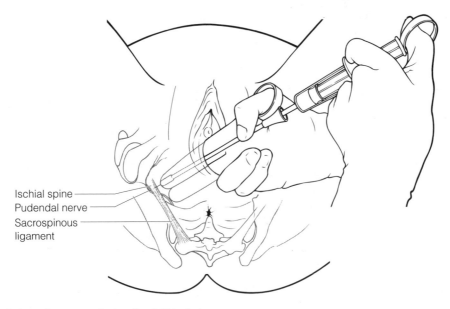

Ischial spine
Pudendal nerve
Sacrospinous ligament

Figure 4-19 • Technique for transvaginal pudendal block.

initial bolus of anesthetic is given and a continuous infusion is started. Again, the epidural does not commonly remove all sensation and can actually be detrimental to the stage 2 if it does so. However, if the patient requires cesarean delivery, the epidural can be bolused and usually provides adequate anesthesia.

Spinal anesthesia provides anesthesia over a region similar to that of an epidural, but differs in that it is given in a one-time dose. It is used more commonly for cesarean section than vaginal delivery. A common complication of both forms of anesthesia is maternal hypotension secondary to decreased systemic vascular resistance, which can lead to decreased placental perfusion and fetal bradycardia. A more serious complication can be maternal respiratory depression if the anesthetic reaches a level high enough to affect diaphragmatic innervation. A spinal headache due to the loss of cerebrospinal fluid is a postpartum complication seen in less than 1% of patients.

General Anesthesia

Although general anesthesia is rarely used for vaginal delivery, it may be used for cesarean section, particularly in the emergent setting. For less urgent cesarean sections, epidural or spinal anesthesia is usually preferred. The two principal concerns of general anesthesia are the risk of maternal aspiration and the risk of hypoxia to mother and fetus during induction. Thus, when choosing the route of anesthesia for a cesarean section, the urgency of the delivery must be assessed. Common reasons for an emergent cesarean section are abruption, fetal bradycardia, uterine rupture, and hemorrhage from a placenta previa.

KEY POINTS

1. Obstetrical anesthesia allows for more patient comfort throughout labor.
2. Epidurals are commonly used during labor, whereas spinals are used more often for cesarean section.
3. Epidural anesthesia leads to a longer stage 2 of labor, but offers better control during crowning.
4. Occasionally, general anesthesia is used in the emergent setting.

Obstetric hemorrhage is a leading cause of maternal death in the United States and one of the leading causes of perinatal morbidity and mortality. Bleeding during pregnancy has different etiologies depending on the trimester. As discussed in Chapter 2, first-trimester bleeding is associated with spontaneous abortion, ectopic pregnancy, and even normal pregnancies. Third-trimester vaginal bleeding occurs in 3% to 4% of pregnancies and may be obstetric or nonobstetric (Table 5-1). Hemorrhage can occur antepartum or postpartum (Chapter 12), with the major causes of antepartum hemorrhage including placenta previa (20%) and placental abruption (30%).

■ PLACENTA PREVIA

Pathogenesis

Placenta previa is defined as abnormal implantation of the placenta over the internal cervical os (Figure 5-1). **Complete previa** occurs when the placenta completely covers the internal os. **Partial previa** occurs when the placenta covers a portion of the internal os. **Marginal previa** occurs when the edge of the placenta reaches the margin of the os. A low-lying placenta is one that is implanted in the lower uterine segment but does not extend to the internal os.

Bleeding from a placenta previa results from small disruptions in the placental attachment during normal development and thinning of the lower uterine segment during the third trimester. As a result, profuse hemorrhage and shock can occur, leading to significant maternal and fetal mortality and morbidity. Although the maternal and perinatal mortality from placenta previa has dropped rapidly in the United States over the past few decades, the perinatal mortality rate is still 10 times that in the general population. Most risk to the fetus comes from premature delivery, which is responsible for 60% of perinatal deaths. Other fetal risks associated with placenta previa are listed in Table 5-2.

Placenta previa may also be complicated by an associated placenta accreta (placenta previa accreta). **Placenta accreta** is defined as the abnormal invasion of the placenta into the uterine wall. An **accreta** is defined as the superficial invasion of the placenta into the uterine myometrium. An **increta** occurs when the placenta invades the myometrium. A **percreta** occurs when the placenta invades through the myometrium to the uterine serosa.

Placenta accreta causes an inability of the placenta to separate from the uterine wall after delivery of the fetus. This can result in profuse hemorrhage and shock with substantial maternal morbidity and mortality. Two-thirds of women with both a placenta previa and an associated accreta require a hysterectomy at the time of delivery (puerperal hysterectomy). Table 5-3 summarizes the abnormalities of placentation.

Epidemiology

Placenta previa occurs in 0.5% of pregnancies (1 : 200 births) and accounts for nearly 20% of all antepartum hemorrhages. It is seen in as many as 1% to 4% of women with prior cesarean sections. Placenta previa can also be complicated by an associated placenta accreta (placenta previa accreta) in 5% to 15% of cases. The risk of accreta is also increased in women with prior cesarean section and has been seen in 25% to 30% of women with one prior cesarean section and placenta previa in 50% to 65% of women with multiple prior cesarean sections.

TABLE 5-1

Differential Diagnosis of Antepartum Bleeding

Obstetric causes	
Placental	Placenta previa, placental abruption, vasa previa
Maternal	Uterine rupture
Fetal	Fetal vessel rupture
Nonobstetric causes	
Cervical	Severe cervicitis, polyps, cervical cancer
Vaginal/Vulvar	Lacerations, varices, cancer
Other	Hemorrhoids, congenital bleeding disorder, abdominal or pelvic trauma, hematuria

Source: Adapted from Hacker N and Moore JG. Essentials of Obstetrics and Gynecology. Philadelphia: WB Saunders, 1992:155.

TABLE 5-2

Fetal Complications Associated with Placenta Previa

Preterm delivery and its complications

Preterm premature rupture of membranes

Intrauterine growth restriction

Malpresentation

Vasa previa

Congenital abnormalities

Adapted from Hacker N and Moore JG. Essentials of Obstetrics and Gynecology. Philadelphia: WB Saunders, 1992:155.

Abnormalities in placentation are the result of events that prevent normal migration of the placenta during normal progressive development of the lower uterine segment during pregnancy (Table 5-4). Previous placental implantations and prior uterine scars are thought to contribute to abnormal placentation in subsequent pregnancies. Thus, placenta previa appears to be increased in patients with other prior uterine surgery such as myomectomy, uterine anomalies, multiple gestations, multiparity, advanced maternal age, smoking, and previous placenta previa. Of note, because many patients receive a routine obstetric ultrasound, marginal previa or low-lying placenta are not uncommonly seen in the second trimester. Most of these will resolve on repeat ultrasound by moving up and away from the cervix during the third trimester as the lower uterine segment develops.

TABLE 5-3

Abnormalities of Placentation

Circumvallate placenta	Occurs when the membranes double back over the edge of the placenta, forming a dense ring around the periphery of the placenta. Often considered a variant of placental abruption, it is a major cause of second-trimester hemorrhage.
Placenta previa	Occurs when the placenta develops over the internal cervical os. Types include complete, partial, and marginal.
Placenta accreta	Abnormal adherence of part or all of the placenta to the uterine wall. May be associated with a placenta in normal locations, but incidence increases in placenta previa.
Placenta increta	Abnormal placentation where the placenta invades the myometrium.
Placenta percreta	Abnormal placentation where the placenta invades through the myometrium to the uterine serosa. Occasionally, placentas may invade into adjacent organs such as the bladder or rectum.
Vasa previa	Occurs when a velamentous cord insertion causes the fetal vessels to pass over the internal cervical os. Seen also with velamentous and succenturiate placenta.
Velamentous placenta	Occurs when the blood vessels insert between the amnion and the chorion, away from the margin of the placenta. This leaves the vessels largely unprotected and vulnerable to compression or injury.
Succenturiate placenta	An extra lobe of the placenta that is implanted at some distance away from the rest of the placenta. Fetal vessels may course between the two lobes, possibly over the cervix, leaving these blood vessels unprotected and at risk for rupture.

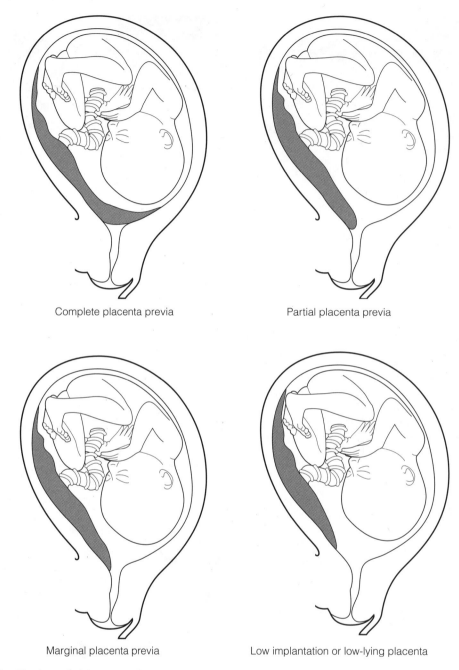

Complete placenta previa

Partial placenta previa

Marginal placenta previa

Low implantation or low-lying placenta

Figure 5-1 • Classifications of placenta previa.

■ CLINICAL MANIFESTATIONS

History

Patients with placenta previa classically present with sudden and profuse **painless vaginal bleeding**. The first episode of bleeding—the "sentinel" bleed— usually occurs after 28 weeks of gestation. During this time, the lower uterine segment develops and thins, disrupting the placental attachment and resulting in bleeding. Placenta accreta is usually asymptomatic. On rare occasions, however, a patient with a percreta into the bladder or rectum may present with hematuria or rectal bleeding.

TABLE 5-4
Predisposing Factors for Placenta Previa
Prior cesarean section, uterine surgery such as myomectomy
Multiparity
Multiple gestation
Erythroblastosis
Smoking
History of placenta previa
Increasing maternal age

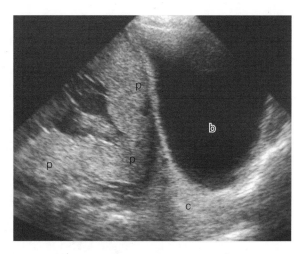

Figure 5-2 • Complete placenta previa. p = placenta, c = cervix, b = bladder.

Physical Examination

Vaginal examination is contraindicated in placenta previa because the digital examination can cause further separation of the placenta and trigger catastrophic hemorrhage. Because many patients have an ultrasound exam that can, among other things, diagnose placenta previa, examination of the placenta previa is uncommon today. In the rare setting of a patient who is misdiagnosed, the cervical exam may reveal soft, spongy tissue just inside the cervix. Because of the increased vascularity, there may be notable varices in the lower uterine segment or cervix that can be seen on speculum exam or palpated. A marginal previa can be palpated at the edge of, or quite near, the internal os.

Diagnostic Evaluation

The diagnosis of placenta previa can be made via ultrasonography with a sensitivity of greater than 95% (Figure 5-2). If it is made before the third trimester in pregnancy, a follow-up ultrasound is often obtained in the third trimester to see if the previa has resolved. In patients with a known or suspected previa, transvaginal sonography is usually avoided. Transabdominal or translabial views can usually be used to determine the extent of placentation. If the ultrasound is performed with a full maternal bladder, placenta previa may be overdiagnosed secondary to compression of the lower uterine segment, resembling a longer cervix. It is therefore important to have the bladder entirely emptied before this portion of the ultrasound is performed if a previa is in question.

Treatment

Management of patients with placenta previa varies between providers. Commonly, antepartum patients with a placenta previa are managed with strict pelvic rest (i.e., no intercourse) and modified bed rest. However, some clinicians will not institute this conservative management until the patient presents with the sentinel bleed. Similarly, hospitalized bed rest is sometimes prescribed after the sentinel bleed by some clinicians, whereas others wait until the patient has a large bleed by history, exam, or drop in hematocrit higher than 3 points.

Unstoppable labor, fetal distress, and life-threatening hemorrhage are all indications for immediate cesarean delivery regardless of gestational age. In the case of preterm pregnancy, if the bleeding is not profuse, fetal survival can be enhanced by aggressive expectant management. However, 70% of patients with placenta previa have a recurring bleeding episode and will require delivery before week 36. For patients who make it to week 36, typical management involves amniocentesis to determine fetal lung maturity and delivery by cesarean section between 36 and 37 weeks after confirmation of lung maturity.

The following should be done in the case of vaginal bleeding and suspected placenta previa.

1. **Stabilize the patient.** Every patient with vaginal bleeding and a known or suspected previa should be hospitalized, placed on fetal monitoring, and have IV access established. If the patient presents with a particularly large bleed, two large bore IVs

will commonly be placed. The labs that are sent include a hematocrit, type and cross, and, if the bleeding has been large or a coagulopathy is suspected, PT, PTT, d-dimer or fibrin split products, and fibrinogen. For an Rh-negative woman, a Kleihauer-Betke test should be performed to determine the extent of any fetomaternal transfusion so that the appropriate amount of RhoGAM can be administered to prevent alloimmunization.

2. **Prepare for catastrophic hemorrhage.** Expectant management in the stabilized patient includes hospitalization, bed rest, and hematocrit monitoring. Two or more units of blood should be typed, cross-matched, and made available. Transfusions are usually given to maintain a hematocrit of 25% or greater.

3. **Prepare for preterm delivery.** Prior to 34 weeks of gestation, betamethasone is administered to promote fetal lung maturity. Tocolysis is also used to assist in prolonging the pregnancy up to 34 weeks of gestation. Occasionally, tocolysis is used past week 34 to help control the bleeding.

KEY POINTS

1. Placenta previa accounts for 20% of antepartum hemorrhage, and is associated with placenta accreta at least 5% of the time.
2. It occurs more often in patients with prior placenta previa, uterine scars, or multiple gestations.
3. It should be diagnosed by transabdominal or translabial ultrasound, not by vaginal exam.
4. The classic presentation of placenta previa is painless vaginal bleeding in the third trimester.
5. Placenta previa is associated with antepartum hemorrhage, preterm delivery, preterm premature rupture of membranes (PPROM), and intrauterine growth restriction (IUGR), and increases the risk of puerperal hysterectomy.
6. Patients are delivered by cesarean section in the case of unstoppable preterm labor, large hemorrhage, or nonreassuring fetal testing, or at week 36 with mature lung indices.
7. Placenta accreta is the abnormal attachment of the placenta to the uterus. Invasion into the myometrium is placenta increta, whereas invasion through the myometrium and to the serosa is placenta percreta.

■ PLACENTAL ABRUPTION

Pathogenesis

Placental abruption (abruptio placentae) is the premature separation of the normally implanted placenta from the uterine wall, resulting in hemorrhage between the uterine wall and the placenta. Fifty percent of abruptions occur before labor and after the 30th week of gestation, 15% occur during labor, and 30% are identified only on placental inspection after delivery. Large placental separations may result in premature delivery, uterine tetany, disseminated intravascular coagulation (DIC), and hypovolemic shock.

The primary cause of placental abruption is unknown, although it is associated with a variety of predisposing and precipitating factors (Table 5-5).

■ TABLE 5-5

Predisposing and Precipitating Factors for Placental Abruption

Predisposing factors
Hypertension
Previous placental abruption
Advanced maternal age
Multiparity
Uterine distension
Multiple pregnancy
Hydramnios
Vascular deficiency
Diabetes mellitus
Collagen vascular disease
Cocaine use
Cigarette smoking
Alcohol use (>14 drinks/wk)
Circumvallate placenta
Short umbilical cord
Precipitating factors
Trauma
External/internal version
Motor vehicle accident
Abdominal trauma
Sudden uterine volume loss
Delivery of first twin
Rupture of membranes with polyhdromnios
Preterm premature rupture of membranes

These factors include maternal hypertension, prior history of placental abruption, maternal cocaine use, external maternal trauma, and rapid decompression of the overdistended uterus.

At the initial point of separation, nonclotted blood courses from the injury site. The enlarging collection of blood may cause further separation of the placenta. In 20% of placental separations, bleeding is confined within the uterine cavity and is referred to as a **concealed hemorrhage** (Figure 5-3). In the remaining 80% of placental separations, the blood dissects downward toward the cervix, resulting in a **revealed** or **external hemorrhage**. Because there is an

egress for the blood, revealed hemorrhages are less likely to result in larger retroplacental clots, which are associated with fetal demise. The result of hemorrhage from torn placental vessels can vary from maternal anemia in mild cases to shock, acute renal failure, and maternal death in severe cases.

Global maternal mortality from placental abruption varies from 0.5% to 5.0%. Most deaths are due to hemorrhage, cardiac failure, or renal failure. Fetal mortality occurs in about 35% of all clinically relevant antepartum placental abruptions and can be as high as 50% to 80% in cases of severe placental abruption. The cause of demise is due to hypoxia resulting from decreased placental surface area and maternal hemorrhage.

Epidemiology

Placental abruption occurs in about 0.5% to 1.5% of pregnancies and is responsible for 30% of cases of third-trimester bleeding and 15% of perinatal mortality. The predisposing and precipitating factors for placental abruption are listed in Table 5-5. The most common factor associated with increased incidence of abruption is hypertension, whether it is chronic or a result of preeclampsia. In cases of abruption that are severe enough to cause fetal death, 50% are due to hypertension: 25% of these are from chronic hypertension and 25% are from preeclampsia. The risk of abruption in future pregnancy is 10% after one abruption and 25% after two prior abruptions.

Clinical Manifestations

History

The classic presentation of placental abruption is third-trimester vaginal bleeding associated with severe abdominal pain and/or frequent, strong contractions. However, about 30% of placental separations are small with few or no symptoms and are identified only after inspection of the placenta at delivery. The symptoms of abruption and their rate of occurrence are listed in Table 5-6.

Physical Examination

On physical examination, a patient with placental abruption will often have vaginal bleeding and a firm, tender uterus. On tocometer, small frequent contractions are usually seen as well as tetanic contractions. On fetal monitoring, nonreassuring fetal heart tracing may be seen secondary to hypoxia. A classic sign of placental abruption that can only be seen at

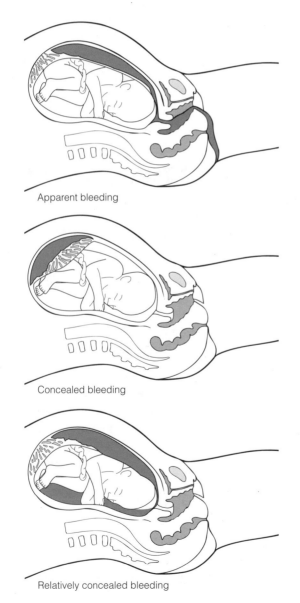

Apparent bleeding

Concealed bleeding

Relatively concealed bleeding

Figure 5-3 • Types of placental separation.

TABLE 5-6

Presentation of Abruptio Placentae

Symptom	Occurrence (%)
Vaginal bleeding	80
Uterine tenderness/abdominal or back pain	67
Abnormal contractions/increased uterine tone	34
Fetal distress	50
Fetal demise	15

the time of cesarean delivery is the Couvelaire uterus. If enough blood from the abruption penetrates into the uterine musculature, it can be seen subserosally when the uterus is removed from the abdomen during repair of the hysterotomy.

Diagnostic Evaluation

The diagnosis of placental abruption is primarily clinical. Only 2% of abruptions are picked up by ultrasound (evidenced by a retroplacental clot). However, because abruption can present similarly to placenta previa, ultrasonography is routinely performed to rule out previa in cases of suspected abruption. The diagnosis of abruption may be confirmed by inspection of the placenta at delivery. The presence of a retroplacental clot with overlying placental destruction confirms the diagnosis.

Treatment

The potential for rapid deterioration (e.g., hemorrhage, DIC, fetal hypoxia) necessitates delivery in some cases of placental abruption. However, most abruptions are small and noncatastrophic, and do not therefore necessitate immediate delivery.

The following should be done in the case of suspected placental abruption.

1. **Stabilize the patient.** When placental abruption is known or suspected, the patient should be hospitalized, IV access gained, and fetal monitoring should be started. Labs ordered should include CBC, type and cross, PT/PTT, and d-dimer or fibrin split products. For an Rh-negative woman, RhoGAM should be administered to prevent alloimmunization.
2. **Prepare for the possibility of future hemorrhage.** Standard antishock measures should be taken, including placement of large-bore intravenous catheters, infusion of lactated Ringer's solution,

and preparation of units of crossed-matched blood (whole or packed red blood cells). Blood loss due to placental abruption is commonly grossly underestimated due to the possibility of concealed bleeding.

3. **Prepare for preterm delivery.** In the preterm pregnancy, betamethasone may be given to promote fetal lung maturity and tocolysis may be given to assist in prolonging the pregnancy to week 34.
4. **Deliver if bleeding is life threatening or fetal testing is nonreassuring.** Delivery should be performed in patients with a life-threatening hemorrhage. This is a clinical determination, but any patient whose vital signs are unstable or has a coagulopathy should be delivered. Vaginal delivery is preferred as long as bleeding is controlled and there are no signs of fetal distress. Because the uterus is typically hyperactive in patients with an abruption, a rapid labor and delivery should be expected. If the fetal heart rate (FHR) tracing is nonreassuring, delivery should occur for fetal indications.

KEY POINTS

1. Placental abruption accounts for 30% of all third-trimester hemorrhages.
2. Fetal mortality rate can be as high as 35%.
3. Patients usually present with vaginal bleeding, painful contractions, and a firm, tender uterus; 20% of cases present with no bleeding (concealed hemorrhages).
4. Major risk factors include hypertension (chronic or gestational) and previous history of abruption.
5. Placental abruption can be complicated by hypovolemic shock, DIC, and preterm delivery.
6. Patients can be delivered vaginally if they are stable; cesarean delivery is necessary in the unstable patient or when fetal testing is nonreassuring.
7. Risk of recurrence increases in subsequent pregnancies.

▪ UTERINE RUPTURE

Pathogenesis

Uterine rupture represents a potential obstetric catastrophe and can lead to both maternal and fetal death. Most complete uterine ruptures occur during the course of labor. Over 90% of all uterine ruptures are associated with a prior uterine scar either from cesarean section or other uterine surgery. In the remaining less than 10% of cases, no prior scarring is present. These ruptures may be related to an abdominal trauma (e.g., auto accidents, external or internal version procedures), associated with labor or delivery (e.g., improper oxytocin use or excessive fundal pressure), or spontaneously initiated (e.g., placenta percreta, multiple gestation, grand multiparity, invasive mole, or choriocarcinoma).

The primary maternal complications from a ruptured uterus include hemorrhage and hypovolemic shock. The overall maternal mortality for uterine rupture is less than 1%, but if it occurs in the antepartum patient at home, it is likely to be higher. The perinatal mortality for uterine rupture ranges from 1% to 15%, again depending on where the patient is when the uterine rupture occurs.

Epidemiology

Uterine rupture is rare, occurring in an estimated 1:15,000 deliveries of patients with no prior uterine surgery. In women with a prior cesarean delivery, it is estimated to occur in 0.5% to 0.1% of deliveries. Risk factors for uterine rupture are conditions that predispose to a weakened uterine wall, including uterine scars, overdistension, inappropriately aggressive use of uterotonic agents, maternal congenital uterine anomalies, and abnormal placentation (Table 5-7).

Clinical Manifestations

The presentation of uterine rupture is highly variable. Typically, it is characterized by the sudden onset of intense abdominal pain. Vaginal bleeding, if present, may vary from spotting to severe hemorrhage. Nonreassuring fetal testing, abnormal abdominal contour, cessation of uterine contractions, disappearance of fetal heart tones, and regression of the presenting part are other signs of uterine rupture.

Treatment

Management of uterine rupture requires immediate laparotomy and delivery of the fetus. If feasible, the rupture site should be repaired and hemostasis obtained. In cases of large rupture extensions, repair may not be feasible and the patient may require a hysterectomy. Patients are usually discouraged to attempt future pregnancies given the high risk of recurrent rupture. Trial of labor would be avoided in any subsequent pregnancy, and the patient would commonly be delivered via repeat cesarean section at week 36 with documentation of fetal lung maturity.

KEY POINTS

1. Uterine rupture is a rare obstetric catastrophe.
2. Maternal and fetal morbidity and mortality are increased in the setting of uterine rupture.
3. It is associated with prior uterine scarring in more than 90% of cases.
4. Patients present with the sudden onset of intense abdominal pain.
5. Uterine rupture requires immediate laparotomy, delivery of the fetus, and either repair of the rupture site or hysterectomy.

■ FETAL VESSEL RUPTURE

Pathogenesis

Most pregnancies complicated by rupture of a fetal vessel are due to **velamentous cord insertion** where the blood vessels insert between the amnion and chorion away from the placenta instead of inserting directly into the chorionic plate (Table 5-3). Because the vessels course unprotected through the membranes before inserting on the placental margin, they are vulnerable to rupture, shearing, or laceration. In addition, these unprotected vessels may cross over the internal cervical os (**vasa previa**), making them vulnerable to compression by the presenting fetal part or to being torn when the membranes are ruptured. Although vasa previa is rare, perinatal mortality is high and increases if the membranes are also ruptured.

■ TABLE 5-7

Risk Factors for Uterine Rupture

Prior uterine scarring

Injudicious use of oxytocin

Grand multiparity

Marked uterine distension

Abnormall fetal lie

Large fetus

External version

Trauma

Unprotected fetal vessels and vasa previa can also be seen with a **succenturiate placenta** or accessory lobe. In this case, the bulk of the placenta is implanted in one portion of the uterine wall, but a small lobe of the placenta is implanted in another location. The vessels that connect these two portions of the placenta are unprotected and may course over the cervix and present as a vasa previa.

Epidemiology

Only 0.1% to 0.8% of pregnancies are complicated by the rupture of a fetal vessel. The incidence of vasa previa is 1:5000 pregnancies. Risk factors for fetal vessel rupture include abnormal placentation leading to succenturiate lobes as well as multiple gestation that increases the risk of velamentous insertion. Although the rate of velamentous insertion is only 1% in singleton gestations, it increases to 10% for twin gestations and 50% for triplet gestations.

Clinical Manifestations

In fortunate cases, the fetal vessels are palpated and recognized through the dilated cervix. More commonly, the presentation of a fetal vessel rupture is vaginal bleeding associated with a sinusoidal variation of the FHR indicative of fetal anemia.

Diagnosis

Unfortunately, diagnosis is often made after a large bleed and fetal compromise have already occurred. With advancing capabilities of ultrasound, velamentous insertion of the umbilical cord and succenturiate placental lobes can be diagnosed antepartum. Further, with the use of color Doppler, vasa previa may also be diagnosed antepartum, but the sensitivity and specificity of these diagnoses have not as yet been determined. Diagnosis at the time of vaginal bleeding can be accomplished by the **Apt test** or examination of the blood for nucleated (fetal) red blood cells. The Apt test, involves diluting the blood with water, collecting the supernatant and combining it with 1% NaOH. If the resulting mixture is pink it indicates fetal blood, a yellow-brown color is seen with maternal blood.

Treatment

Given the high risk of fetal exsanguination and death (the vascular volume of the term fetus is less than 250 mL), the treatment for a ruptured fetal vessel is emergent cesarean delivery. Now that vasa previa can occasionally be diagnosed antepartum, these patients are often given the option of elective cesarean delivery, although there is little data as to the fetal risk. If they elect to undergo a trial of labor, artificial rupture of membranes (AROM) is contraindicated.

KEY POINTS

1. Fetal vessel rupture is a rare obstetric complication, usually associated with multiple gestation.
2. It is due primarily to velamentous cord insertion.
3. It is associated with a perinatal mortality of 50%.
4. Patients may present with vaginal bleeding and a sinusoidal FHR pattern.
5. Fetal vessel rupture usually requires an emergency cesarean section.

■ NONOBSTETRIC CAUSES OF ANTEPARTUM HEMORRHAGE

Nonobstetric causes of antepartum hemorrhage are listed in Table 5-1. Patients with these conditions usually present with spotting rather than frank bleeding. Typically, there are no uterine contractions or abdominal pain. The diagnosis is usually made by speculum examination, Pap smear, cultures, or colposcopy as indicated. Other than advanced maternal neoplasia, which is associated with poor maternal outcome, most nonobstetric causes of antepartum hemorrhage require relatively simple management and have good outcomes. Vaginal lacerations and varices can be located and repaired. Infections may be treated with appropriate agents, cervical polyps can be removed, and benign neoplasms usually require simple treatment.

KEY POINTS

1. Nonobstetric causes of antepartum hemorrhage include cervical and vaginal lacerations, hemorrhoids, infections, and neoplasms.
2. Patients typically present with spotting rather than frank bleeding.
3. Nonobstetric causes of antepartum hemorrhage generally require simple management and have good outcomes.

Complications of Labor and Delivery

PRETERM LABOR (PTL)

Labor that occurs before week 37 is called **preterm labor** (PTL). Many patients present with preterm contractions, but only those who have changes in the cervix are diagnosed as having preterm labor. PTL differs from **incompetent cervix**, which is a silent, painless dilation of the cervix. Both can result in preterm delivery, which is the leading cause of fetal morbidity and mortality in the United States. The incidence of preterm delivery increased to over 10% of all births in 1993, and was approximately 11% in 2001.

Preterm Delivery

Infants born before week 37 are termed premature and have higher rates of morbidity and mortality. Infants are also at risk when they are born weighing less than 2500 g, and are termed **low birth weight** (LBW) infants. Infants who have not grown appropriately for their gestational age are termed **intrauterine growth restricted** (IUGR). Thus, an IUGR infant can be born after week 37 but still be LBW. Prematurity places infants at increased risk of respiratory distress syndrome (RDS) or hyaline membrane disease, intraventricular hemorrhage, sepsis, and necrotizing enterocolitis. Morbidity and mortality of preterm infants are dramatically affected by gestational age and birth weight. Infants born on the cusp of viability at 24 weeks gestation have a greater than 50% mortality rate, whereas infants born after week 36 have a mortality rate similar to that of full-term infants.

Etiology and Risk Factors

The defining physiologic mechanism that causes the onset of labor is unknown. However, various risk factors have been associated with preterm labor (PTL). These include preterm rupture of membranes (PROM); chorioamnionitis; multiple gestations; uterine anomalies such as a bicornuate uterus; previous preterm delivery; maternal prepregnancy weight less than 50 kg; placental abruption; maternal disease including preeclampsia, infections, intra-abdominal disease or surgery; and low socioeconomic status.

Tocolysis

Tocolysis is the attempt to prevent contractions and the progression of labor. Many tocolytics are used in the United States, but only ritodrine—a beta-mimetic agent—is FDA approved for this purpose. Because most patients and clinicians are unwilling to allow contractions to proceed without some tocolytic therapy, it is difficult to do placebo-controlled studies of new tocolytics. Thus, many of the current trials compare currently used tocolytics to other tocolytics. Many of the tocolytics used have only been shown to make a difference in prolonging gestation for 48 hours.

The principal benefit from gaining 48 hours in a pregnancy is to allow treatment with steroids to enhance fetal lung maturity when preterm delivery is threatened. **Betamethasone**, a glucocorticoid, has been shown to reduce the incidence of RDS and other complications from preterm delivery. Thus, prior to 34 weeks of gestation, the advantage of treating with steroids needs to be weighed against the risk of prolonging the pregnancy. In fact, there are many situations in which preterm labor should be allowed to progress. Chorioamnionitis, nonreassuring fetal testing, and significant placental abruption are absolute indications to allow labor to progress, and often to hasten delivery. With many other issues such as maternal disease—particularly preeclampsia or poor placental perfusion—an assessment of the severity of the situation, the precipitous nature of the complication, and the risks from prematurity all contribute to the decision of whether or not to tocolyze. In addition, because evidence for the efficacy of tocolytics is unclear, institutions and practitioners vary widely in practice.

Tocolytics

The goal of a tocolytic is to decrease or halt the cervical change resulting from contractions. In the case of preterm contractions without cervical change, hydration can often decrease the number and strength of the contractions. This operates along the principle that a dehydrated patient has increased levels of vasopressin or **antidiuretic hormone** (ADH), the octapeptide synthesized in the hypothalamus along with oxytocin. ADH may cross-react with oxytocin receptors and lead to contractions. Thus, hydration, which decreases the level of ADH, may also decrease the number of contractions. For patients who do not respond to hydration or whose cervices are actively changing, a variety of tocolytics may be used.

Beta-mimetics

Uterine myometrium is composed of smooth muscle fibers. The contraction of these fibers is regulated by myosin light chain kinase that is activated by calcium ions through their interaction with calmodulin (Figure 6-1). Thus, by increasing the level of cAMP, the level of free calcium ions decreases, likely by sequestration in the sarcoplasmic reticulum, and uterine contractions may be decreased. Conversion of ATP to cAMP is increased by β-agonists that bind and activate β_2 receptors on myometrial cells.

The two **beta-mimetics** commonly used for preterm labor are **ritodrine** and **terbutaline**. Although both are certainly effective in halting preterm contractions, in randomized controlled studies where patients were truly in preterm labor, β-agonists gained an average of only 24 to 48 hours further gestation over hydration and bed rest alone. Side effects of these drugs include tachycardia, headaches, and anxiety. More seriously, pulmonary edema may occur and, in rare cases, maternal death. Ritodrine is given as continuous IV therapy, whereas terbutaline is usually given as 0.25 mg SC, loaded Q 20 min × 3 doses and then Q 3–4 h maintenance.

Magnesium Sulfate

Magnesium decreases uterine tone and contractions by acting as a calcium antagonist and a membrane stabilizer. Although magnesium can stop contractions, in small placebo-controlled trials it has not been shown to change gestational age of delivery. In larger trials, the efficacy of magnesium did not vary significantly from that of beta mimetics. Side effects such as flushing, headaches, fatigue, and diplopia are seen, but they are generally considered to be less severe than those seen with ritodrine and terbutaline. At toxic levels of magnesium (>10 mg/dL), respiratory depression, hypoxia, and cardiac arrest have been seen. Since deep tendon reflexes (DTR) are depressed and then lost at levels <10 mg/dL, the best way to rule out magnesium toxicity is with serial reflex checks rather than serum levels. Pulmonary edema has also been seen in women treated with magnesium sulfate, although it may be secondary to the concomitant fluid given to patients in preterm labor. Generally, magnesium sulfate should be loaded as a 6 g bolus over 15 to 30 minutes, then maintained with a 2–3 g/hr continuous infusion. Because it is renally cleared, a slower infusion should be used in the case of renal insufficiency.

Calcium Channel Blockers

Calcium channel blockers decrease the influx of calcium into smooth muscle cells thereby diminishing uterine contractions. These have definitely been shown to decrease myometrial contractions in vitro. In clinical studies, **nifedipine** has been the principal drug studied and seems to have comparable efficacy to that of ritodrine and magnesium. Side effects include headaches, flushing, and dizziness. Nifedipine is given orally and, as with other tocolytics, should be loaded. A 10 mg dose Q 15 min for the first hour or until contractions have ceased is usually used. This is followed by a maintenance dose of 10–30 mg Q 4–6 h as tolerated by the patient's blood pressure. Long-acting preparations of nifedipine in small studies seem to have similar efficacy to the quick-release doses and can be used for long-term therapy to increase compliance and decrease side effects.

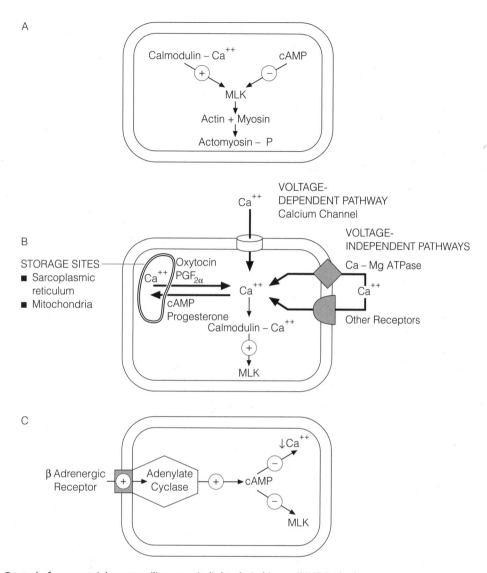

Figure 6-1 • Control of myometrial contractility: myosin light-chain kinase (MLK) is the key enzyme.

Prostaglandin Inhibitors

Prostaglandins increase the intracellular levels of calcium, thereby increasing myometrial contractions. Further, these have been shown to enhance myometrial gap junction formation and are commonly used to induce labor and to heighten contractions in postpartum patients with uterine atony. Thus, antiprostaglandin agents should theoretically inhibit contractions and possibly halt labor. **Indomethacin**, a nonsteroidal anti-inflammatory drug (NSAID) that blocks the enzyme cyclooxygenase and decreases the level of prostaglandins, is used as a tocolytic. In clinical trials, it has been shown to effectively decrease contractions and forestall labor with minimal maternal side effects. However, it has been associated with a variety of fetal complications. These include premature constriction of the ductus arteriosus, pulmonary hypertension, and oligohydramnios secondary to renal failure. Furthermore, in one study, extremely premature fetuses that had been exposed to indomethacin within 48 hours of delivery had an increased risk of necrotizing enterocolitis and intraventricular hemorrhage. Therefore, even though indomethacin is a promising tocolytic, many practitioners shy away from its use.

Oxytocin Antagonists

Currently, oxytocin antagonists are being studied as tocolytics. These have been shown to decrease uterine myometrial contractions, but clinical studies have been small thus far. In theory, these seem to be an obvious choice for an effective tocolytic and should have minimal side effects. Current clinical use has been limited to experimental trials that have shown no difference from the other commonly used tocolytics.

KEY POINTS

1. Preterm delivery occurs in greater than 10% of all pregnancies.
2. PTL is treated with tocolytics including beta-agonists, magnesium, calcium channel blockers, and NSAIDs.
3. Current tocolytics are only marginally effective, but may buy time for a course of betamethasone to accelerate fetal lung maturity.

■ PRETERM AND PREMATURE RUPTURE OF MEMBRANES

Rupture of membranes (ROM) occurring before week 37 is considered **preterm rupture of the membranes**, whereas rupture of membranes occurring before the onset of labor is termed **premature rupture of the membranes** (PROM). If the two occur together it is termed **preterm premature rupture of the membranes** (PPROM). Anytime rupture of membranes lasts longer than 18 hours before delivery, it is described as **prolonged rupture of membranes**.

Preterm Rupture of Membranes

Spontaneous rupture of the fetal membranes before week 37 is a common cause of preterm labor, preterm delivery, and chorioamnionitis. Without intervention, approximately 50% of patients who have ROM will go into labor within 24 hours, and up to 75% will do so within 48 hours. These rates are inversely correlated to gestational age at ROM; thus, patients with ROM prior to 26 weeks gestational age are more likely to gain an additional week than those greater than 30 weeks gestational age. While maintaining the pregnancy to gain further fetal maturity would seem beneficial, prolonged PPROM has been correlated with increased risk of chorioamnionitis, abruption, and cord prolapse.

Diagnosis

Commonly, a patient complains of a gush of fluid from the vagina. However, any increased vaginal discharge or complaints of stress incontinence should be evaluated to rule out PROM. The diagnosis is made by obtaining a history of leaking vaginal fluid, pooling on speculum examination, and positive nitrazine and fern tests. If these tests are equivocal, an ultrasound can be performed to examine the level of amniotic fluid. If the diagnosis is still unconfirmed, the amnio/dye test can be performed with injection of a dye via amniocentesis and observation of whether or not the dye leaks into the vagina. This is also known as the **tampon test** because the dye is usually identified by its absorption into a tampon. If there is concern for chorioamnionitis, maternal temperature and white blood count, uterine tenderness, and the fetal heart tracing should all be checked for signs of infection.

Treatment

The management of preterm rupture of membranes varies depending on the gestational age of the fetus. The reasoning behind the management of PPROM is that at some gestational age, the risk from prematurity is equal to the risk of infection. That point is somewhere between week 32 and week 36; thus, up to this point, the risk of prematurity drives management, whereas after it the risk of infection motivates delivery. There is debate regarding the point at which the risk of infection is greater. Some practitioners prefer to wait until week 36, whereas others prefer to test for fetal lung maturity starting at week 32 and deliver when mature, while still others would deliver at 32 to 34 weeks gestation without fetal lung maturity testing.

There is strong evidence that the use of antibiotics in PPROM leads to a longer latency period prior to the onset of labor. Thus, ampicillin with or without erythromycin is recommended in the setting of PPROM. There is debate surrounding the use of tocolysis and corticosteroids in the setting of PPROM. Tocolysis seems to be of little benefit in PPROM, and may even be harmful in the case of chorioamnionitis. However, at many institutions tocolysis is used for 48 hours, particularly at earlier gestational ages, in order to gain time to administer a course of corticosteroids. Currently, the recommendation is to use corticosteroids in the setting of PPROM despite any concern regarding immunosuppression because of the fetal benefits.

■ PREMATURE RUPTURE OF THE MEMBRANES (PROM)

The most common concern of premature rupture of the membranes (PROM) is that of chorioamnionitis, the risk of which increases with the length of ROM. If ROM is expected to last beyond 18 hours, it is termed prolonged rupture of the membranes and is treated with antibiotics during labor. Commonly, if ROM occurs anytime after 34 to 36 weeks, labor is induced. However, the risks of infection with prolonged PROM versus cesarean section for failed induction should be discussed with patients before any decision is made. Some patients may elect to bear the risk of increased infection to await the onset of spontaneous labor.

KEY POINTS

1. Preterm rupture of membranes is when ROM occurs before 37 weeks of gestation; premature rupture of membranes (PROM) is ROM that occurs before the onset of labor.
2. The latency period prior to the onset of labor is inversely correlated with gestational age in PPROM.
3. Once ROM is confirmed, the therapeutic course depends on gestational age, concern for risk of infection, and fetal lung maturity.
4. Any patient who shows signs of infection or fetal distress needs to be delivered.

■ OBSTRUCTION, MALPRESENTATION, AND MALPOSITION

Although the most common form of delivery is the spontaneous vertex vaginal delivery, other presentations and deliveries also occur. Many of the malpresentations lead to cesarean section.

Cephalopelvic Disproportion

One of the most common indications for cesarean section is failure to progress (FTP) in labor, most often caused by **cephalopelvic disproportion** (CPD). The three "Ps"—pelvis, passenger, and power—are primarily responsible for a vaginal delivery. If the pelvis is too small, the fetal presenting part is too large, or the contractions are inadequate, there will be FTP. The strength of uterine contractions can be measured with an intrauterine pressure catheter (IUPC) and augmented with pitocin, but little can be done about the other two factors that make up CPD.

Diagnosis

The maternal pelvis is described as one of four dominant types: **gynecoid**, **android**, **anthropoid**, and **platypelloid** (Figure 6-2). Further, many pelvises have characteristics from more than one of these types. Common measurements of the pelvis include those of the pelvic inlet, the midpelvis, and the pelvic outlet. The **obstetric conjugate**, which is the distance between the sacral promontory and the midpoint of the symphysis pubis, is the shortest anteroposterior diameter of the pelvic inlet. The anteroposterior diameter of the pelvic outlet, which measures from the tip of the sacrum to the inferior margin of the pubic symphysis, ranges from 9.5–11.5 cm. These measurements are performed with both clinical and x-ray pelvimetry, but it is rare to assume CPD based on measurements alone.

The fetal skull is composed of the face, the base, and the vault. The face and base are composed of fused bones that do not change during labor; however, the bones of the vault are not fused and can undergo molding to conform to the maternal pelvis. The vault is composed of five bones: two frontal, two parietal, and one occipital. The spaces between the bones are known as sutures; the two places where the sutures intersect are the **anterior** and **posterior fontanelles**. How the fetal head presents to the maternal pelvis is important in accomplishing a vaginal delivery. There is great variation in the diameter of the skull at various levels and with various inclinations. When the fetal skull is properly flexed, the suboccipitobregmatic diameter presenting to the pelvis averages 9.5 cm in a term infant. When the sagittal suture is not located midline in the pelvis (asynclitism), the diameter of the skull being accommodated is effectively increased.

Treatment

Even if cephalopelvic disproportion is suspected, it is still often worthwhile to attempt a trial of labor. In the case of fetal macrosomia, elective induction of labor may be chosen before the opportunity for vaginal delivery passes. This practice leads to a similar cesarean section rate but as a result of failed induction rather than CPD.

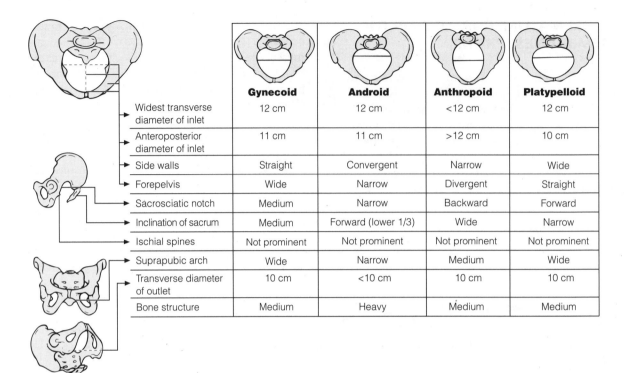

	Gynecoid	Android	Anthropoid	Platypelloid
Widest transverse diameter of inlet	12 cm	12 cm	<12 cm	12 cm
Anteroposterior diameter of inlet	11 cm	11 cm	>12 cm	10 cm
Side walls	Straight	Convergent	Narrow	Wide
Forepelvis	Wide	Narrow	Divergent	Straight
Sacrosciatic notch	Medium	Narrow	Backward	Forward
Inclination of sacrum	Medium	Forward (lower 1/3)	Wide	Narrow
Ischial spines	Not prominent	Not prominent	Not prominent	Not prominent
Suprapubic arch	Wide	Narrow	Medium	Wide
Transverse diameter of outlet	10 cm	<10 cm	10 cm	10 cm
Bone structure	Medium	Heavy	Medium	Medium

Figure 6-2 • Characteristics of four types of pelvises.

KEY POINTS

1. If the fetal head is too large to pass through the maternal pelvis, it is deemed cephalopelvic disproportion (CPD).
2. Unless ultrasound and CT have been used to document a fetal head larger than the maternal pelvis, in the case of suspected CPD, a trial of labor is often attempted.

■ BREECH PRESENTATION

Breech presentation, or buttocks first, occurs in 3% to 4% of all singleton deliveries. Factors associated with breech presentation include previous breech delivery, uterine anomalies, polyhydramnios, oligohydramnios, multiple gestations, PPROM, hydrocephalus, and anencephalus. Persistent breech presentation is also associated with placenta previa and fetal anomalies. Complications of a vaginal breech delivery include prolapsed cord and entrapment of the head.

Types of Breech

There are three categories of the breech presentation (Figure 6-3): **frank**, **complete**, and **incomplete** or **footling**. The frank breech has flexed hips and extended knees and thus the feet are near the fetal head. The complete breech has flexed hips, but one or both knees are flexed as well, with at least one foot near the breech. The incomplete or footling breech has one or both of the hips not flexed so that the foot or knee lies below the breech in the birth canal.

Diagnosis

The breech presentation may be diagnosed in several ways. With abdominal examination using the Leopold maneuvers, the fetal head can be palpated near the fundus while the breech is palpated in the pelvis. With vaginal examination, the breech can be palpated, the common landmarks being the gluteal cleft and the anus or, in the case of an incomplete breech, the fetal lower extremity. Diagnosis is often made or confirmed with ultrasound. On ultrasound, it is easy to confirm breech and then to determine the type of breech.

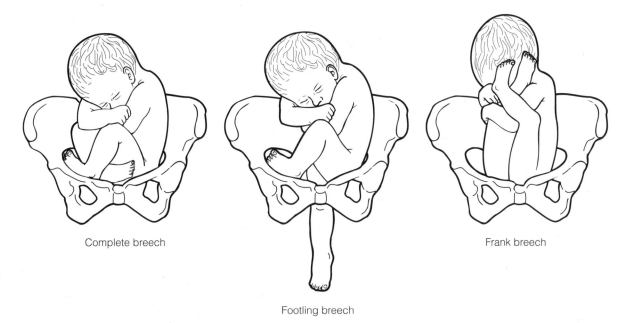

Complete breech

Footling breech

Frank breech

Figure 6-3 • Types of breech presentations.

Treatment

How a breech presentation is managed depends on the experience of the obstetrician and the patient's wishes. The three options are external version of the breech, trial of breech vaginal delivery, and elective cesarean section. External version consists of manipulation of the breech infant into a vertex presentation. It is rarely performed before week 37 because of the likelihood of spontaneous version before this point and the risk of delivery after version secondary to abruption or rupture of membranes.

Trial of breech vaginal delivery can be attempted in the proper setting. A favorable pelvis (by clinical or CT pelvimetry), a flexed head, estimated fetal weight between 2000 and 3800 g, and frank or complete breech are common criteria used for trial of labor of breech presentation. Relative contraindications include nulliparity, incomplete breech presentation, and estimated fetal weight greater than 3800 g. Patients with these contraindications are usually offered a cesarean delivery. However, if a patient insists on attempting vaginal delivery, careful monitoring of the fetus and progress of labor is imperative.

KEY POINTS

1. There are three types of breech: frank, complete, and incomplete or footling.
2. Breech presentations may be managed by version to vertex, trial of labor, or cesarean section.
3. The complications of labor and delivery of breech presentation include cord prolapse and entrapment of the fetal head.

■ MALPRESENTATION OF VERTEX

Malpresentation can occur even in the setting of a cephalic or vertex presentation. The face, brow, persistent occiput posterior (OP), or a compound presentation with a fetal upper extremity can complicate the vertex presentation. In addition, the shoulder can present in the setting of a transverse lie.

Face

The diagnosis of face presentation (Figure 6-4) can be made with vaginal examination and palpation of the nose, mouth, eyes, or chin (mentum). If the fetus is mentum anterior, vaginal delivery will often ensue. However, with a mentum posterior or transverse, the fetus must rotate to mentum anterior to deliver

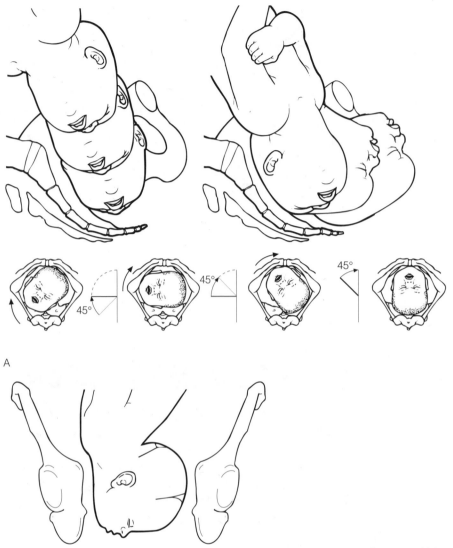

A

Face presentation

B

Figure 6-4 • A: Mechanisms of labor for right mentum posterior position with subsequent rotation of mentum anterior and delivery. **B:** Face presentation. Well engaged in the mentolateral position.

vaginally. Of note, many anencephalic fetuses have a face presentation. Augmentation is used only sparingly with a face presentation as the pressure on the face leads to edema.

Brow

Brow presentation (Figure 6-5) occurs when the portion of the fetal skull just above the orbital ridge presents. With the brow presenting, a larger diameter must pass through the pelvis. Therefore, unless the fetal head is particularly small or the pelvis is particularly large, the brow presentation must convert to vertex or face to deliver.

Shoulder

If the fetus is in a transverse lie, often the shoulder is presenting to the pelvic inlet. Diagnosis of this malpresentation can be made with abdominal or vaginal examination and ultrasound confirmation. Unless there is spontaneous conversion to vertex, shoulder presentations are delivered via cesarean section because of the increased risk of cord prolapse, increased risk for uterine rupture, and the difficulty of vaginal delivery.

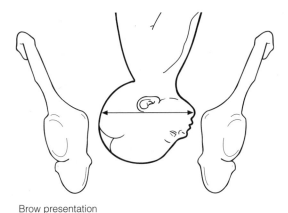

Brow presentation

Figure 6-5 • Brow presentation with mentovertex diameter presenting.

Compound Presentation

A fetal extremity presenting alongside the vertex or breech is considered a compound presentation (Figure 6-6). This occurs in less than 1:1000 pregnancies. The rate increases with prematurity, multiple gestations, polyhydramnios, and CPD. A common complication of compound presentation is umbilical cord prolapse. The diagnosis is often made with vaginal examination when the fetal extremity is palpated alongside the presenting part. At this point it should be determined whether the prolapsed fetal part is a hand or foot. Ultrasound may be used to determine the type of extremity presenting.

Treatment

Often times, if an upper extremity is presenting alongside the vertex, the part may be gently reduced. However, prolapse of a lower extremity in vertex presentation is far less likely to deliver vaginally. Compound presentation of a lower extremity with a breech is considered a footling or incomplete breech presentation and calls for cesarean section. In all cases of compound presentation, umbilical cord prolapse should be suspected and careful monitoring with continuous fetal heart tracings and frequent vaginal examinations should ensue.

Persistent Occiput Transverse and Posterior Position

The most common position of the fetus at the onset of labor is either left occiput transverse (LOT) or right occiput transverse (ROT). From the transverse position, the cardinal movement of internal rotation

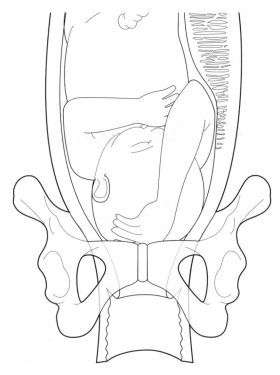

Figure 6-6 • Compound presentation. The left hand is lying in front of the vertex. With further labor, the hand and arm may retract from the birth canal and the head may then descend normally.

usually converts the fetus to the occiput anterior (OA) position. However, it is not uncommon for the fetus to stay in the occiput transverse (OT) position, or rotate to the occiput posterior (OP) position. If this occurs, the progress of labor may be arrested. Diagnosis is made by palpation of the fetal sutures and fontanelles and following the progress of labor.

A persistent OT position leading to transverse arrest of labor is more common in women with a platypelloid pelvis. If the cervix is not fully dilated, an attempt may be made at manual rotation to the OA position. If the cervix is fully dilated, rotation to the OA position can be attempted manually or with forceps. Additionally, an attempt at vacuum delivery may be effective as the traction on the fetal scalp may lead to autorotation to the OA position.

Usually, during descent, OP positions will rotate to OA, although this does not always occur and can slow progress in labor. The management is similar to that for OA position: patiently watch and wait. However, spontaneous vaginal delivery will occur less often. If stage 2 of labor is prolonged, the options include delivery of the fetus with forceps or vacuum in the OP position, rotation with forceps, or manual rotation. In either the OT or OP position, if the attempt at rotation or operative vaginal delivery fails, cesarean delivery is required.

KEY POINTS

1. Vertex malpresentations include face, brow, compound, and persistent OP.
2. These presentations will often deliver vaginally but need closer monitoring and sometimes require different maneuvers.

■ OBSTETRIC EMERGENCIES

Fetal Bradycardia

One of the most common events on labor and delivery that leads to much anxiety among both the practitioners and the patients is fetal heart rate (FHR) bradycardia. Any time the fetal heart rate is below 100–120 for longer than 2 minutes it is called a prolonged deceleration. Longer than 10 minutes is bradycardia. Older terminology deemed a deceleration lasting longer than 2 minutes a bradycardia, so this is commonly used on labor and delivery in the setting of prolonged decelerations. Either way, these FHR decelerations are associated with a number of other complications such as placental abruption, cord prolapse, tetanic contraction, uterine rupture, pulmonary embolus (PE), amniotic fluid embolus (AFE), and seizure. They have also been associated with poor fetal outcome.

The etiology of prolonged FHR decelerations can be considered to be pre-uterine, utero-placental, or postplacental. Pre-uterine issues would be any event leading to maternal hypotension or hypoxia. These would include seizure, AFE, PE, MI, respiratory failure, or recent epidural or spinal placement. Uteroplacental issues include placental abruption, infarction, and previa, as well as uterine hyperstimulation. Postplacental etiologies include cord prolapse, cord compression, and rupture of a fetal vessel.

Diagnosis

FHR decelerations are usually not subtle. However, the FHR should be differentiated from the maternal heart rate, which is commonly in the 60s to 100s in these settings. This can be done by having a fetal scalp electrode (FSE) on the fetus and more importantly an O_2 sat monitor on the mother. In facilities without access to these tools, palpation of the maternal pulse while listening to the FHR can usually differentiate between the two.

Diagnosis of the etiology of the bradycardia is often more important than the diagnosis of bradycardia, which is relatively straightforward in the era of continuous fetal monitoring. A simple algorithm follows.

1. *Look at the mother for signs of respiratory compromise or change in mental status.* This should commonly diagnose seizures, PE, and AFE.
2. *While putting on a glove for a cervical examination, assess the maternal blood pressure and heart rate.* This will diagnose maternal hypotension, commonly seen after epidural placement and a potential cause of FHR decelerations. This will also aid in determining whether the FHR being recorded could be maternal.
3. *Immediately before the examination look to see how much vaginal blood is passing.* With increased vaginal bleeding, placental abruption and uterine rupture should be considered. If placentation is unknown, placenta previa is also a possibility. Rarely, vaginal bleeding is secondary to rupture of a fetal vessel as in vasa previa.
4. *Examine the patient with one hand on the maternal abdomen and one hand vaginally feeling for cervical dilation, fetal station, and prolapsed umbilical cord.* The abdominal hand should feel for uterine tetany and fetal parts outside the uterus. If the fetal station is dramatically lower than expected, then the prolonged FHR deceleration may be due to rapid descent and vagal stimulation. If the fetal station is much higher than expected, uterine rupture should be suspected. If the cervix is fully dilated and the fetus in the pelvis, operative vaginal delivery can be performed if the FHR deceleration does not resolve in a timely fashion.

Treatment

In the setting of prolonged FHR deceleration, the initial management is standardized. The patient is moved from one side to the other in case the FHR deceleration is secondary to compression of the inferior vena cava (IVC) leading to decreased preload or more commonly a compressed umbilical cord by the fetus. Oxygen by face mask is commonly administered to the mother in case hypoxia is an issue. The examination is performed as described above, and the individual etiologies treated appropriately. In the setting of maternal hypotension, the patient can be given aggressive IV hydration and ephedrine. The management of seizure, AFE, uterine rupture, and PE are discussed elsewhere. Tetanic uterine contraction is treated with nitroglycerin, usually administered via a sublingual spray, and/or terbutaline a β-agonist tocolytic. If umbilical cord prolapse is identified, there have been case reports of it being replaced into the uterus, but most commonly this requires an emergent cesarean section, performed with the examining clinician lifting the fetal head off of the prolapsed cord. In the setting of previa, cesarean delivery should be expedited as well. If abruption is suspected, and the patient is remote from delivery, cesarean section may be necessary.

It is imperative that the timing of these events is followed very closely. Further, clinicians need to know the capabilities of their labor and delivery units and the rapidity of response of the anesthesiologists. Commonly, a patient is moved from the labor room to the OR after 4 to 5 minutes of FHR deceleration. If the FHR is checked in the OR (at this time, usually 8 minutes) and still found to be down, plans for emergent cesarean delivery should proceed. This delivery may not follow all of the most common sterile techniques usually used because delivery of the fetus within the next 2 to 4 minutes is the goal.

KEY POINTS

1. Prolonged fetal heart rate decelerations may have a variety of etiologies and can be thought of as pre-uterine, uteroplacental, and postplacental.
2. A quick examination and verification of vital signs will often determine the etiology of a prolonged deceleration.
3. If there is no sign of resolution of the FHR deceleration in 4 to 5 minutes, the patient should either be delivered vaginally or moved to the OR for cesarean.

Shoulder Dystocia

Once the head of the fetus is delivered, difficulty in delivering the shoulders, particularly because of impaction of the anterior shoulder behind the pubic symphysis, is termed **shoulder dystocia**. Risk factors for shoulder dystocia include fetal macrosomia, gestational diabetes, previous shoulder dystocia, maternal obesity, postdate pregnancy, and prolonged stage 2 of labor. Increased morbidity and mortality are associated with shoulder dystocia. Fetal complications include fractures of the humerus and clavicle, brachial plexus nerve injuries (Erb's palsy), hypoxic brain injury, and death.

Diagnosis

The actual diagnosis of a shoulder dystocia is made when routine obstetric maneuvers fail to deliver the infant. When antepartum risk factors are present, shoulder dystocia can be predicted, prepared for, and possibly even prevented. Preparation for a shoulder dystocia includes placing the patient in the dorsal lithotomy position, having adequate anesthesia, cutting a generous episiotomy, and having several experienced clinicians present at the birth. At the time of delivery, suspicion is increased with prolonged crowning of the head and then with the "turtle" sign of either incomplete delivery of the head or the chin tucking up against the maternal perineum.

Treatment

The series of maneuvers for delivering an infant with a shoulder dystocia are as follows.

- **McRoberts maneuver:** Sharp flexion of the maternal hips that decreases the inclination of the pelvis and can free the anterior shoulder (Figure 6-7).
- **Suprapubic pressure:** This is to dislodge the anterior shoulder from behind the pubic symphysis and should be directed at an oblique angle (Figure 6-8).
- **Rubin maneuver:** Place pressure on an accessible shoulder to push it toward the anterior chest wall of the fetus to decrease the bisacromial diameter and free the impacted shoulder (Figure 6-9).
- **Wood's corkscrew maneuver:** Apply pressure behind the posterior shoulder to rotate the infant and dislodge the anterior shoulder.
- **Delivery of the posterior arm/shoulder:** By sweeping the posterior arm across the chest and deliver-

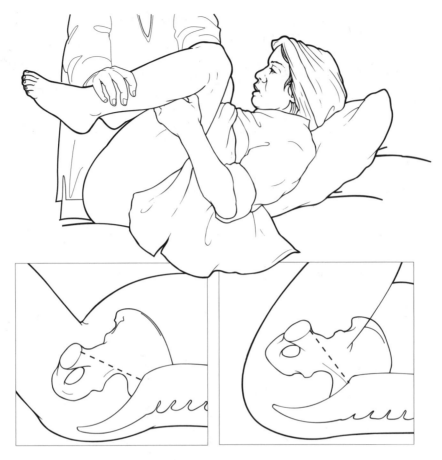

Figure 6-7 • Sharp ventral rotation of both maternal hips (McRoberts maneuver) brings the pelvic inlet and outlet into a more vertical alignment, facilitating delivery of the fetal shoulders.

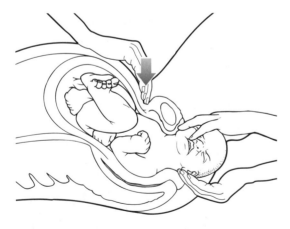

Figure 6-8 • Moderate suprapubic pressure is often the only additional maneuver necessary to free the anterior fetal shoulder.

ing it, the bisacromial diameter can then be rotated to an oblique diameter of the pelvis and the anterior shoulder is freed.

If these maneuvers are unsuccessful, they may be performed again. If the infant is still undelivered, there are several other maneuvers that can be performed. Cutting or fracturing the fetal clavicle or cutting the maternal pubic symphysis will often release the infant. Symphysiotomy is a morbid procedure often complicated by infection, failure to heal, and chronic pain, and thus should be reserved for the true emergency. If none of these maneuvers are successful, the **Zavanelli** maneuver, which involves placing the infant's head back into the pelvis and performing cesarean delivery, can be attempted.

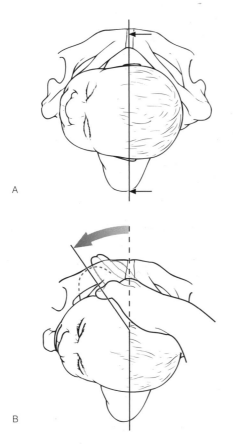

Figure 6-9 • Rubin maneuver. A: The shoulder-to-shoulder diameter is shown as the distance between the two small arrows. B: The most easily accessible fetal shoulder (the anterior is shown here) is pushed toward the anterior chest wall of the fetus. Most often, this results in abduction of both shoulders, reducing the shoulder-to-shoulder diameter and freeing the impacted anterior shoulder.

KEY POINTS

1. Shoulder dystocias can result in fetal fractures, nerve damage, and hypoxia.
2. Risk factors for shoulder dystocia include fetal macrosomia, diabetes, previous dystocia, maternal obesity, postdate deliveries, and prolonged stage 2 of labor.
3. The maneuvers to reduce a shoulder dystocia include suprapubic pressure, McRoberts maneuver, Rubin maneuver, Wood's corkscrew, delivery of posterior arm, fracture or cutting the clavicle or pubic symphysis, and the Zavanelli maneuver.

Uterine Rupture

Uterine rupture is seen in one in 10,000 to 20,000 deliveries in patients with unscarred uteri. Associated complications in these patients include uterine fibroids, uterine malformations, obstructed labor, and the use of uterotonic agents like oxytocin and prostaglandins. In patients who have had a prior uterine scar from myomectomy or cesarean delivery, the risk of uterine rupture is theoretically 0.5% to 1.0%. The risk is increased in patients who have more than one cesarean scar, have a "classical" or high vertical scar, undergo labor induction, and/or are treated with uterotonic agents.

Uterine rupture is suspected in the setting of FHR decelerations in patients with prior scars on their uterus. Patients may feel a "popping" sensation or experience sudden abdominal pain. On physical examination, the fetus may be palpable extrauterine, there may be vaginal bleeding, and commonly the fetal presenting part is suddenly much higher than it had been. If a uterine rupture is strongly suspected, the patient should be brought to the OR for immediate cesarean delivery and exploratory laparotomy.

Maternal Hypotension

Pregnant patients commonly have blood pressures in the 90/50 range. BPs much lower than the 80/40 range is unusual and can lead to poor maternal and uterine perfusion. Common etiologies of maternal hypotension include vasovagal events, regional anesthesia, overtreatment with antihypertensive drugs, hemorrhage, anaphylaxis, and AFE. Most of these events can be differentiated from each other quickly and by the clinical scenario.

Treatment of maternal hypotension may vary based on the etiology, but the mainstays are aggressive IV hydration and adrenergic medications to clamp down peripheral vessels and increase both the preload and the afterload. If the event does occur in close proximity to medication administration, benadryl and even epinephrine should be considered for a possible anaphylactic reaction. If the patient has an AFE, the mortality rate is quite high. The definitive diagnosis of AFE is the finding of fetal cells in the pulmonary vasculature at autopsy.

Seizure

Seizures on labor and delivery are usually quite startling and can be dangerous. In patients with a history of a seizure disorder as well as preeclamptics, careful observation for particular seizure precursors is maintained. However, many patients who seize on labor and delivery have no history and may be normotensive.

Many vasovagal events are misdiagnosed as a seizure because the patient may have several tonic-clonic movements. One of the key ways to differentiate between the two is the presence of a postictal period after the event. To help sort out the etiology, patients should have a full preeclamptic work-up and, when it is safe for the patient to leave the floor, obtain a head CT. A neurology consult on these patients is also indicated. Acutely, the patients should be managed with the ABCs of resuscitation and with antiseizure medications (Table 6-1). In pregnancy, magnesium sulfate is the antiseizure medication of choice.

■ TABLE 6-1

Management of a Pregnant Patient with Seizures or in Status Epilepticus

Assess and establish airway and vital signs including oxygenation

Assess FHR or fetal status

Bolus magnesium sulfate, or give 10 g IM

Bolus with lorazepam 0.1 mg/kg, 5.0–10.00 mg at no more than 2.0 mg/min

Load phenytoin 20 mg/kg, usually 1–2 g at no more than 50 mg/min

If not successful, load phenobarbital 20 mg/kg, usually 1–2 g at no more than 100 mg/min

Labs include electrolytes, AED levels, glucose, and toxicology screen

If fetal testing is not reassuring, move to emergent delivery

KEY POINTS

1. Uterine rupture is uncommon in patients with no prior uterine scar; it is seen in 0.5% to 1.0% of patients who labor with a prior cesarean delivery.
2. Maternal hypotension may have a variety of etiologies including regional anesthesia, hemorrhage, vasovagal events, AFE, and anaphylaxis.
3. Patients with seizures in pregnancy are managed first line with IV or IM magnesium sulfate.

Fetal Complications of Pregnancy

■ DISORDERS OF FETAL GROWTH

Newborns with birth weight less than the 10th percentile or greater than the 90th percentile are easily identified. However, the accuracy of antepartum estimates of fetal weight can vary. Ultrasound is the most commonly used modality to estimate fetal weight. Fetuses whose estimated fetal weight (EFW) is less than the 10th percentile are termed **small for gestational age** (SGA). Those whose EFW is greater than the 90th percentile are termed **large for gestational age** (LGA). SGA fetuses are further described as either symmetric or asymmetric. *Symmetric* implies that the fetus is proportionally small. *Asymmetric* implies that certain organs of the fetus are disproportionally small. Classically, an asymmetric infant will have wasting of the torso and extremities while preserving the brain. Thus, the skull will be at a greater percentile than the rest of the body. Screening for disorders of fetal growth is done during routine prenatal care. Once the fetus is at or greater than 20 weeks gestational age, the uterine fundal height (in cm) should be approximately equal to the gestational age (in weeks). Fetal growth can therefore be followed by serial examinations of the fundal height. Before making the diagnosis of either SGA or LGA, it is imperative that accurate dating of the pregnancy is ascertained. If the fundal height varies by more than 3 cm from the gestational age, ultrasound is usually obtained.

Small for Gestational Age (SGA)

SGA infants are associated with higher rates of mortality and morbidity for their gestational age. However, they do better than infants with the same weight delivered at earlier gestational ages. SGA babies born at 34 weeks that weigh the same as 28-week infants will have lower morbidity and mortality rates. Factors that can result in infants being SGA can be divided into those that lead to **decreased growth potential** and those that lead to **intrauterine growth restriction** (IUGR) (Table 7-1).

Decreased Growth Potential

Congenital abnormalities account for approximately 10% to 15% of SGA infants. Trisomy 21 (Down syndrome), trisomy 18 (Edwards' syndrome), and trisomy 13 (Patau's syndrome) all lead to SGA babies. Turner's syndrome (45,XO) leads to a decrease in birth weight. Infants with osteogenesis imperfecta, achondroplasia, neural tube defects, anencephaly, and a variety of autosomal recessive syndromes may all be SGA.

All intrauterine infections—particularly **cytomegalovirus** (CMV) and **rubella**—lead to SGA infants. These probably account for 10% to 15% of all SGA babies. Exposure to **teratogens**, most chemotherapeutic agents, and other drugs during pregnancy can also lead to decreased growth potential. The two most common teratogens causing SGA are alcohol and cigarettes. Up to 10% of SGA fetuses are constitutionally small based purely on parental stature.

Intrauterine Growth Restricted (IUGR)

Fetal growth can be divided into two phases. Prior to week 20, growth is primarily hyperplastic (increasing number of cells); after week 20, it is primarily hypertrophic. Because of this, an insult leading to growth restriction occurring prior to 20 weeks will most likely result in symmetric growth restriction, whereas insults occurring after 20 weeks in a prolonged fashion result in asymmetric growth. Asymmetric

TABLE 7-1

Risk Factors for SGA Infants

Decreased growth potential
Genetic and chromosomal abnormalities

Intrauterine infections

Teratogenic exposure

Substance abuse

Radiation exposure

Small maternal stature

Pregnancy at high altitudes

Female fetus

Intrauterine growth restricted (IUGR)
Maternal factors including hypertension, anemia, chronic renal disease, malnutrition, and severe diabetes

Placental factors including placenta previa, chronic abruption, placental infarction, multiple gestations

growth most likely results from decreased nutrition and oxygen being transmitted across the placenta, which is then shunted to the fetal brain. Two-thirds of the time, growth restriction is asymmetric and can be identified by increased head to abdominal measurements.

Maternal risk factors include baseline hypertension, anemia, chronic renal disease, antiphospholipid antibody syndrome, systemic lupus erythematosus (SLE), and severe malnutrition. Severe diabetes with extensive vascular disease may also lead to IUGR. Placental factors leading to diminished placental blood flow may lead to IUGR. These factors include placenta previa, marginal cord insertion, and placental thrombosis with or without infarction. Multiple gestations often lead to lower birth weights because of earlier delivery and SGA infants. In twins, SGA infants are seen particularly in the twin-twin transfusion syndrome.

Diagnosis

The risk of having an SGA baby increases in mothers with a previous SGA baby or with any of the above etiologies. These fetuses should be followed carefully for intrauterine growth. Fundal height is measured at each prenatal visit. Oligohydramnios and SGA fetuses have fundal heights less than expected. Anytime a fundal height is 3 cm less than expected, fetal growth should be estimated via ultrasound.

If SGA is suspected, the accuracy of the pregnancy's dating should be verified. Any infant at risk for IUGR or being SGA is followed with serial ultrasound scans for growth. A fetus with decreased growth potential will usually start small and stay small, whereas one with IUGR will fall off the growth curve.

Treatment

For patients with a history of SGA infants, the underlying etiology should be explored. If malnutrition or drugs like alcohol or cigarettes were issues in a prior pregnancy, these should be dealt with at each prenatal visit. Patients with a history of placental insufficiency, preeclampsia, collagen vascular disorders, or vascular disease are often treated with low-dose aspirin. Patients with prior placental thrombosis, thrombophilias, or antiphospholipid antibody syndrome have been treated with heparin and corticosteroids as well, with mixed results.

There is no indication to expedite delivery in SGA fetuses who have consistently been small throughout the pregnancy. However, the risk of prematurity is likely to be lower than that of remaining in the intrauterine environment for SGA fetuses near term that have fallen off the growth curve. This is assessed with fetal testing such as a nonstress test (NST), oxytocin challenge test (OCT), biophysical profile (BPP), and/or umbilical Doppler velocimetry. If fetal testing is nonreassuring, the fetus should be delivered. The decision of whether to deliver SGA fetuses remote from term is based on how the infant will do in a neonatal intensive care unit versus how it will be maintained in the intrauterine environment. For those left undelivered, frequent antenatal testing with NSTs, OCTs, and BPPs; weekly ultrasounds for fetal growth; and possibly, admission to the hospital for continuous monitoring may be indicated.

KEY POINTS

1. Fetuses whose EFW is less than the 10th percentile are small for gestational age (SGA).
2. Common causes of decreased growth potential include congenital abnormalities, drugs, infections, radiation, and small maternal stature.
3. IUGR infants are commonly born to women with systemic diseases leading to poor placental blood flow.

Large for Gestational Age (LGA) and Fetal Macrosomia

An LGA fetus is defined as having an EFW greater than the 90th percentile. However, LGA is less important than the diagnosis of fetal macrosomia. Although definitions of macrosomia vary, the American College of Obstetricians and Gynecologists use **a birth weight greater than 4500 g**. Birth weights of greater than 4000 g or 4200 g are also used by many clinicians and researchers to define macrosomia. Macrosomic fetuses have a higher risk of shoulder dystocia and birth trauma with resultant brachial plexus injuries with vaginal deliveries. Other neonatal risks include low Apgar scores, hypoglycemia, polycythemia, hypocalcemia, and jaundice. LGA infants are at a higher risk for childhood leukemia, Wilms' tumor, and osteosarcoma.

Mothers with LGA macrosomic fetuses are at increased risk for cesarean section, perineal trauma, and postpartum hemorrhage. There is a higher rate of cesarean section for macrosomic infants due to failure to progress in labor and electively because of suspected increased risk for shoulder dystocia.

Etiology

The most classically associated risk factor for fetal macrosomia is gestational or preexisting diabetes. **Maternal obesity**—weight greater than 90 kg—is also correlated with an increased risk for fetal macrosomia. This correlation is seemingly independent of maternal stature and gestational diabetes. Any woman who has previously delivered an LGA infant is at increased risk in ensuing pregnancies for fetal macrosomia. **Postterm pregnancies** have an increased rate of macrosomic infants. **Multiparity** and **advanced maternal age** are also risk factors (Table 7-2), but these are mostly secondary to the increased prevalence of diabetes and obesity.

Diagnosis

Upon routine prenatal care, patients with macrosomic infants will often be of a size greater than dates on measurement of the fundal height and, by the late third trimester, Leopold's examination reveals a fetus that seems large. Patients whose fetuses are a size greater than dates by 3 cm or more are referred to ultrasound for EFW. Ultrasound uses the biparietal diameter, femur length, and abdominal circumference to estimate fetal weight. These estimates are usually accurate to within 10% to 15%. As with SGA

TABLE 7-2
Risk Factors for Macrosomic Infants
Diabetes
Maternal obesity
Postterm pregnancy
Previous LGA or macrosomic infant
Maternal stature
Multiparity
AMA
Male infant
Beckwith-Wiedemann syndrome (pancreatic islet-cell hyperplasia)

fetuses, pregnancy dating should be verified. At many institutions, any patient with diabetes or a previous LGA infant merits an estimated fetal weight by ultrasound in the late third trimester.

Treatment

Management of LGA and macrosomic infants includes prevention, surveillance, and—in some cases—induction of labor before the attainment of macrosomia. Patients with type I and II diabetes require tight control of blood glucose during pregnancy. Well-controlled sugars are thought to decrease the incidence of macrosomic infants in this population, although this has not been confirmed by large randomized studies. Studies of gestational diabetes have demonstrated a decrease in birth weight when women maintained good control of blood glucose.

Obese patients can be counseled to lose weight before conception. Once pregnant, these patients are advised to gain less weight (but never to lose weight) than the average patient and should be referred to a nutritionist for assistance in maintaining adequate nutrition with some control of caloric intake.

Because of the risk for birth trauma and failure to progress in labor secondary to cephalopelvic disproportion, LGA pregnancies are often induced before the fetus can attain macrosomic status. The risks of this course of action are increased rate of cesarean section for failed induction and prematurity in a poorly dated pregnancy. Thus, induction should be used primarily when the cervix is favorable for induction and there is either excellent dating or lung maturity as assessed via amniocentesis. Prospective studies of the practice of induction for impending macrosomia have not shown to decrease cesarean delivery rates. Vaginal delivery of the suspected macrosomic infant involves preparing for a shoulder dystocia. Operative vaginal delivery with forceps or vacuum is generally not advised because such a delivery increases the risk of shoulder dystocia.

KEY POINTS

1. An LGA fetus has an EFW greater than the 90th percentile.
2. Both 4000 g and 4500 g have been used as the threshold for defining fetal macrosomia.
3. LGA and macrosomic fetuses are at greater risk for birth trauma, hypoglycemia, jaundice, lower Apgar scores, and childhood tumors.
4. Increased size in the fetus is seen with maternal diabetes, maternal obesity, increased maternal height, postterm pregnancies, multiparity, advanced maternal age, and male sex.

■ DISORDERS OF AMNIOTIC FLUID

The amniotic fluid reaches its maximum volume of about 800 mL at about 28 weeks. This volume is maintained until close to term when it begins to fall to about 500 mL at week 40. The balance of fluid is maintained by production of the fetal kidneys and lungs and resorption by fetal swallowing and the interface between the membranes and the placenta. A disturbance in any of these functions may lead to a pathologic change in amniotic fluid volume.

Ultrasound can be used to evaluate the amniotic fluid volume. The classic measure of amniotic fluid is the **amniotic fluid index** (AFI). The AFI is calculated by dividing the maternal abdomen into quadrants, measuring the largest vertical pocket of fluid in each quadrant in cm, and summing them. An AFI of less than 5 is considered **oligohydramnios**. An AFI greater than 20 or 25 is used to diagnose **polyhydramnios**, depending on gestational age.

Oligohydramnios

Oligohydramnios in the absence of rupture of membranes is associated with a 40-fold increase in perinatal mortality. This is partially because without the amniotic fluid to cushion it, the umbilical cord is more susceptible to compression leading to fetal asphyxiation. It is also associated with congenital anomalies, particularly of the genitourinary system, and growth restriction. In labor, nonreactive nonstress tests, fetal heart rate (FHR) decelerations, meconium, and cesarean section due to nonreassuring fetal testing are all associated with an AFI of less than 5.

Etiology

The cause of oligohydramnios can be thought of as either decreased production or increased withdrawal. Amniotic fluid is produced by the fetal kidneys and lungs. It can be resorbed by the placenta, swallowed by the fetus, or leaked out into the vagina. Chronic uteroplacental insufficiency (UPI) can lead to oligohydramnios because the fetus likely does not have the nutrients or blood volume to maintain an adequate glomerular filtration rate. UPI is commonly associated with growth-restricted infants.

Congenital abnormalities of the genitourinary tract can lead to decreased urine production. These malformations include renal agenesis (Potter's syndrome), polycystic kidney disease, or obstruction of the genitourinary system. The most common cause of oligohydramnios is rupture of membranes. Even without a history of leaking fluid, the patient should be examined to rule out this possibility.

Diagnosis

Diagnosis of oligohydramnios is made by AFI less than 5 as measured by ultrasound. Patients screened for oligohydramnios include those measuring size less than dates, with a history of ruptured membranes, with suspicion of IUGR, and who have a postterm pregnancy. Once the diagnosis of oligohydramnios is made, the etiology also needs to be determined prior to creating a management plan.

Treatment

Management of oligohydramnios is entirely dependent upon the underlying etiology. In pregnancies that are IUGR, a host of other data needs consideration, including the rest of the biophysical profile (BPP), cord Doppler flow, gestational age, and the cause of the IUGR. Labor is usually induced in the case of a pregnancy at term or postdate. In the case of a fetus with congenital abnormalities, the patient should be referred to genetic counseling. A plan for delivery should be made in coordination with the pediatricians and pediatric surgeons. Severely preterm patients with no other etiology are usually managed expectantly with frequent antenatal fetal testing.

Labor is induced in patients with rupture of membranes at term if they are not already in labor. If there is meconium or frequent decelerations in the FHR, an amnio infusion may be performed to increase the AFI. Amnioinfusion is performed to dilute any meconium present in the amniotic fluid and theoretically to decrease the number of variable decelerations caused by cord compression. Preterm premature rupture of membranes (PPROM) is discussed in Chapter 6.

KEY POINTS

1. Oligohydramnios is defined by an AFI of less than 5.
2. Oligohydramnios can be caused by decreased placental perfusion, decreased fluid production by the fetus, and rupture of membranes.
3. Pregnancies at term complicated by oligohydramnios should be delivered.

Polyhydramnios

Polyhydramnios, defined by an AFI greater than 20 or 25, is present in 2% to 3% of pregnancies. Fetal structural and chromosomal abnormalities are more common in polyhydramnios. It is associated with maternal diabetes and malformations such as neural tube defects, obstruction of the fetal alimentary canal, and hydrops.

Etiology

Polyhydramnios is not as ominous a sign as oligohydramnios. However, it is associated with an increase in congenital anomalies. It is also more common in pregnancies complicated by diabetes, hydrops, and multiple gestation. An obstruction of the gastrointestinal tract may render the infant unable to swallow the amniotic fluid, leading to polyhydramnios. Just as in other diabetic patients, the increased levels of circulating glucose can act as an osmotic diuretic in the fetus leading to polyhydramnios. Hydrops secondary to high output cardiac failure is generally associated with polyhydramnios. Monozygotic multiple gestations can lead to twin-to-twin transfusion syndrome with polyhydramnios around one fetus and oligohydramnios around the other.

Diagnosis

Polyhydramnios is diagnosed by ultrasound in patients being scanned for size greater than dates,

routine screening of diabetic or multiple gestation pregnancies, or as an unsuspected finding on an ultrasound performed for other reasons.

Treatment

As in oligohydramnios, the particular setting of polyhydramnios dictates the management of the pregnancy. Patients with polyhydramnios are at risk for malpresentation and should be carefully evaluated during labor. There is an increased risk of cord prolapse with polyhydramnios. Thus, rupture of membranes should be performed in a controlled setting if possible and only if the head is truly engaged in the pelvis. Upon spontaneous rupture of membranes, a sterile vaginal examination should be performed to verify fetal presentation and rule out cord prolapse.

KEY POINTS

1. Polyhydramnios is diagnosed by an AFI greater than 20 on ultrasound.
2. Polyhydramnios is associated with diabetes, multiple gestations, hydrops, and congenital abnormalities.
3. Obstetric management of polyhydramnios should include careful verification of presentation and observation for cord prolapse.

Rh Incompatibility and Alloimmunization

If a woman is Rh negative and her fetus is Rh positive, she may be sensitized to the Rh antigen and develop antibodies. These antibodies cross the placenta and cause hemolysis of fetal red blood cells. The incidence of Rh negativity varies among race (Table 7-3), with the highest incidence of 30% seen among individuals in the Basque region of Spain. Commonly, most individuals only become sensitized during pregnancy and blood transfusion. In the United States, the incidence of sensitization is decreasing from both causes due to careful management of transfusions and the use of Rh immunoglobulin (RhoGAM) in pregnancy. Interestingly, because there is some transplacental passage of fetal cells in all pregnancies, ABO incompatibility actually decreases the risk of Rh sensitization because of destruction of these fetal cells by anti-A or anti-B antibodies.

■ TABLE 7-3

Prevalence of Rh Negativity by Race and Ethnicity

Race and Ethnicity	Percent Rh Negative
Caucasian	15
African American	8
African	4
Native American	1
Asian	<1

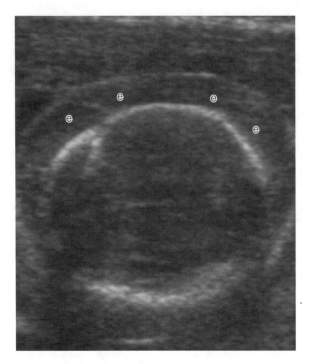

Figure 7-1 • Scalp edema (e).

In sensitized patients with Rh positive fetuses, the antibodies cross the placenta and cause hemolysis leading to disastrous complications in the fetus. The anemia caused by hemolysis leads to increased extramedullary production of fetal red cells. **Erythroblastosis fetalis**, or fetal hydrops, a syndrome that includes a hyperdynamic state, heart failure, diffuse edema (Figure 7-1), ascites (Figure 7-2), and pericardial effusion, is the result of serious anemia. Bilirubin, a breakdown product of red blood cells, is cleared by the placenta before birth but can lead to jaundice and neurotoxic effects in the neonate.

The Unsensitized Rh Negative Patient

If a patient is Rh negative but has a negative antibody screen, the goal during pregnancy is to keep her from becoming sensitized. Any time during the pregnancy that there is a possibility that a patient may be exposed to fetal blood, such as during amniocentesis, miscarriage, vaginal bleeding, abruption, and delivery, she should be given RhoGAM, an anti-D immunoglobulin (Rh IgG). An antibody screen is performed at the initial visit to detect prior sensitization. RhoGAM should be administered at 28 weeks and postpartum if the neonate is Rh positive.

A standard dose of RhoGAM, 0.3 mg of Rh IgG, will eradicate 15 mL of fetal red blood cells (30 mL of fetal blood with a hematocrit of 50). This dose is adequate for a routine pregnancy. However, in the setting of placental abruption or any antepartum bleeding, a Kleihauer-Betke test for amount of fetal red blood cells in the maternal circulation can be sent. If the amount of fetal red blood cells is more than can be eliminated by the single RhoGAM dose, additional doses can be given.

The Sensitized Rh Negative Patient

If the antibody screen for Rh comes back positive during the initial prenatal visit, the titer is checked

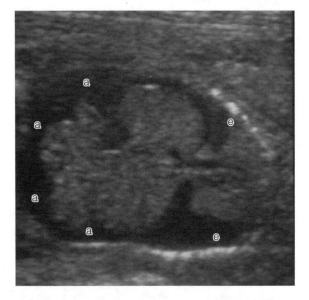

Figure 7-2 • Note the large ascites (a) and pleural effusions (e) in this fetus with hydrops.

as well. Antibody titers of 1 : 16 and greater have been associated with fetal hydrops. If paternity is not in question, blood type can be performed on the father of the baby to determine whether the fetus is at risk. However, because approximately 5% of all pregnancies have unknown or incorrect paternity, the safest course is to treat all pregnancies as if the fetus is at risk.

Throughout pregnancy, the antibody titer is followed approximately every 4 weeks. As long as it remains less than 1 : 16, the pregnancy can be managed expectantly. However, if it becomes 1 : 16 or greater, serial amniocentesis is begun as early as 16 to 20 weeks. At the first amniocentesis, fetal cells can be collected and analyzed for the Rh antigen. If negative, the pregnancy can be followed expectantly. However, if the fetus is Rh positive, serial amniocenteses are done and the amniotic fluid is analyzed by a spectrophotometer that measures the light absorption (ΔOD_{450}) by bilirubin, which will accumulate in the amniotic fluid with increasing fetal hemolysis. These measurements are plotted on the Liley curve (Figure 7-3), which predicts the severity of disease. The curve is divided into three zones.

Zone 1 is suggestive of a mildly affected fetus, and follow-up amniocentesis can be performed approximately every 2 to 3 weeks. Zone 2 is suggestive of a moderately affected fetus, and amniocentesis should be repeated every 1 to 2 weeks. The severely affected fetus will fall into zone 3. Once in zone 3, it is likely that the fetus has anemia, and percutaneous umbili-

cal blood sampling (PUBS) is usually the next step. PUBS can be used to obtain a fetal hematocrit and to perform an intrauterine transfusion (IUT). If a PUBS or IUT cannot be performed, fetal intraperitoneal transfusion has also been utilized.

Other Causes of Immune Hydrops

There are a variety of other red blood cell antigens including the **ABO** blood type, antigens **CDE** in which D is the Rh antigen, **Kell**, **Duffy**, and **Lewis**. Some may cause fetal hydrops (e.g., Kell and Duffy), whereas others may lead to a mild hemolysis but not severe immune hydrops (e.g., ABO, Lewis). With the advent of treatment with RhoGAM, the incidence of Rh isoimmunization has decreased and the other causes of immune-related fetal hydrops now account for a greater percentage of cases. Sensitized patients are managed similarly to Rh negative patients with antibody titers, amniocentesis, PUBS, and transfusions.

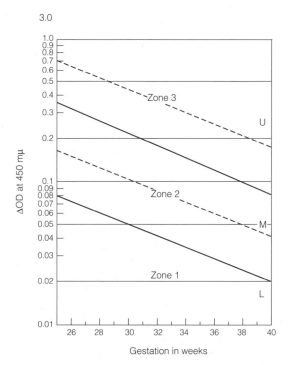

Figure 7-3 • Liley curve used to predict severity of fetal hemolysis with red cell isoimmunization.

KEY POINTS

1. Rh sensitized women with Rh positive fetuses have antibodies that cross the placenta, leading to hemolysis and anemia in the fetuses. If the anemia is severe enough, hydrops develops with edema, ascites, and heart failure.
2. Rh negative patients who are not sensitized should be treated with antepartum RhoGAM to prevent sensitization. Postpartum, they should receive another dose of RhoGAM if the fetus is Rh positive.
3. Rh negative patients undergoing miscarriage, abruption, amniocentesis, ectopic pregnancy, and vaginal bleeding should also be given RhoGAM.
4. Rh negative patients who are sensitized are followed closely with serial ultrasounds and amniocentesis. The amniocentesis is done to measure the amount of bilirubin in the fluid, which is indicative of the amount of hemolysis.

Fetal Demise

Intrauterine fetal demise (IUFD) is a rare but disastrous occurrence, occurring in approximately 1 : 1000 births. It is increased with a variety of medical and obstetric complications of pregnancy, including abruption, congenital abnormalities, and postterm pregnancy. Chronic placental insufficiency secondary to rheumatologic, vascular, or hypertensive disease may lead to IUGR and eventually IUFD. When there is no explanation for a fetal demise, it is usually attributed to a "cord accident." A retained IUFD greater than 3 to 4 weeks can lead to hypofibrinogenemia secondary to the release of thromboplastic substances from the decomposing fetus. In some cases, full-blown disseminated intravascular coagulation (DIC) can result.

Diagnosis

Early in pregnancy, before 20 weeks, the diagnosis of fetal death (missed abortion) is suspected by lack of uterine growth or cessation of symptoms of pregnancy. Diagnosis is confirmed with serially falling human chorionic gonadotropin (hCG) and ultrasound documentation. After week 20, fetal death is suspected with absence of fetal movement noted by the mother and absence of uterine growth. Diagnosis can be confirmed by ultrasound.

Treatment

Because of the risk of DIC with retained IUFD, the best treatment is delivery. Early gestations can be terminated by dilation and evacuation. After 20 weeks, the pregnancy is usually terminated by induction of labor with prostaglandins or high-dose oxytocin. Helping patients understand what may have caused the fetal death is imperative to helping them cope with the situation. Tests for causes of fetal death include screening for collagen vascular disease or hypercoagulable state, fetal karyotype, and often TORCH titers (i.e., toxoplasmosis, RPR, CMV, and HSV). It is extremely important to get an autopsy on the fetus, which can contribute valuable information. Despite this extensive battery of tests, the etiology of fetal demise will likely remain unknown greater than 90% of the time.

KEY POINTS

1. IUFD is more common with disorders of the placenta.
2. The cause of IUFD is usually unknown but is often attributed to cord accidents.
3. Retained IUFD can lead to DIC; thus, delivery soon after diagnosis is indicated.

Postterm Pregnancy

A postterm pregnancy is defined as one that goes beyond 42 weeks gestational age or greater than 294 days past the last menstrual period (LMP). It is estimated that 3% to 10% of all pregnancies will go postterm. This is an important obstetric issue because of the increased risk of macrosomic infants, oligohydramnios, meconium aspiration, intrauterine fetal death, and dysmaturity syndrome. There is also greater risk to the mother because of a greater rate of cesarean sections (approximately doubled) and delivery of large infants. With improved dating, there are an increasing number of studies that show these complications of pregnancy may increase after 40 or 41 weeks of gestation.

Etiology

The most common reason for the diagnosis of postterm pregnancy is inaccurate dating; accurate dating is therefore imperative. Because the physiologic basis for the onset of labor is poorly understood, the mechanisms for preterm or postterm labor are also unclear. There are a few rare conditions of the fetus associated with postterm pregnancy. These include anencephaly, fetal adrenal hypoplasia, and absent fetal pituitary. All are notable for diminished levels of circulating estrogens.

Diagnosis

Again, the diagnosis is made by accurate dating. Because ultrasound can be off by as much as 3 weeks near term, this cannot be used to confirm dating. Accurate dating is made by a certain LMP consistent with a bimanual examination in the first trimester or a first-trimester ultrasound. Dating by a second-trimester ultrasound or unsure LMP is more suspect.

Treatment

The varying approaches to the postterm pregnancy generally involve more frequent visits, increased fetal testing, and plans for eventual induction. A typical plan for following a postterm pregnancy is outlined below.

Patients whose pregnancies go past week 40 usually receive an NST during week 41. Induction is indicated with nonreassuring fetal testing. During week 42, the patient should be seen twice and receive a BPP at one of the visits and NST at the other. Alternatively, many practitioners use the modified BPP (an NST and AFI) for fetal testing at each visit past the due date. Induction is indicated with nonreassuring fetal testing or electively with an inducible cervix (Bishop score > 6). After week 42, the patient is often induced regardless of cervical examination. Increasingly, patients are induced between 41 and 42 weeks, as a result of improved dating by ultrasound, patient demand, as well as the risk-averse environment of obstetrics.

KEY POINTS

1. Postterm pregnancy is defined as greater than 42 weeks gestational age.
2. Postterm pregnancies are at increased risk for fetal demise, macrosomia, meconium aspiration, and oligohydramnios.
3. Increased fetal surveillance and labor induction are the most common management options for postterm pregnancies.

Multiple Gestations

If a fertilized ovum divides into two separate ova, monozygotic, or "identical," twins result. If ovulation produces two ova and both are fertilized, dizygotic twins result. Without assisted fertility, the rate of twinning is approximately 1:80 pregnancies, with 30% of those monozygotic. The rate of naturally occurring triplets is approximately 1:7000–8000 pregnancies. However, with ovulation-enhancing drugs and in vitro fertilization (IVF), the incidence of multiple gestations is increasing.

Complications of Multiple Gestation

Multiple gestations result in an increase in a variety of obstetric complications including preterm labor, placenta previa, cord prolapse, postpartum hemorrhage, cervical incompetence, gestational diabetes, and preeclampsia. The fetuses are at increased risk for preterm delivery, congenital abnormalities, SGA, and malpresentation. The average gestational age of delivery for twins is between 36 and 37 weeks; for triplets it is 33 to 34 weeks. Monochorionic (one placenta), diamnionic (two amniotic sacs) twins, also referred to as MoDi twins, often have placental vascular communications and can develop **twin-to-twin transfusion syndrome** (TTTS). Monochorionic, monoamnionic (Mo-Mo) twins have an extremely high mortality rate (40% to 60%) secondary to cord accidents from entanglement.

Pathogenesis

Monozygotic twinning results from division of the fertilized ovum or cells in the embryonic disk. If separation occurs before the differentiation of the trophoblast, two chorions and two amnions (Di-Di) result. After trophoblast differentiation and before amnion formation (days 3 to 8), separation leads to a single placenta, one chorion, and two amnions (Mo-Di). Division after amnion formation leads to a single placenta, one chorion, and one amnion (Mo-Mo) (days 8 to 13) and rarely, conjoined or "Siamese" twins (days 13 to 15). Division of cells beyond day 15 or 16 will result in a singleton fetus. Monozygotic twinning does not follow any inheritable pattern and, historically, the only risk factor ever identified is a slight increase with advancing maternal age. In the 1990s it was determined that assisted reproductive techniques, while increasing the risk of dizygotic twins, also increases the risk of monozygotic twins.

Dizygotic twins primarily result from fertilization of two ova by two sperm. There are varying risk factors associated with dizygotic twinning. Dizygotic twins tend to run in families and are more common in people of African descent. Globally, the rate of dizygotic twins ranges from 1:1000 in Japan to 1:20 in several Nigerian tribes. The rate of all multiple gestations has increased sharply since the onset of medical treatment of infertility. Clomiphene citrate, a fertility-enhancing drug, increases the rate of dizygotic twinning up to 8%.

Diagnosis

Multiple gestations are usually diagnosed by ultrasound. Multiple gestations are indicated by rapid uterine growth, excessive maternal weight gain, or palpation of three or more fetal large parts (cranium and breech) on Leopold's. The level of β-hCG, human placental lactogen (HPL), and maternal serum α-fetoprotein (MSAFP) are all elevated for gestational age. Rarely, diagnosis will be made after delivery of the first fetus with palpation of the after-coming fetus(es).

Treatment

Because of the increased risk of complications, multiple-gestation pregnancies are managed as high-risk pregnancies, usually in conjunction with a perinatologist. Aside from the antenatal management of the complications, the principal issue in multiple gestations is mode of delivery.

Twin-to-Twin Transfusion Syndrome (TTTS)

Polyhydramnios-oligohydramnios (poly-oli) sequence or TTTS has been described for several centuries and results in a small, anemic twin and a large, plethoric, polycythemic, and occasionally hydropic twin. The etiology of TTTS appears to be secondary to unequal flow within vascular communications between the twins in their shared placenta leading to one twin becoming a donor and the other a recipient of this unequal blood flow. This can result in one fetus with hypervolemia, cardiomegaly, glomerulotubal hypertrophy, edema, and ascites and the other with hypovolemia, growth restriction, and oligohydramnios. Because of the risk of this syndrome in Mo-Di twins, serial ultrasounds examining the amniotic fluid and fetal growth should be obtained every 2 weeks after diagnosis.

TTTS has historically been managed with serial amnioreduction, which can reduce preterm contractions secondary to uterine distension and maternal symptoms, but only occasionally actually cures the fetal syndrome. More recently, as these vascular connections have been identified as the etiology of the syndrome, coagulating these vessels has been proposed as the treatment of choice in more severe cases. This is accomplished by fetal surgeons using a fetoscopically placed laser to coagulate the vessels.

Mono-Mono Twins

Because of the risk of cord entanglement and IUFD, Mo-Mo twins are often managed with frequent antenatal testing and early delivery. Unfortunately, frequent antenatal testing has not in and of itself appeared to make a difference in the rate of IUFD in these cases. Because of this, some patients are offered admission to the hospital and continuous electronic fetal monitoring from weeks 28 to 34, at which time delivery is performed via cesarean section. Mo-Mo and conjoined twins are almost always delivered via cesarean section.

Delivery of Twins

There are four possibilities for twin presentation: both vertex (40%), both breech, vertex then breech (40%), and breech then vertex. When deciding mode of delivery, all breech presenting twins (20%) are considered together.

Vertex/vertex twins should undergo a trial of labor with cesarean section reserved for the usual indications. Vertex/nonvertex twins can also undergo a trial of labor if the twins are concordant or the presenting twin is larger. The twins should be between 2000 g and 3500 g by classic criteria, although current data suggest that delivery is safe above 1500 g. Either external version to vertex of the second twin or breech extraction is used for delivery of the second twin. Internal podalic version has been used for delivery of the second twin, but has been correlated with a worsened fetal outcome. Nonvertex presenting twins are usually delivered via cesarean section.

Delivery of Triplets

Most triplet gestations are delivered via cesarean section. Rarely, triplets will be concordant, with vertex presenting, all greater than 1500 g to 2000 g and a vaginal delivery can be attempted. Multiple gestations beyond triplets are all delivered via cesarean section if possible.

KEY POINTS

1. Monozygotic twins carry identical genetic material, whereas dizygotic twins are from separate ova and sperm.
2. Multiple gestations are at increased risk for preterm labor and delivery, placenta previa, postpartum hemorrhage, preeclampsia, cord prolapse, malpresentation, and congenital abnormalities.
3. There is a genetic predisposition for dizygotic twinning, whereas the rate of monozygotic twinning is the same throughout all races and families.
4. Monozygotic twins are at risk for TTTS, and should have frequent ultrasound examinations to diagnose this early.
5. Vaginal delivery of vertex/vertex presenting twins is preferred and is possible with vertex/nonvertex twins under the right circumstances. Nonvertex presenting twins are delivered by cesarean section.

Hypertension and Pregnancy

Blood pressure in pregnancy is usually decreased. As a result of decreased vascular resistance, the blood pressure decreases in the latter half of the first trimester reaching its nadir in the mid-second trimester. During the third trimester, blood pressure will usually increase, but should not be higher than prepregnancy. Hypertension may be present before pregnancy—as with chronic hypertension, or may be induced by pregnancy—as with gestational hypertension (GH), preeclampsia, and eclampsia (Table 8-1). Liver injury is seen in a small percentage of patients with preeclampsia and is associated with two diseases in pregnancy with high morbidity and mortality: HELLP syndrome (hemolysis, elevated liver enzymes, low platelets) and acute fatty liver of pregnancy. Complications from these disorders are consistently among the leading causes of maternal death in developed countries. Because treatment is delivery, these disorders are also leading causes of premature delivery.

▆ PREECLAMPSIA

Pathogenesis

Preeclampsia is the presence of nondependent edema, hypertension, and proteinuria in the pregnant woman. The classic presentation is of a nulliparous woman in her third trimester. Although no definitive cause for preeclampsia has been determined, it is well accepted that the underlying pathophysiology involves a **generalized arteriolar constriction** (vasospasm) and intravascular depletion secondary to a generalized transudative edema that can produce symptoms related to ischemia, necrosis, and hemorrhage of organs. Thus, one of the fundamental aspects of the disease is vascular damage. It is theorized that

this is primarily related to circulating antibodies or antigen-antibody complexes (not unlike systemic lupus erythematosus) that damage the lining of vessel walls leading to exposure of the underlying collagen structure. The hyperdynamic state of pregnancy has also been proposed to cause this underlying vascular injury rather than an immunogenic phenomenon.

As outlined in Table 8-2, major fetal complications of preeclampsia are due to prematurity. Also, the generalized vasoconstriction of preeclampsia can result in decreased blood flow to the placenta. This may manifest as acute uteroplacental insufficiency, resulting in abruption or fetal distress. The uteroplacental insufficiency may also be chronic in nature and result in an intrauterine growth restricted (IUGR) fetus.

Maternal complications associated with preeclampsia (Table 8-3) are related to the generalized arteriolar vasoconstriction that affects the brain (seizure and stroke), kidneys (oliguria and renal failure), lungs (pulmonary edema), liver (edema and subcapsular hematoma), and small blood vessels (thrombocytopenia and disseminated intravascular coagulation [DIC]). Severe preeclampsia is diagnosed with severely elevated blood pressure or the presence of any of the above findings.

About 10% of patients with severe preeclampsia develop HELLP syndrome. **HELLP syndrome** is a subcategory of preeclampsia in which the patient presents with hemolysis, elevated liver enzymes, and low platelets. Hypertension and proteinuria may be minimal in these patients. HELLP syndrome is uncommon, but patients who experience it decline rapidly, resulting in poor maternal and fetal outcomes. Despite careful management, HELLP syndrome results in a high rate of stillbirth (10% to 15%) and neonatal death (20% to 25%).

■ TABLE 8-1
Hypertensive States of Pregnancy
Pregnancy-induced (or gestational) hypertension
Preeclampsia
Severe preeclampsia
Chronic hypertension
Chronic hypertension w/superimposed preeclampsia
HELLP syndrome
AFLP

■ TABLE 8-2
Fetal Complications of Preeclampsia
Complications related to prematurity (if early delivery is necessary)
Acute uteroplacental insufficiency
Placental infarct and/or abruption
Intrapartum fetal distress
Stillbirth (in severe cases)
Chronic uteroplacental insufficiency
Asymmetric and symmetric SGA fetuses
IUGR
Oligohydramnios

■ TABLE 8-3
Maternal Complications of Preeclampsia
Medical manifestations
Seizure
Cerebral hemorrhage
DIC and thrombocytopenia
Renal failure
Hepatic rupture or failure
Pulmonary edema
Obstetrical complications
Uteroplacental insufficiency
Placental abruption
Increased premature deliveries
Increased cesarean section deliveries

Epidemiology

Preeclampsia occurs in 5% to 6% of all live births and can develop any time after the 20th week, but is most commonly seen in the third trimester near term. When hypertension is seen in the early second trimester (14 to 20 weeks), a hydatidiform mole or previously undiagnosed chronic hypertension should be considered. Unlike other preeclamptic patients, the patient with HELLP is more likely to be less than 36 weeks gestation at the time of presentation. Although 80% of patients develop HELLP after being diagnosed with preeclampsia (30% with mild preeclampsia; 50% with severe preeclampsia), 20% of patients with HELLP have no previous history of hypertension before their diagnosis, and will present merely with the symptom of right upper-quadrant pain.

Risk Factors

Risk factors for preeclampsia fall essentially into two categories: those related to the manifestations of the disease (like chronic hypertension or renal disease), and those related to the immunogenic nature of preeclampsia (Table 8-4). These latter risk factors are quite interesting. For example, it has been shown that in addition to a family history in the parturient, if the mother of the father of her baby (mother-in-law) had preeclampsia, the patient is at greater risk of developing preeclampsia. While multiparous women who have not had preeclampsia in the past have a decreased risk, if a woman conceives with a new

■ TABLE 8-4
Risk Factors for Preeclampsia
Primarily disease related
Chronic hypertension
Chronic renal disease
Collagen vascular disease (e.g., SLE)
Pregestational diabetes
African American
Maternal age (<20 or >35)
Primarily immunogenic related
Nulliparity
Previous preeclampsia
Multiple gestation
Abnormal placentation
New paternity
Family history
Female relatives of parturient
Mother-in-law
Cohabitation less than 1 year

father of her baby, her risk increases back to that of a nullipara. A tolerance effect is seen in women who cohabitate with the father of the baby longer than 1 year prior to conceiving in comparison to women who conceive sooner. These risk factors support the theory that preeclampsia has an alloimmunogenic pathophysiology.

Clinical Manifestations and Diagnoses

Gestational Hypertension

Blood pressures elevated above 140/90 or an increase of 30 mm Hg above prepregnancy systolic BP or 15 mm Hg above prepregnancy diastolic BP are necessary to diagnose GH or pregnancy-induced hypertension (PIH). Blood pressures should be elevated on at least two occasions 4 to 6 hours apart and taken while the patient is seated. If the patient's 24-hour urinary protein total is <300 mg, then preeclampsia is ruled out and the patient can be managed expectantly. Because it is believed that preeclampsia is a continuum from PIH through severe disease, these patients are at risk for developing preeclampsia and should be followed closely with frequent blood pressure checks, laboratory tests, and antenatal fetal testing.

Mild Preeclampsia

As shown in Table 8-5, mild preeclampsia is classically defined as a third-trimester **blood pressure** greater than 140 mm Hg systolic or 90 mm Hg diastolic on two occasions at least 6 hours apart (or a 30 mm Hg rise in systolic or 15 mm Hg rise in diastolic pressure above previous levels) accompanied by **proteinuria** greater than 300 mg/24 h and **nondependent edema** (face and/or hands). It has been determined that edema is not essential to the diagnosis of preeclampsia, but the occurrence of hypertension and proteinuria are diagnostic. If a diagnosis is being made in the acute setting, proteinuria of 2+ or greater on two occasions has been used to assess proteinuria. In one study, more than two-thirds of patients with 1+ and 2+ protein and all patients with 3+ and 4+ protein had significant proteinuria. A better predictor of significant proteinuria is the urine protein to creatinine ratio. Because creatinine excretion is relatively constant, this ratio gives a rough estimate of the amount of protein that will be excreted over a 24-hour period. A ratio of >0.3 has been used as a threshold.

■ TABLE 8-5

Criteria for Diagnosis of Gestational Hypertension, Preeclampsia, and Eclampsia

Gestational Hypertension
Blood Pressure: >140/90 or increase over prepregnancy BP of >30/15

Mild Preeclampsia
Blood Pressure: >140/90 or increase over prepregnancy BP of >30/15

Proteinuria: >300 mg/24 hr or >1–2 plus on dipstick

Nondependent Edema

Severe Preeclampsia (by systems)
Neuro: Severe headache (not relieved by acetaminophen)
    Visual changes; scotomata

Cardiovascular: BP > 160/110

Pulmonary: Pulmonary edema

Renal: Acute renal failure with rising creatinine
    Oliguria < 400 mL/24 h or < 30 mL/h

GI: Right upper-quadrant pain
    Elevation of transaminases, AST and ALT

Heme: Hemolytic anemia
    Thrombocytopenia
    DIC

Fetal: IUGR, abnormal umbilical dopplers

Eclampsia
Seizure

Severe Preeclampsia

Criteria for severe preeclampsia (Table 8-5) include blood pressure greater than 160 mm Hg systolic or 110 mm Hg diastolic on two occasions at least 6 hours apart, accompanied by proteinuria greater than 5 g/24 h (or 3–4+ protein on dipstick on two occasions). A woman with mild preeclampsia by blood pressure and proteinuria parameters would be diagnosed with severe preeclampsia if she also developed certain associated conditions. These include altered consciousness, headache or visual changes, epigastric or right upper-quadrant pain, significantly impaired liver function (>2 times normal), oliguria (<400 mL in 24 h), pulmonary edema, and significant thrombocytopenia (<100,000/mm^3). Many clinical manifestations of preeclampsia are explained by vasospasm leading to necrosis and hemorrhage of organs.

HELLP Syndrome

The disorder is characterized by rapidly deteriorating liver function and thrombocytopenia. In addition, a number of patients will develop DIC. The criteria for diagnosis and relevant laboratory tests are outlined in Table 8-6. Liver capsule distension produces epigastric pain, often with progressive nausea and vomiting, and can lead to hepatic rupture. Patients with HELLP syndrome should be screened for acute fatty liver of pregnancy (AFLP) that presents with frank hepatic failure.

Acute Fatty Liver of Pregnancy (AFLP)

It is unclear whether AFLP is truly in the spectrum of preeclamptic syndromes or an entirely separate entity with similar signs and symptoms. More than 50% of patients with AFLP will also have hypertension and proteinuria. It presents in approximately 1:10,000 pregnancies and has a high mortality rate. Interestingly, it has been found that a number of AFLP patients will have fetuses with long-chain hydroxyacyl-CoA dehydrogenase (LCHAD) deficiency.

To differentiate AFLP from HELLP, labs associated with liver failure such as an elevated ammonia level, blood glucose less than 50, and markedly reduced fibrinogen and antithrombin III levels have been associated with AFLP. Management of these patients is supportive and, while liver transplant has been used, in some studies, it appears that it will resolve in many patients without this aggressive intervention.

Treatment

Mild Preeclampsia

Because delivery is the ultimate treatment for preeclampsia, induction of labor is the treatment of choice for pregnancies at term, unstable preterm pregnancies, or pregnancies where there is evidence of fetal lung maturity. In these cases, vaginal delivery may be attempted with the assistance of prostaglandins, pitocin, or amniotomy as needed. Cesarean delivery need only be performed for obstetric indications. For stable preterm patients, bed rest and expectant management, commonly in the hospital, is used. Betamethasone is given to enhance fetal lung maturity.

Patients with mild preeclampsia are often started on magnesium sulfate therapy for seizure prophylaxis (4 g load and 2 g/h maintenance) during labor and delivery and should be continued for 12 to 24 hours after delivery.

Severe Preeclampsia

The goals of treatment in severe preeclampsia are to prevent eclampsia, control maternal blood pressure, and deliver the fetus. However, management varies based on gestational age. Initially, patients with severe preeclampsia should be stabilized using magnesium sulfate for seizure prophylaxis and hydralazine (a direct arteriolar dilator) for blood pressure control. Once the patient is stabilized, if the gestational age is between 24 and 32 weeks, expectant management to gain treatment with betamethasone and further fetal maturity is often used. Beyond week 32 or in a severe preeclamptic with signs of renal failure, pulmonary edema, hepatic injury, HELLP syndrome, or DIC, delivery should ensue immediately.

Even though delivery is the cure for preeclampsia, patients can have lingering effects for up to several weeks. In fact, some patients will worsen acutely in the immediate postpartum period, possibly related to the increased placental antigen exposure during labor and delivery. Because of this, seizure prophylaxis is usually continued 24 hours postpartum, or until the patient improves markedly. In the setting of chronically elevated blood pressures, antihypertensive medications (most commonly labetolol and nifedipine) should be used and, in some cases, patients may need continue medications for several weeks after release to home. Patients with HELLP syndrome may have worsening thrombocytopenia, and it has been shown that corticosteroid treatment can decrease the amount of time until the nadir and return to normal levels.

Follow-Up

Women who develop preeclampsia during their first pregnancy will have a 25% to 33% recurrence rate in subsequent pregnancies. In patients with both

TABLE 8-6

Diagnosis of HELLP Syndrome

Hemolytic anemia
Schistocytes on peripheral blood smear
Elevated lactate dehydrogenase
Elevated total bilirubin

Elevated liver enzymes
Increase in aspartate aminotransferase
Increase in alanine aminotransferase

Low platelets
Thrombocytopenia

chronic hypertension and preeclampsia, the risk of recurrence is 70%. Low doses of aspirin prior to and during subsequent pregnancies to decrease the risk of preeclampsia, IUGR, and preterm deliveries has been studied. While this appeared to be a promising treatment in smaller, nonrandomized studies, larger studies have shown mixed outcomes.

KEY POINTS

1. Preeclampsia is the presence of hypertension (>140/90 mm Hg), proteinuria (>300 mg/day), and significant nondependent edema after 20 weeks gestation.
2. It has an incidence of 5% to 6% of all live births and occurs most commonly in nulliparous women in their third trimester.
3. Preeclampsia is characterized by a generalized multiorgan vasospasm that can lead to seizure, stroke, renal failure, liver damage, DIC, or fetal demise.
4. Risk factors include nulliparity, multiple gestation, and chronic hypertension.
5. Preeclampsia is ultimately treated with vaginal delivery, using magnesium sulfate and hydralazine as indicated.

▪ ECLAMPSIA

Eclampsia is the occurrence of grand mal seizures in the preeclamptic patient not attributed to other causes (Table 8-5). Although patients with severe preeclampsia are at greater risk for developing seizures, 25% of women with eclampsia were originally found to have only mild preeclampsia before the onset of seizures. Of note, eclampsia may also occur without proteinuria. Complications of eclampsia include cerebral hemorrhage, aspiration pneumonia, hypoxic encephalopathy, and thromboembolic events.

Clinical Manifestations

Seizures in the eclamptic patient are tonic-clonic in nature and may or may not be preceded by an aura. These seizures may develop before labor (25%), during labor (50%), or after delivery (25%). Most postpartum seizures occur within the first 48 hours after delivery, but will occasionally occur as late as several weeks after delivery.

Treatment

Treatment strategy for eclamptic patients includes seizure management, blood pressure control, and prophylaxis against further convulsions. Hypertension management can usually be achieved using hydralazine to lower the blood pressure. For seizure control and prophylaxis, eclamptic patients are treated with magnesium sulfate ($MgSO_4$) to decrease hyperreflexia and prevent further seizures by raising the seizure threshold. In prospective, randomized studies, magnesium has been found to be as good as or better than phenytoin, carbamazepine, and phenobarbital in the prevention of recurrent seizures in eclamptic patients.

In eclampsia, $MgSO_4$ therapy is initiated at the time of diagnosis and continued for 12 to 24 hours after delivery. The goal of magnesium sulfate therapy is to reach a therapeutic level while avoiding toxicity through careful clinical monitoring (Table 8-7). In the case of overdose, 10 mL 10% calcium chloride or calcium gluconate should be rapidly administered intravenously for cardiac protection.

Delivery should only be initiated after the eclamptic patient has been stabilized and convulsions have been controlled. In the case of eclampsia, the best way to treat the fetus is to stabilize the mother. Cesarean delivery should be reserved for obstetric indications.

▪ TABLE 8-7

Clinical Response to Serum Magnesium Sulfate Concentrations

Serum Concentration $MgSO_4$ (mg/mL)	Clinical Response
4.8–8.4	Therapeutic seizure prophylaxis
8	Central nervous system depression
10	Loss of deep tendon reflexes
15	Respiratory depression/paralysis
17	Coma
20–25	Cardiac arrest

CHRONIC HYPERTENSION

Pathogenesis

Chronic hypertension is defined as hypertension present before conception, before 20 weeks gestation, or persisting more than 6 weeks postpartum. Approximately one-third of patients with chronic hypertension in pregnancy will develop superimposed preeclampsia. Because of poor vascular development, the fetus may suffer from IUGR and the mother is at increased risk for superimposed preeclampsia, premature delivery, and abruptio placentae.

Treatment

Treatment of mild chronic hypertension is controversial. However, mothers with controlled blood pressures tend to have fewer problems. Patients with chronic hypertension whose blood pressures in early pregnancy are consistently 140/90 and less can be managed expectantly. With persistent elevated blood pressures or in patients who were on an antihypertensive agent prior to pregnancy, antihypertensive medications are used. The two most common medications used are labetolol (a beta-blocker with concomitant alpha blockade) and nifedipine (a peripheral calcium channel blocker). In retrospective studies, beta-blocker use has been associated with decreased birth weight. However, these studies are likely biased by the severity of disease. Methyldopa (a central alpha-adrenergic agonist) has been the drug of choice in these patients for several decades. It has not been shown to effectively manage blood pressure or change outcomes, so its usage has therefore decreased.

Because these patients are at risk for other complications of chronic hypertension, a baseline ECG and 24-hour urine collection for creatinine clearance and protein should be obtained. This will also help differentiate superimposed preeclampsia from chronic renal disease later in pregnancy. Low-dose aspirin may decrease the risk of developing superimposed preeclampsia and is used by some practitioners.

Superimposed Preeclampsia

One-third or more of patients with chronic hypertension will develop superimposed preeclampsia. Because the hypertension is longstanding, complications such as IUGR and placental abruption are also more common. The diagnosis can sometimes be difficult to make because many of these patients will have concomitant renal disease at baseline. An increase in the systolic BP of 30 mmHg or in the diastolic BP of 15 mmHg over prepregnancy blood pressure is indicative of superimposed preeclampsia. If a 24-hour urine protein is now elevated, the diagnosis is made; if not, then the blood pressure can be managed with increasing doses of medications. In patients who have baseline renal disease as well, an elevated uric acid above 6.0 to 6.5 has been used to differentiate preeclampsia from exacerbation of hypertension.

Diabetes During Pregnancy

Diabetes during pregnancy encompasses a range of disease entities including gestational diabetes and overt diabetes mellitus (Table 9-1). Nonpregnant diabetics are divided into two types based on the pathophysiology of their disease, whereas diabetes in pregnancy is usually divided into pregestational and gestational diabetes. Pregestational diabetics include all patients with type 1 and type 2 diabetes diagnosed prior to pregnancy. Gestational diabetics are those diagnosed in pregnancy. Because of lack of screening in many nonpregnant women, this latter group may occasionally contain undiagnosed pregestational diabetic women.

■ GESTATIONAL DIABETES

True gestational diabetes mellitus (GDM) is an impairment in carbohydrate metabolism that first manifests during pregnancy. These patients may have borderline carbohydrate metabolism impairment at baseline or be entirely normal. In pregnancy, placental hormones, human placental lactogen for example, act as anti-insulin agents leading to increased insulin resistance and generalized carbohydrate intolerance. Because the carbohydrate metabolism abnormalities usually don't appear until the third trimester, these patients generally are not at increased risk for congenital anomalies like the pregestational diabetics. They do, however, carry an increased risk of fetal macrosomia and birth injuries as well as neonatal hypoglycemia. These women are at a four- to tenfold increased risk of developing type 2 diabetes during their lifetime.

Epidemiology

The incidence of GDM ranges from 1% to 12% of pregnant women depending on the population. Gestational diabetes is seen in women of Hispanic, Southeast Asian, Native American, and African American descent, increasing maternal age, obesity, family history of diabetes, previous infant weighing more than 4000 g, and previous stillborn infant.

Diagnostic Evaluation

The best time to screen for diabetes during pregnancy is at the end of the second trimester between 24 and 28 weeks gestation. Patients with one or more risk factors for developing gestational diabetes should be screened at their first prenatal visit and during each subsequent trimester.

There are a variety of proposed methods of screening for diabetes during pregnancy (Table 9-2). The most common screening test consists of giving a 50-g glucose load and then measuring the plasma glucose 1 hour later. If the 1-hour glucose level is greater than 140 mg/dL, then the test is positive and glucose tolerance testing is necessary. Recently, a screening threshold of 135 mg/dL has been proposed that would increase the sensitivity of the test at a cost of increasing the number of false positives. The optimal threshold still needs further elucidation.

Women with a positive screening test are diagnosed with a 3-hour oral glucose tolerance test (GTT) to evaluate their carbohydrate metabolism (Table 9-3). The GTT involves the administration of 100 mg of oral glucose given after an 8-hour overnight fast preceded by a 3-day special carbohydrate diet. Glucose levels are measured immediately before glucose administration and again at 1, 2, and

TABLE 9-1

White Classification for Diabetes During Pregnancy

Classification	Description
Class A_1	Gestational diabetes; diet controlled
Class A_2	Gestational diabetes; insulin controlled
Class B	Onset: age 20 or older or Duration: less than 10 years
Class C	Onset: age 10–19 or Duration: 10–19 years
Class D	Onset: before age 10 or Duration: greater than 20 years
Class F	Diabetic nephropathy
Class R	Proliferative retinopathy
Class RF	Retinopathy and nephropathy
Class H	Ischemic heart disease
Class T	Prior renal transplantation

TABLE 9-2

Glucose Screening Tests During Pregnancy

Test	Normal Glucose Level (mg/dL)
Fasting	<105
1 h after a 50-g glucose load	<140

TABLE 9-3

Three-Hour Glucose Tolerance Test: Venous and Plasma Criteria for GDM*

Timing of Glucose Measurement	Normal Whole Venous Blood Glucose (mg/dL)	Normal Plasma Glucose (mg/dL)
Fasting	90	105
1 h	165	190
2 h	145	165
3 h	125	145

Notes: *Results reflect upper limits of normal. Diagnosis of gestational diabetes is made if fasting value or any two values are exceeded.

3 hours after the dose. If either the fasting glucose or two or more of the postprandial values are elevated, a diagnosis of gestational diabetes is made. The values shown in Table 9-3 reflect recently lowered values that will increase the number of women diagnosed with gestational diabetes.

Treatment

Once the diagnosis of gestational diabetes is made, the patient is usually started on a diabetic diet. An American Diabetic Association (ADA) diet of 2200 calories per day is recommended for all patients with diabetes during pregnancy, although the total carbohydrate intake is more important. Both the timing and content of meals are important; therefore, a meal plan based on intake of 30–35 kcal/kg of ideal body weight is suggested. Patients are taught to count carbohydrates and meals are designed to contain between 30–45 g of carbohydrates at breakfast, with 45–60 g of carbohydrates for lunch and dinner, and 15 g snacks. While on this diet, the patient also monitors her blood glucose levels four times per day, which includes a fasting and three postprandial values.

If the diabetic diet controls the blood sugars (fasting values <90 and 1 hour postprandial values <140 or 2 hour postprandial values <120) then this management is continued throughout the pregnancy. These patients are classified as class A_1 or diet-controlled diabetics in the **White classification of gestational diabetes**. This classification is used as a prognostic tool to determine the likely severity of a woman's diabetes and its interaction with pregnancy. It was originally designed to predict perinatal survival. However, if more than 25% to 30% of a patient's blood sugar values are elevated, medication —usually insulin or an oral hypoglycemic agent— is indicated. These individuals are considered class A_2 or medication-controlled diabetics. In true gestational diabetics, fasting values are commonly normal while postprandial values are elevated. These patients can be started on short-acting insulin in combination with an intermediate-acting insulin in the morning (to cover breakfast and lunch) and a short-acting insulin at dinner. Commonly, the short-acting insulin is humalog or Lispro, but some providers still use regular insulin; the intermediate insulin is NPH.

Historically, the oral hypoglycemic agents were not used in pregnancy because of concerns regarding fetal hypoglycemia. However, recent studies indicate that adequate blood glucose control is achieved without particular harm to the fetus. Because of the ease of patient administration and possibly improved compliance, oral agents such as glyburide are now being used by some institutions. Long-term results are not as yet available.

Fetal Monitoring

In patients started on insulin or an oral hypoglycemic agent, fetal monitoring via nonstress test (NST) or modified biophysical profile (BPP) is typically begun between 32 and 36 weeks gestation and continued until delivery on a weekly or biweekly basis. Because of the increased risk of macrosomia, these patients commonly receive an obstetric ultrasound for an estimated fetal weight (EFW) between 34 and 37 weeks. It is not common to offer fetal monitoring to patients who are well controlled on diet alone. The decision to offer these patients an ultrasound for EFW varies among practitioners.

Delivery Management

The intrapartum management of diet-controlled gestational diabetics does not differ from that of nondiabetic women, provided an admission random glucose does not reveal significant hyperglycemia that should be corrected to avoid neonatal hypoglycemia. It is unclear whether well-controlled gestational diabetics have any particular increased risk for peripartum complications other than the theoretical risk of macrosomia. A closer evaluation of fetal weight at term may be prudent in patients going past their due date.

Scheduled delivery (typically via induction of labor) between weeks 39 and 40 is common in patients on insulin or a hypoglycemic agent (class A2 gestational diabetes). One concern about allowing their pregnancies to proceed is that there may be an increased risk of hypoglycemia as their placental function decreases toward the end of pregnancy. These patients are commonly brought in to labor and delivery between weeks 39 and 40, where their long-term agents are discontinued and blood sugars monitored every hour. Dextrose and insulin drips are used if necessary to maintain blood sugars within normal limits. Patients with poor blood sugar control are offered delivery between weeks 37 and 39 after verification of fetal lung maturity. Patients who have an estimated fetal weight above 4000 g have increased risks of shoulder dystocia and their labor curves should be followed closely. Some clinicians offer these patients an elective caesarean birth but, more commonly, elective cesarean delivery is offered to those with an EFW greater than 4500 g.

At the time of delivery, forceps and vacuum are generally not used because of the increased risk of shoulder dystocia, except in the case of true outlet forceps for nonreassuring fetal monitoring. To prepare for a possible shoulder dystocia, there should be at least one experienced obstetrician in the delivery room and usually an extra nurse. This allows one nurse to perform suprapubic pressure while the other is available to time events and function as an assistant.

Follow-Up

Among patients who develop GDM during pregnancy, 50% will experience GDM in subsequent pregnancies and 25% to 35% will go on to develop overt diabetes within 5 years. The infants of patients with GDM have an increased incidence of childhood obesity and type II diabetes during early adulthood and later in life.

KEY POINTS

1. Gestational diabetes occurs in 1% to 12% of pregnant women.
2. Risk factors for gestational diabetes include Hispanic, Asian American, Native American, and African American ethnicity, obesity, family history of diabetes, and prior pregnancy complicated by gestational diabetes, macrosomia, shoulder dystocia, or fetal death.
3. All pregnant women should be screened for diabetes between weeks 24 and 28. High-risk women should also be screened at their first prenatal visit.
4. Fetal complications of gestational diabetes include macrosomia, shoulder dystocia, and neonatal hypoglycemia.
5. Pregnancy management should include frequent health care visits, thorough patient education, American Diabetic Association diet, glucose monitoring, fetal monitoring, and insulin or an oral hypoglycemic agent as indicated.
6. Patients should generally be induced between 39 and 40 weeks gestation. Intrapartum insulin and dextrose are used to maintain tight control during delivery. Cesarean section is offered if fetal weight is over 4500 g.

◼ PREGESTATIONAL DIABETES

Diabetes during pregnancy can have devastating effects on both mother (Table 9-4) and fetus (Table 9-5). Diabetic women are four times more likely to develop preeclampsia or eclampsia than nondiabetic women and twice as likely to have a spontaneous abortion. Similarly, the rates of infection, hydramnios, postpartum hemorrhage, and cesarean section are all increased for diabetic mothers. Major fetal effects include a fivefold increase in perinatal death and a two- to threefold increase in the rate of congenital malformations.

Control of maternal glucose levels in overtly diabetic women is an important factor in determining fetal outcome. In older studies, with minimal diabetic management in the setting of pregnancy, the perinatal mortality rate was as high as 30%. However, with careful management by specialists, this rate can be reduced to less than 1%. The fetuses of diabetic mothers are more likely to develop congenital anomalies, both cardiac anomalies, and most dramatically, caudal regression syndrome. The fetus is also at risk for fetal growth abnormalities and sudden intrauterine fetal demise (IUFD).

Epidemiology

Less than 1% of pregnant women have pregestational diabetes. However, with improved management of type 1 diabetics and increased rates of type 2 diabetics, the number of women with pregestational diabetes who become pregnant is increasing.

Risk Factors

The White classification system was originally designed to prognosticate perinatal survival; with changing management of diabetes as a chronic disease, it has, however, become less useful. The length of illness used to differentiate classes B, C, and D has little predictive value at this point because there are likely some class B patients with poor control and many class D patients with excellent control. However, the severity of illness as reflected by classes R (retinopathy), F (nephropathy), and H (heart disease) is certainly predictive of worsened perinatal outcomes in these patients. Along with the White classification, other prognostic factors include hypertension, pyelonephritis, ketoacidosis, and poor glucose control. Glucose control is measured by a HgbA$_1$c, which gives an estimate of the

◼ **TABLE 9-4**

Maternal Complications of Diabetes During Pregnancy

Obstetric complications
Polyhydramnios
Preeclampsia
Miscarriage
Infection
Postpartum hemorrhage
Increased cesarean section

Diabetic emergencies
Hypoglycemia
Ketoacidosis
Diabetic coma

Vascular and end organ involvement
Cardiac
Renal
Ophthalmic
Peripheral vascular

Neurologic
Peripheral neuropathy
Gastrointestinal disturbance

◼ **TABLE 9-5**

Fetal Complications of Diabetes Mellitus

Macrosomia
Traumatic delivery
Shoulder dystocia
Erb's palsy

Delayed organ maturity
Pulmonary
Hepatic
Neurologic
Pituitary-thyroid axis

Congenital malformations
Cardiovascular defects
Neural tube defects
Caudal regression syndrome
Situs inversus
Duplex renal ureter

IUGR
Intrauterine death

average glucose control over the prior 8 to 12 weeks. Patients with an $HgbA_1c$ <6.5 generally have good outcomes, whereas patients with an $HgbA_1c$ of 12 or greater are estimated to have a 25% rate of congenital anomalies.

Treatment

The goals of managing the diabetic patient include thorough patient education, control of maternal glucose, and careful maternal and fetal monitoring and testing. To achieve these goals, tight glucose control should be maintained prior to conception and throughout the pregnancy. Studies now show that stricter control of serum glucose levels during pregnancy can decrease the rate of maternal and neonatal complications. To achieve euglycemia, diet, insulin, and exercise must all be regulated.

Diabetic patients have become increasingly aware of the differences that tight control can make as well as the importance of this management during pregnancy. Ideally, these patients should be seen prepregnancy to discuss the risks and benefits of pregnancy. In these visits, a diabetic woman can be counseled regarding the risks to her health, particularly in the setting of chronic renal disease that has been shown to worsen during pregnancy. The patient can also be counseled about the risk of congenital anomalies in the fetus based on her $HgbA_1c$. If she is not in optimal control, this can be tightened to prepare for pregnancy. Because these patients are at higher risk of neural tube defects, they are also placed on 4 mg of folate daily.

It has been standard for patients to use the American Diabetic Association diet of 2200 calories per day. More recently, however, the focus on diabetic diet management has focused on total carbohydrate intake rather than caloric intake. Generally, patients keep their carbohydrate intake at 30–45 g at breakfast and 45–60 g at lunch and dinner with 15-g snacks. Patients can increase or decrease protein and fat based on whether they need more or less calories to gain or maintain weight. These carbohydrate-focused diets should be maintained during pregnancy, although the total caloric intake is usually about 300 kcal higher than in nonpregnant patients.

Type 1 Diabetes

Historically, these patients had extremely poor maternal and perinatal outcomes, many of which can be attributed to longstanding and poorly managed disease. Currently, many type 1 diabetics are checking their blood sugars seven or more times per day, doing carbohydrate counting, and maintaining their $HgbA_1c$ below 6.0–6.5. When patients are able to maintain tight control prior to and during their pregnancies, the rates of microvascular disease, renal disease, and hypertension are significantly decreased. These lower rates of baseline disease lead to fewer complications during pregnancy.

Because of the correlation of outcome with prepregnant disease, patients are extensively screened at their first visit (if not preconceptionally). Routinely, patients should obtain an ECG, particularly those with longstanding disease, hypertension, advanced maternal age (AMA) or renal disease. A 24-hour urine collection for creatinine clearance and protein should be sent to assess baseline renal function. An $HgbA_1c$ is ordered to assess baseline glucose management as well as a TSH since these patients are at risk for other endocrinopathies. In addition, a referral to an ophthalmologist should be made to check for baseline retinopathy.

Because type 1 diabetics require insulin, they are usually very experienced at managing their disease. However, this experience may not be applicable during pregnancy, which can be dramatically different. During the first half of pregnancy, the patient's prior dosing regimen is usually increased slightly, but can increase substantially during the latter half of pregnancy as insulin resistance increases. If patients have been managed on an insulin pump, that practice should be continued. In fact, because an insulin pump can help maintain patients in tight control, it is often begun either immediately prepregnancy for patients planning to conceive or after the first trimester in patients who are becoming increasingly difficult to manage with NPH and humalog insulin shots.

Table 9-6 demonstrates the relationship between the time of insulin dose, the time of glucose testing, and the target blood glucose levels. When adjusting a patient's dosing schedule, it is important to consider other factors that may alter insulin requirements, such as diet, exercise, stress, and infection. When insulin changes become necessary, there are a few simple rules that aid in the process (Table 9-7). In addition to the schedules given in Table 9-6 and Table 9-7, patients on insulin pumps should also check premeal glucose values throughout the day to get a sense of how well blood sugars are being managed at baseline.

Because the level of physical activity affects the

TABLE 9-6

Glucose Monitoring and Insulin Dosing During Pregnancy

Insulin Type and Dose Time	Time Impact Seen	Target Glucose Level (mg/dL)
Evening NPH	Fasting	70–90
Morning Humalog	Post breakfast	100–139
Morning NPH	Post lunch	100–139
Evening Humalog	Post dinner	100–139

TABLE 9-7

Instructions for Adjusting Insulin Dosage

1. Establish a fasting glucose level between 70–90 mg/dL.
2. Only adjust one dosing level at a time.
3. Do not change any dosage by more than 20% per day.
4. Wait 24 h between dosage changes to evaluate the response.

plasma glucose level, consistent levels of physical activity are suggested. Keep in mind that a hospitalized patient who achieves euglycemia in the context of relatively low activity may encounter bouts of hypoglycemia when at home on the same insulin regime because her physical activity level increases, thus lowering the need for insulin. Physical activity can also be used to help manage blood glucose. If a patient consistently has an elevated postmeal blood glucose, the premeal insulin or postmeal activity can be increased. It is also important to consider differences between weekday and weekend activity. Some patients will require entirely different insulin regimens on the weekends.

Type 2 Diabetes

The pathophysiology of type 2 diabetics differs from type 1 diabetics. Type 1 diabetics have had autoimmune destruction of their pancreatic islet cells resulting in diminished or absent insulin production, whereas type 2 diabetics have insulin resistance. Many type 2 diabetics are managed prior to pregnancy with oral hypoglycemic agents or diet alone.

However, in pregnancy, most will require insulin. Oral hypoglycemic agents have not generally been used during pregnancy because of concerns regarding fetal hypoglycemia or potential teratogenicity, but recent studies have not shown a difference in fetal outcomes or demonstrated any particular association with congenital anomalies, and patients are now managed on these medications during pregnancy. Of note, compliance with these medications may be better than with potentially complicated insulin regimens.

When oral hypoglycemic agents do not adequately maintain glucose control during pregnancy, insulin can be substituted or supplemented. In general, insulin is started as NPH in the AM and at bedtime to provide a longer acting substrate throughout the day. A short acting insulin, usually Humalog (although regular insulin has been used traditionally) is used at meals to control immediate carbohydrate intake. Once patients are started on insulin, management is very similar to that of type 1 diabetics, although the doses are often higher depending on the patient's degree of insulin resistance.

Fetal Testing and Delivery

In the patient with pregestational diabetes, antenatal testing to evaluate the growth and well-being of the fetus usually begins at week 32. Earlier testing is recommended in the setting of poor glucose control. Testing regimens vary, but may resemble the following. Antenatal fetal assessment consisting of weekly NSTs until week 36, at which time biweekly testing is implemented, which includes weekly NST alternating with weekly modified BPP to assess amniotic fluid measurement as well. In addition to the weekly testing, an ultrasound to assess fetal growth is usually obtained between 32 and 36 weeks gestation.

In general, well-controlled pregestational insulin-dependent diabetics with no complications are offered fetal lung maturity testing at 37 weeks gestation and delivered if mature. Many patients may decline this management, and are instead offered induction of labor between 39 to 40 weeks gestation without fetal lung maturity testing. Indications for earlier delivery include nonreassuring fetal testing, poor glucose control, worsening or uncontrolled hypertension, worsening renal disease, or poor fetal growth.

Blood sugars can be extremely difficult to manage in the laboring diabetic woman. The physical effort of labor and delivery decreases the overall insulin requirements. Patients are usually begun on dextrose and insulin drips to maintain blood sugars between 100–120 mg/dL. If the blood sugar increases above 120, the insulin can be increased. Conversely, if the blood sugar drops to between 80–100, an infusion of dextrose can be started or increased.

After delivery, maternal insulin requirements decrease significantly because of the removal of the placenta, which contains many insulin antagonists. In fact, insulin requirements may go below prepregnant levels during the puerperium, particularly in breast-feeding women. Type 2 diabetics may require no insulin during this period. However, type 1 diabetics should always be maintained on at least a small amount of insulin because they do not produce any endogenously.

Follow-Up

In the puerperal period, pregestational diabetics should resume their prepregnancy regimens. Patients who were on oral hypoglycemic agents, however, should not use them if breast-feeding because of concerns regarding neonatal hypoglycemia. In patients with preexisting renal disease, a 24-hour urine collection for creatinine clearance and protein is usually done at 6 weeks postpartum to assess worsening of disease. In addition, an ophthalmologic appointment is usually scheduled 12 to 14 weeks postpartum. After 6 to 8 weeks postpartum, management of the patients' diabetes should be transferred back to their primary physician or endocrinologist.

KEY POINTS

1. Maternal complications of diabetes during pregnancy include hyperglycemia, hypoglycemia, urinary tract infection, worsening renal disease, hypertension, and retinopathy.
2. Fetal complications of diabetes during pregnancy include spontaneous abortion, congenital anomalies, macrosomia, IUGR, neonatal hypoglycemia, respiratory distress syndrome, and perinatal death.
3. Pregnancy management is optimized by a preconceptional visit, early prenatal care, thorough patient education, tight glucose monitoring and management with insulin, fetal monitoring, and thoughtful plan for delivery.
4. Motivated type 1 diabetics can usually maintain tighter control on an insulin pump. Management in labor and delivery usually requires an insulin drip; however, insulin requirements decrease dramatically postpartum.

Chapter 1

Infectious Diseases in Pregnancy

As with other diseases in pregnancy, one must think about the effect of an infectious disease on the parturient (mom) and the fetus (baby) as well as the interaction between the two. In this chapter we discuss common infections that increase or whose complications increase in pregnancy, infections specific to pregnancy, and infections that can affect the fetus (Table 10-1). The infectious complications that are common to the puerperium such as endomyometritis and wound infections are discussed in Chapter 12.

■ URINARY TRACT INFECTIONS (UTIS)

The incidence of urinary tract infections (UTIs), particularly the more serious UTIs, increases during pregnancy. Multiple studies show that asymptomatic bacteriuria with greater than 100,000 colonies on culture occurs in roughly 5% of all pregnancies. Although this is similar to the rate of occurrence in the nonpregnant population, it can lead to episodes of cystitis and pyelonephritis at higher rates than in nonpregnant women. Asymptomatic bacteriuria will proceed to UTI, cystitis, or pyelonephritis in 25% of patients. Of the cases of pyelonephritis, 15% will be complicated by bacteremia, sepsis, or adult respiratory distress syndrome (ARDS). In sickle cell patients, the rate of asymptomatic bacteriuria doubles to 10%.

Pathogenesis

A number of factors can contribute to a higher incidence of cystitis and pyelonephritis in pregnancy.

During pregnancy, the smooth muscle relaxation effects of progesterone decrease bladder tone and cause ureteral dilation. In addition, mechanical compression from the enlarged uterus can cause obstruction of the ureters, leading to stasis. Both cystitis and vesicoureteral reflux are increased, leading to more ascending infections.

Diagnosis

UTIs are diagnosed with clinical signs and symptoms of dysuria, urinary frequency, and urinary urgency in conjunction with a positive urine culture. Because urine cultures may take 3 to 4 days to become positive, a urinalysis is often used as a proxy during initial evaluation. The urinalysis will be positive for leukocyte esterase and nitrites, and the urine sediment will have elevated white blood cells and bacteria. Cystitis is diagnosed with suprapubic tenderness upon palpation and complaints of lower abdominal pain in the setting of a UTI.

Treatment

Escherichia coli accounts for greater than 70% of all UTIs. The remainder are usually due to *Klebsiella*, *Enterococcus*, *Proteus*, coagulase negative *Staphylococcus*, and group B *Streptococcus*. Because most UTIs are caused by *E. coli*, initial treatment of asymptomatic bacteriuria is usually with amoxicillin, Macrodantin, or Bactrim. Symptomatic UTIs and cystitis are also treated in this fashion, with adjustment of medication based on culture-sensitivity results. Because an asymptomatic bacteriuria may persist, a test of cure culture should be obtained 1 to 2 weeks after treatment has begun.

■ TABLE 10-1

Infectious Diseases in Pregnancy

Infections whose complications increase during pregnancy
UTIs
Bacterial vaginosis
Surgical wound
Group B *Strep*

Infections more common in pregnancy and the puerperium
Pyelonephritis
Endomyometritis
Mastitis
Toxic shock syndrome (TSS)

Infections specific to pregnancy
Chorioamnionitis
Septic pelvic thrombophlebitis
Episiotomy or perineal lacerations

Infections that affect the fetus
Neonatal sepsis (e.g., Group B *Strep, E. coli*)
HSV
VZV
Parvovirus B19
CMV
Rubella
HIV
Hepatitis B & C
Gonorrhea
Chlamydia
Syphilis
Toxoplasmosis

Pyelonephritis

The most common complication of a lower UTI is an ascending infection to the kidneys, or **pyelonephritis**. Pyelonephritis is estimated to complicate as many as 1% to 2% of pregnancies and has particularly serious associated complications including septic shock and ARDS. Because of these risks, pyelonephritis during pregnancy is usually treated aggressively with hospital admission, IV hydration, and intravenous (IV) antibiotics—often ampicillin and gentamicin—until the patient is afebrile and asymptomatic for 24 to 48 hours. Once per day dosing of gentamicin is not used during pregnancy because of case reports of fetal ototoxicity. There have been small trials that have examined the possibility of treating these patients with a single dose of IV antibiotics and continuing with oral antibiotics or treating with oral antibiotics alone as an outpatient. While

these treatments seem to be effective, selecting entirely compliant patients with social support is imperative.

KEY POINTS

1. Five percent of pregnant women have asymptomatic bacteriuria and are at increased risk for cystitis and pyelonephritis.
2. Lower UTIs can be treated with oral antibiotics, whereas pyelonephritis in pregnancy is treated with IV antibiotics.
3. Pyelonephritis may be complicated by septic shock and ARDS.

■ BACTERIAL VAGINOSIS IN PREGNANCY

Studies have demonstrated that **bacterial vaginosis** (BV) increases the risk for preterm premature rupture of membranes (PPROM), preterm delivery, and puerperal infections. Because of this, it has been proposed that patients with BV be treated and followed up with a test of cure to decrease their risk of preterm delivery. Initial smaller studies supporting this have led to screening programs where women are screened for BV using the diagnostic techniques discussed below and subsequently treated. However, these larger screening programs find that treatment does not appear to decrease the risk of preterm delivery and in fact may even increase the risk of preterm labor among the patients treated for asymptomatic BV, perhaps as a result of intolerance of the treatment.

Diagnosis and Treatment

Common symptoms are a malodorous discharge or vaginal irritation, although many patients with BV may be asymptomatic. Diagnosis can be made with an amine odor on the "whiff" test (see Chapter 16), pH of 5–6, examination of slides for clue cells, or upon culture of the vaginal discharge. Common organisms include *Gardnerella vaginalis*, *Bacteroides*, and *Mycoplasma hominis*. Metronidazole (Flagyl) is the treatment of choice and is often used as a vaginal gel to avoid increasing nausea during pregnancy. Clindamycin orally or as a vaginal gel can also be used. In pregnancy, because of the high rate of asymptomatic patients, a test of cure is usually performed.

GROUP B *STREPTOCOCCUS*

Group B *Streptococcus* is commonly responsible for UTIs, chorioamnionitis, and endomyometritis during pregnancy. It is also a major pathogen in neonatal sepsis, which has severe implications. Although sepsis occurs in only two to three per 1000 live births, the mortality rate with group B streptococcal sepsis ranges from 25% to 50%. Various studies have demonstrated a wide range of asymptomatic colonization in pregnant women, from 10% to 35%. To protect infants from group B *Streptococcus* infections, widespread screening programs have been implemented utilizing a rectovaginal culture for group B *Strep* colonization between weeks 36 and 37. Large, prospective studies have shown that these screening programs do decrease the rate of neonatal sepsis from group B *Strep*. Of note, there are concerns that the increase in prophylactic antibiotics given to these patients will increase widespread antibiotic resistance.

Diagnosis and Treatment

Group B *Strep* is commonly screened for by a culture of the perianal area and vagina, which may be self-administered. Screening usually occurs between weeks 36 and 37. Women with positive group B *Strep* cultures are subsequently treated with IV penicillin G when in labor. Women with an unknown group B *Strep* status who are delivering before 37 weeks gestation or have rupture of membranes greater than 18 hours are also treated with penicillin G until delivery. Because of the difficulty of obtaining the correct doses of penicillin G, ampicillin is commonly used in its stead. This is more likely to increase antibiotic resistance.

CHORIOAMNIONITIS

Chorioamnionitis is an infection of the membranes and amniotic fluid surrounding the fetus. It is frequently associated with preterm and prolonged rupture of membranes (ROM) but can also occur without ROM. It is the most common precursor of neonatal sepsis, which has a high rate of fetal mortality. It has maternal sequelae of endomyometritis and septic shock.

Diagnosis

The common signs of chorioamnionitis are maternal fever, elevated maternal white blood count, uterine tenderness, and fetal tachycardia. Because this problem is of such great concern, other causes of these signs and symptoms should be excluded. Other loci of maternal infection may cause maternal fever and elevated white blood cell count as well as fetal tachycardia. Elevations in maternal temperature have also been seen in patients undergoing labor induction with prostaglandins as well as those with epidurals. Fetal tachycardia may be congenital. Thus, a prior baseline fetal heart rate (FHR) can be useful. Fetal tachycardia can also be caused by a β-agonist tocolytic. The maternal white blood cell count is elevated in pregnancy and further elevated with the onset of labor. The white blood cell count is also increased by administration of corticosteroids.

In term patients, if the constellation of the above signs exists without any other etiology, the diagnosis should be presumed and treatment begun. In preterm patients whose fetuses would benefit from being in utero for more time, a more aggressive means to reach the diagnosis can be taken if there is any doubt. The gold standard for diagnosis of chorioamnionitis is a culture of the amniotic fluid, which can be obtained via amniocentesis. At the same time, the amniotic fluid can be sent for glucose, white blood cell count, protein, and Gram's stain. Unfortunately, these tests have a sensitivity that ranges from 40% to 70%. The infected fetus has been described to experience a fetal immune response syndrome (FIRS), which results in the release of cytokines. This has led to research that shows that the most sensitive screening test for chorioamnionitis appears to be IL-6 levels in the amniotic fluid that rise prior to changes in many of the other screening tests. This screening test is still used only in experimental protocols at most institutions.

Treatment

When chorioamnionitis is suspected, intravenous antibiotics should be started. Commonly, the causative organisms are those that colonize the vagina and rectum. Thus, broad-spectrum coverage should be used, most commonly a second- or third-generation cephalosporin, gentamicin, and ampicillin or clindamycin. In addition to antibiotics, delivery should be hastened with induction, augmentation, or, in the case of a nonreassuring fetal tracing, by cesarean section.

KEY POINTS

1. Chorioamnionitis is diagnosed by maternal fever, uterine tenderness, elevated maternal white blood cell count, and fetal tachycardia.
2. Although the infection is often polymicrobial, group B *Strep* colonization has a high correlation with both chorioamnionitis and neonatal sepsis.
3. Chorioamnionitis is treated by IV antibiotics and delivery.

■ INFECTIONS THAT AFFECT THE FETUS

Herpes Simplex Virus (HSV)

Herpes simplex virus (HSV) is a DNA virus that has two subtypes: HSV-1 and HSV-2. Genital herpes infections are primarily caused by HSV-2; however, there are extragenital HSV-2 infections and genital HSV-1 infections. Patients with a history of herpes should have their vulva, vagina, and cervix carefully examined for lesions when presenting in labor because of the risk of vertical transmission of HSV to the fetus during vaginal delivery. If lesions are present, cesarean section is the optimal mode of delivery. Patients with an outbreak of HSV during

their pregnancies are usually offered acyclovir prophylaxis from week 36 until delivery to prevent recurrent lesions.

Primary herpes infections in pregnancy have a much higher fetal and neonatal attack rate than secondary lesions. This virus can even be transmitted across the placenta during the viremic segment of the illness. A primary infection can be differentiated from a secondary one by checking antibody titers. A previously infected person will have circulating IgG antibodies. A primary infection transmitted late in the third trimester—particularly close to delivery—is far more dangerous because of the lack of maternal antibodies transmitted to the fetus.

HSV can cause severe infections in the neonate. Herpetic lesions may occur on the skin and mouth of approximately 50% of infected infants. These infections can be diagnosed by viral cultures of the herpetic lesions, oropharynx, or eyes. The infection can progress to a viral sepsis, pneumonia, and herpes encephalitis, which can lead to neurologic devastation and death. Infected infants are treated with IV acyclovir as soon as infection is suspected.

Varicella Zoster Virus (VZV)

Varicella zoster virus (VZV) is a DNA herpes virus that causes chickenpox and can reactivate to cause herpes zoster or shingles. Because it is primarily a disease of childhood, more than 90% of adults are immune to VZV infection. The infection in adults tends to be more serious than in children, with a higher rate of varicella pneumonia. Routine varicella titers are not drawn in pregnancy. However, VZV titers are often ordered for those patients who are unsure about history of exposure. Women who present preconceptually can be screened for VZV titers and, if negative, be immunized prior to conceiving.

Vertical transmission occurs transplacentally. In the first trimester, there is an increased risk of spontaneous abortion and it is thought that VZV may pose some teratogenic threat. Infections near term may lead to a postnatal infection that may range from a benign course (like chickenpox) to a fulminant disseminated infection, leading to death. Other infants may show no signs of infection at birth; however, they will develop shingles at some point later in childhood.

Varicella zoster immune globulin (VZIG) may prevent transmission of the disease. Therefore, any patient without a history of chickenpox with an exposure in pregnancy should receive VZIG within 72 hours of exposure. Infants of mothers who develop varicella disease within 5 days before delivery or 2 to 3 days after should also receive VZIG.

Parvovirus

Parvovirus B19 causes erythema infectiosum (fifth disease). Classically, this mild infection presents with a red macular rash giving the slapped cheek appearance, and usually resolves with minimal intervention. In pregnancy, however, there is concern for maternal-fetal transmission, which has been noted to cause fetal infection and death. First trimester infections have been associated with miscarriage, but midtrimester and later infections are associated with fetal hydrops. The Parvovirus B19 attacks fetal erythrocytes leading to a hemolytic anemia, hydrops and death.

If Parvovirus exposure is suspected in the mother, acute infection can be diagnosed by checking Parvovirus IgM levels. If it is positive, then the fetus can be followed ultrasonographically, most commonly 4 to 6 weeks after the exposure. Because of the risk of fetal anemia, serial ultrasounds and transfusion with evidence of hydrops have been recommended by some perinatologists. This intervention has not been studied in large populations, however, and is of unclear benefit.

Cytomegalovirus (CMV)

Cytomegalovirus (CMV) infections in the mother usually cause either a subclinical or mild viral illness. Only rarely will it lead to hepatitis or a mononucleosis-like syndrome. Thus, maternal infections are rarely diagnosed. CMV causes in utero infections in approximately 1% of all newborns. However, probably less than 10% of these infections will result in a clinically recognized illness.

Infants who are symptomatic can develop cytomegalic inclusion disease manifested by a constellation of findings including hepatomegaly, splenomegaly, thrombocytopenia, jaundice, cerebral calcifications, chorioretinitis, and interstitial pneumonitis. Affected infants have a high mortality rate of up to 30% and may develop mental retardation, sensorineural hearing loss, and neuromuscular disorders. Less than 10% of affected infants will have no sequelae of the disease.

Currently, there is no treatment or prophylaxis for the disease. Antiviral medications have been tried without success. A vaccine for the prevention of disease in the mother is also being investigated.

Rubella Virus

Rubella infection in adults leads to a mild illness with a maculopapular rash, arthritis, arthralgias, and a diffuse lymphadenopathy that lasts 2 to 4 days. The infection can be transmitted to the fetus and cause congenital rubella infection, which may lead to **congenital rubella syndrome** (CRS). The maternal–fetal transmission rate is highest during the first trimester, as are the rates of congenital abnormalities. However, transmission may occur at any time during pregnancy.

The congenital abnormalities associated with CRS include deafness, cardiac abnormalities, cataracts, and mental retardation. However, with rubella infection during organogenesis, any organ system may be affected. There are a variety of latent sequelae including the delayed onset of diabetes, thyroid disease, deafness, ocular disease, and growth hormone deficiency. The diagnosis of rubella infection relies on serologies. IgM titers will result from primary infection and reinfection with rubella. Because IgM does not cross the placenta, titers in the infant are indicative of infection. IgG titers that are elevated over time support the diagnosis of CRS in an infant as well.

Currently, there is no treatment for rubella once acquired. However, the institution of rubella immunization has decreased the number of CRS cases to less than 20 per year. In pregnancy, the rubella titer is checked during the first trimester. Because of theoretic risk of transmission of the live virus in the vaccine, patients do not receive the measles, mumps, and rubella vaccine until postpartum. Women who are known to have low or nonexistent titers should be advised to avoid anyone with possible rubella infections.

Human Immunodeficiency Virus (HIV)

With no treatment, approximately 25% of infants born to **human immunodeficiency virus** (HIV) infected mothers will become infected with HIV. Increased transmission can be seen with higher viral burden or advanced disease in the mother, rupture of the membranes, and events during labor and delivery that increase neonatal exposure to maternal blood. Transmission is believed to occur late in pregnancy or during labor and delivery. Cesarean delivery has been shown to lower transmission rates by roughly two-thirds compared to vaginal delivery in patients on no therapy. Current evidence suggests that zidovudine or AZT administration during the antepartum (after the first trimester), intrapartum, and neonatal period can reduce the risk of maternal–fetal HIV transmission by two-thirds in women with mildly symptomatic HIV disease. There is also evidence that as the viral load decreases, so does the rate of transmission, with several small studies showing a transmission rate less than 1% to 2% with an undetectable viral load. Currently, the standard of care is to maintain HIV-positive women on triple therapy, and even highly active antiretroviral therapy (HAART) in pregnancy to keep their HIV viral load down. Because of the effective interventions in HIV-positive women to decrease vertical transmission, it is recommended that HIV screening be offered to all expectant mothers.

Neisseria gonorrhoeae

Gonococcal infections are transmitted during passage of the neonate through the birth canal. The infection in neonates can be of the eye, oropharynx, external ear, and anorectal mucosa. These infections can become disseminated, causing arthritis and meningitis.

Because there are antibiotic therapies for *N. gonorrhoeae*, it should be screened for in early pregnancy and eradicated. In high-risk populations, third-trimester screening is common as well. The diagnosis is made via culture or by DNA probe. Treatment can be with ceftriaxone or penicillin and probenecid. Patients should be treated with azithromycin or erythromycin for presumed *Chlamydial* infection as well, since the two diseases often co-occur.

Chlamydia trachomatis

Chlamydial infections in the newborn can lead to serious sequelae. The infection is transmitted during delivery from the genital tract to the infant. In infected patients with vaginal deliveries, 40% of infants will develop conjunctivitis and greater than 10% will develop *Chlamydia* pneumonia.

Asymptomatic infection is common, therefore all patients should be screened during pregnancy. Because tetracycline and doxycycline are not advised in pregnancy, the treatment of choice for a positive test is erythromycin or azithromycin. Usually patients who test positive for *Chlamydia* are treated

for gonococcus as well, because the two infections tend to be transmitted together.

Hepatitis B

Viral hepatitis caused by the **hepatitis B** DNA virus can be acquired from sexual contact, exposure to blood products, and transplacentally. The clinical manifestations of the disease range from mild hepatic dysfunction to fulminant liver failure and death. It can be diagnosed using a variety of antibody and antigenic markers.

During the prenatal period, all patients are screened for hepatitis B surface antigen (HBsAg). Those with HBsAg are likely to have chronic disease and are at risk for transmission to the fetus. If patients are exposed during pregnancy, they can be given HepB immunoglobulin, which may be protective. Neonates of mothers who are HBsAg positive should be given HepB immunoglobulin at birth, 3 months, and 6 months. All infants are routinely immunized with the hepatitis B vaccine.

Syphilis

Syphilis is caused by infection with the spirochete *Treponema pallidum* and is usually transmitted via sexual contact or transplacentally to the fetus. Because there must be spirochetemia for vertical transmission to occur, pregnant women with latent syphilis may not transmit the disease, whereas those with primary or secondary syphilis are likely to do so. Despite prenatal screening and readily available treatment, there are still several hundred cases of congenital syphilis annually in the United States.

Syphilis in pregnancy that results in vertical transmission may lead to a late abortion, a stillborn infant, or a congenitally infected infant. Patients with early congenital syphilis present with a systemic illness accompanied by a maculopapular rash, snuffles, hepatomegaly, splenomegaly, hemolysis, lymphadenopathy, and jaundice. Diagnosis can be made by identification of IgM antitreponemal antibodies, which do not cross the placenta. Treatment is with penicillin as discussed in Chapter 16. If early congenital syphilis is untreated, manifestations of late congenital syphilis can develop, including eighth nerve deafness, saber shins, Hutchinson's teeth, and a saddle nose.

Toxoplasmosis

Toxoplasma gondii is a common protozoan parasite that can be found in humans and domestic animals. The infections in immunocompetent hosts are often subclinical. Occasionally, a patient will develop fevers, malaise, lymphadenopathy, and a rash as with most viral infections. A pregnant woman who is infected can transmit the disease transplacentally to the fetus. Transmission is more common when the disease is acquired in the third trimester, although neonatal manifestations are usually mild or subclinical. Infections acquired in the first trimester are transmitted less commonly; however, the infection has far more serious consequences in the fetus. Severe congenital infection can involve fevers, seizures, chorioretinitis, hydro- or microcephaly, hepatosplenomegaly, and jaundice. Thus, the differential diagnosis for this infection includes nearly all other commonly acquired intrauterine infections. Diagnosis of **toxoplasmosis** in the neonate can be made with detection of IgM antibodies, but lack of the antibodies does not necessarily rule out infection.

Because women with previous *Toxoplasma* exposure are likely to be protected from further infections, high-risk patients can be screened with titers for IgG to ascertain whether or not they are at risk for infection. Because the disease is transmitted commonly to and from cats, patients have been advised to avoid cat litter boxes during pregnancy, even though there is minimal evidence to suggest this makes a difference. Toxoplasmosis in pregnancy can be diagnosed maternally with IgM and IgG titers. If the diagnosis is made or suspected early in pregnancy, verification of fetal infection can be made by obtaining fetal blood via percutaneous umbilical blood sampling. Diagnosis may influence the decision of whether to terminate a pregnancy in the first two trimesters. The disease can be treated with spiramycin or, after 14 weeks gestational age, pyrimethamine, and a sulfonamide. Spiramycin is preferable in pregnant women because no teratogenic effects are known.

KEY POINTS

1. It is important to differentiate between infections that are transmitted transplacentally and those that are acquired from passage through the birth canal.
2. Infections during the first trimester during organogenesis are more likely to cause congenital abnormalities and spontaneous abortions.
3. Congenital infections can lead to serious infections in the neonatal period, often with disastrous long-term sequelae, including mental retardation, blindness, and deafness.

Other Medical Complications of Pregnancy

The previous three chapters discussed hypertension, diabetes, and infectious disease in the context of the pregnant patient. In this chapter, a variety of the other common medical complications of pregnancy are discussed. Pregnancy affects every physiologic system in the body as well as many disease states. When considering disease management in pregnancy, the potential teratogenic effects of any treatment or imaging modality must also be taken into consideration.

■ HYPEREMESIS GRAVIDARUM

Nausea and vomiting in pregnancy, or "morning sickness," are common. Seen in 88% of pregnancies, this usually resolves by week 16. Various etiologies have been proposed, including elevated levels of human chorionic gonadotropin, thyroid hormone, or the intrinsic hormones of the gut. There seems to be a disordered motility of the upper gastrointestinal tract that contributes to the problem. Despite the nausea and vomiting, patients are usually able to maintain adequate nutrition. However, patients will occasionally become dehydrated and potentially develop electrolyte abnormalities. When this occurs, the diagnosis of **hyperemesis gravidarum** is given.

Treatment and Prognosis

For patients with true hyperemesis gravidarum, symptoms may persist into the third trimester and, rarely, until term. The goal of therapy is to maintain adequate nutrition. Upon presentation with dehydration, patients should be rehydrated and electrolyte abnormalities corrected. Since a hypochloremic alkalosis often results from extensive vomiting, normal saline with 5% dextrose is commonly used for intravenous hydration. The nausea and vomiting may respond to antiemetics. Compazine, Phenergan, Tigan, and Reglan are commonly used. If these fail, droperidol and Zofran can also be used safely in pregnancy. Antiemetics should be given intravenously, intramuscularly, or as suppositories because oral medications often lead to further emesis.

Long-term management of hyperemesis includes maintaining hydration, adequate nutrition, and symptomatic relief from the nausea and vomiting. Many patients respond to antiemetics and IV hydration. Once they are rehydrated, they will be able to use the antiemetic to control their nausea so that they are able to maintain oral intake. However, a small percentage of patients will require feeding tubes or even parenteral nutrition for the course of the pregnancy. As long as hydration and adequate nutrition are maintained, pregnancy outcomes are usually good.

KEY POINTS

1. Nausea and vomiting in pregnancy are common; however, patients with hyperemesis gravidarum will not be able to maintain adequate hydration and nutrition.
2. Acute management involves IV hydration, electrolyte repletion, and antiemetics.
3. Chronic treatment utilizes antiemetics and occasionally tube feeding or parenteral nutrition.

■ SEIZURE DISORDERS

Approximately 20,000 women with seizure disorders give birth each year. Concerns during these pregnancies include risk of fetal malformations, miscarriage, perinatal death, and increased seizure frequency. Women with epilepsy appear to have a greater baseline risk of fetal malformations that is further increased with the use of antiepileptic drugs (AEDs). During pregnancy, there is both increased volume of distribution (V_D) as well as increased hepatic metabolism of the AEDs. Coupled with decreased compliance of AEDs due to concerns regarding fetal effects, these factors lead to an increase in seizure frequency seen in 17% to 33% of pregnancies. When managing these women in pregnancy the risks of increased seizures versus use of AEDs need to be weighed carefully.

Seizure Frequency

There are a variety of possible etiologies proposed for the increase in seizure frequency that may be seen in pregnancy. Increased levels of circulating estrogen during pregnancy in turn increase the function of the P_{450} enzymes, which leads to more rapid hepatic metabolism of the AEDs. In addition, it is clear that renal function increases during pregnancy with a 50% rise in creatinine clearance that impacts on the metabolism of carbamazepine, primidone, and the benzodiazepines. The increase in total blood volume and concomitant rise in the V_D leads to decreased levels of circulating AEDs. The increased stress, hormonal changes, and decreased sleep during pregnancy likely lower seizure threshold and have been shown to increase seizure frequency in nonpregnant patients. Finally, many women may have decreased compliance with AEDs because of concerns regarding fetal effects.

The increased levels of estrogen and progesterone may both have direct impact on seizure activity during pregnancy. Estrogen has been shown to be epileptogenic, decreasing seizure threshold. Thus, the rising estrogen levels in pregnancy that peak in the third trimester may have some impact on the observed increase in seizure frequency. Conversely, progesterone seems to have an antiepileptic effect. It has been observed that women with seizure disorders have fewer seizures during the luteal phase of the menstrual cycle.

Fetal Congenital Abnormalities and Adverse Outcomes

The earliest reports of congenital malformations associated with AEDs occurred in the 1960s. Since then, unique malformations and syndromes have been ascribed to phenytoin, phenobarbital, primidone, valproate, carbamazepine, and trimethadione. However, there are similarities between most of the congenital abnormalities caused by the AEDs (Table 11-1). There is evidence that epileptic women have an increased risk of fetal malformations even without AED use. Further, while some studies suggest monotherapy does not increase that baseline risk, there are other studies that do show evidence of an increase in fetal malformations with AED polytherapy.

Specific increases in congenital abnormalities seen in infants born to epileptic mothers include a four-fold increase in cleft lip and palate, and a three- to fourfold increase in cardiac anomalies. There is also an increase in the rate of neural tube defects (NTDs) seen in the offspring of epileptic patients who are using carbamazepine or valproic acid. Long-term studies on neurodevelopment show higher rates of abnormal EEG findings, higher rates of developmentally delayed children, and lower IQ scores. There are specific findings that are attributed to particular AEDs.

Mechanisms of Teratogenicity

The mechanisms of teratogenicity of the AEDs have not been fully characterized. Phenobarbital, primidone, and phenytoin act as folate antagonists. Certainly, it appears that folate deficiency can lead to an increase in congenital malformations, particularly NTDs. Folate prior to conception has therefore been recommended for prophylaxis. Since the AEDs all have a similar central mechanism to control seizures, there may be a common pathway—disrupted during embryogenesis—that leads to the similarities in the syndromes described and this may explain why there is an additive effect in polytherapy.

Recent studies in teratogenesis—particularly in the fetal hydantoin syndrome—point to a genetic predilection for the generation of epoxides. These anomalies have been seen at an increased rate in children where the enzyme activity of epoxide hydrolase is one-third less than normal. Anomalies have also been observed in children with low epoxide hydrolase activity in carbamazepine exposure.

■ TABLE 11-1

Fetal Anomalies Associated with Antiepileptic Drugs

Fetal Anomaly	Phenytoin	Phenobarbital	Primidone	Valproate	Carbamazepine	Trimethadione
NTD				X	X	
IUGR	X					X
Microcephaly					X	X
Low IQ	X		X			
Distal digital hypoplasia	X	X	X			
Low-set ears	X	X				X
Epicanthal fold	X	X		X	X	X
Short nose	X	X		X	X	
Long philtrum			X		X	
Lip abnormalities	X	X	X	X		
Hypertelorism	X	X				
Developmental delay		X			X	X
Other	Ptosis	Ptosis	Hirsutism forehead		Hypoplastic nails	Cardiac anomalies

Clinical Management

Because exposure to multiple AEDs seems to be more teratogenic than monotherapy, patients are advised to switch to a single AED prior to conception and taper down to the lowest possible dose. Patients who have been seizure-free for 2 to 5 years may wish to attempt complete withdrawal from AEDs prior to conception. Because there is evidence that high peak plasma levels of valproic acid may be more teratogenic, it should be dosed three to four times per day rather than the standard twice per day dosing. However, epileptic patients should be counseled that they are still at a greater risk (4% to 6% vs. 2% to 3%) for fetal anomalies than the baseline population. Folate has been shown to decrease NTDs in patients without epilepsy, therefore patients should be advised to take supplemental folate prior to conception, particularly those using either valproic acid or carbamazepine.

Because of the increased risk of anomalies a level II fetal survey at 19 to 20 weeks of gestation should be performed with careful attention to the face, central nervous system, and heart (Table 11-2). Due to the increased risk of NTDs, a maternal serum α-fetoprotein (MSAFP) screening test should be

■ TABLE 11-2

Management of Women with Epilepsy During Pregnancy

Check total and free levels of antiepileptic drugs on a monthly basis

Consider early genetic counseling

Check MSAFP

Level II ultrasound for fetal survey at 19 to 20 weeks gestation

Consider amniocentesis for α-fetoprotein and acetylcholinesterase

Supplement with oral vitamin K 20 mg QD starting at 37 weeks until delivery

offered. The decision to perform an amniocentesis routinely for AFP and acetylcholinesterase is controversial. Many practitioners recommend it in the setting of a family history of NTDs or with use of valproic acid or carbamazepine since the sensitivity of amniocentesis is higher than either maternal serum α-fetoprotein (MSAFP) or ultrasound for NTDs.

Recent studies of seizure frequency show less of an increase than older studies, which suggests that the practice of closer monitoring of AED dosing and levels may have some impact on the number of seizures during pregnancy. A recent study shows that 38% of pregnant patients with epilepsy require changes in their AED dosing to achieve seizure control. Assuming that monotherapy with one of the AEDs has been achieved preconceptionally, total and free levels of the AED that keep the patient seizure-free should be obtained on a monthly basis (see Table 11-2).

Labor and Delivery

Management of the epileptic patient on labor and delivery should involve preparation and close monitoring. All care providers—obstetricians, neurology, nursing, anesthesia, and pediatrics—should be informed about an epileptic patient in labor and delivery. AED levels should be checked upon admission. If the level is low, patients may be given extra dosing or switched to intravenous benzodiazepines or phenytoin, bearing in mind that benzodiazepines can cause respiratory depression in both the mother and newborn. Since trauma and hypoxia from a seizure can put both the mother and fetus at risk, treatment of seizures should be discussed a priori with the group of practitioners caring for the patient. Management of seizures on labor and delivery is discussed in Chapter 6. One difference is that the drug of choice in patients with a known seizure disorder is usually phenytoin compared to magnesium used in preeclamptic patients.

There have been reports of increased risk of spontaneous hemorrhage in newborns because of the inhibition of vitamin K dependent clotting factors (i.e., II, VII, IX, X) secondary to increased vitamin K metabolism and inhibition of placental transport of vitamin K by AEDs. While the risk is small, conservative management is to overcome this theoretical vitamin K deficiency by aggressive supplementation with vitamin K toward the end of pregnancy. Upon delivery, clotting studies can be performed on the cord blood and vitamin K administered to the infant. If the cord blood is deficient in clotting factors, fresh frozen plasma may be required to protect the newborn.

KEY POINTS

1. The increase in seizure frequency may be related to increased metabolism of AEDs, decreased patient compliance, lower seizure threshold, and/or hormonal changes in pregnancy.
2. Whereas patients with seizure disorders have an increased baseline risk for congenital anomalies, this risk is likely increased with the use of AEDs, particularly in cases of polytherapy.
3. Because of the risk for congenital anomalies, all patients should have a Level II ultrasound.
4. Patients should be followed frequently in pregnancy with monthly AED level checks.

■ MATERNAL CARDIAC DISEASE

The cardiovascular system undergoes a number of dramatic changes in pregnancy with a 50% increase in blood volume, decrease in systemic vascular resistance, increase in cardiac stroke volume, and actual remodeling of the myocardium to accommodate some of these changes. When caring for patients with cardiac disease preconceptionally or during pregnancy, these changes are paramount when counseling them regarding their options and managing their disease. In particular, patients with primary pulmonary hypertension, Eisenmenger's physiology, severe mitral or aortic stenosis, and Marfan's syndrome are at a high risk of maternal mortality in pregnancy reportedly ranging from 15% to 70% in small case series.

Principles of Management

Cardiac diseases vary widely but the principles of management are similar. Many of the diseases are stable prior to pregnancy with medical management, but during pregnancy can become quite unstable in response to the physiologic changes. One reason is that the medications being used may be different. In particular, many of the newest antihypertensives and antiarrhythmics have had little experience in pregnancy, and are thus commonly avoided. Of the more common agents, ACE inhibitors, diuretics, and Coumadin have all been associated with congenital anomalies and other fetal effects and are usually discontinued in pregnancy. Other aspects of medical management may include rest. However, even when resting, the cardiac output is increased in pregnancy leading to increased stress on the heart. In patients with cardiac anomalies, SBE prophylaxis should be used during labor.

In patients who would benefit from surgical repair of a lesion as in mitral or aortic stenosis, it is often best to recommend that the surgical repair is performed a year or more prior to becoming pregnant. In the high-risk patients listed above, recommending a termination of pregnancy because of the high risk to them is the first line of management. For patients who decline, preparing them and their families for the possibilities of disabling morbidity and mortality is important. In most cardiac patients, the stress of labor and delivery is minimized with an early epidural to diminish pain response, and an assisted vaginal delivery to diminish the effects from valsalva.

Cardiovascular Disease

Because of the rising average maternal age in pregnancy, there will be an increasing number of patients with a history of a myocardial infarction (MI) who become pregnant. If these patients have been optimally managed, there are small case series that show they do relatively well in pregnancy. A baseline ECG and adjustment of medications if necessary, should be performed at the initial visit. Throughout pregnancy and on labor and delivery, it is important to diminish the workload on the heart.

Eisenmenger's Syndrome and Pulmonary Hypertension (PH)

Patients with right-to-left shunts and PH are among the sickest in pregnancy, with mortality rates estimated at 50% and higher. The most common causes of right-to-left shunts are patent ductus arteriosus (PDA) and ventricular septal defect (VSD). These result from Eisenmenger's physiology that occurs when the initial left-to-right shunt leads to right ventricular hypertrophy and pulmonary hypertension and eventually a right-to-left shunt.

These patients are chronically hypoxic secondary to the mixing of deoxygenated blood and are encouraged to terminate their pregnancies. Patients who elect to continue are followed with serial echocardiograms to measure the pulmonary pressures and cardiac function. Some have been managed with inhaled nitric oxide, but this has not been shown to significantly improve the measured clinical indicators of disease or the outcomes. These patients often decompensate in the third trimester of pregnancy.

Delivery via labor and assisted delivery is preferable to elective cesarean delivery. Perhaps the greatest concentrated risk of morbidity and mortality is in the postpartum period for to 2 to 4 weeks. It has been hypothesized that this risk is secondary to the sudden changes in hormones. Unfortunately, attempts to counter this with progesterone and estrogen supplementation have been tried with little success.

Valvular Disease

While the manifestations of the different valvular diseases vary, one similarity is that, with moderate or severe disease that may increase maternal mortality, it is better to surgically treat or repair the lesion prior to becoming pregnant. Aortic stenosis and aortic insufficiency patients require a decreased afterload to maintain cardiac output, so initially may have diminished symptoms in response to the decreased systemic vascular resistance seen in pregnancy. Patients with mitral stenosis may be unable to meet the increased demands of pregnancy and experience a backup into the pulmonary system leading to congestive heart failure (CHF). Patients with pulmonary stenosis who elect to continue their pregnancy may actually undergo valvuloplasty during the pregnancy if they have severe disease.

Marfan's Syndrome

Patients with Marfan's syndrome have a deficiency in their elastin that leads to a number of valvular cardiac complications as well as dilation of the aortic root. During pregnancy, the hyperdynamic state can increase the risk of aortic dissection and/or rupture, particularly in those patients with an aortic root diameter greater than 4 cm. In order to decrease some of the pressure on the aorta, patients are advised to maintain a sedentary lifestyle and are often placed on beta-blockers to decrease cardiac output.

Peripartum Cardiomyopathy (PPCM)

A small percentage of patients will be found to have heart failure secondary to a dilated cardiomyopathy either immediately before, during, or after delivery. Some of these patients likely have a baseline mild cardiomyopathy, whereas others have a postinfectious dilated cardiomyopathy. However, the epidemiology supports the idea that, at least in some cases, PPCM is specifically caused by pregnancy. Patients present with classic signs and symptoms of heart failure and on echocardiogram have a dilated heart with an ejection fraction far below normal in the 20% to 40% range.

Patients with PPCM should be managed according the gestational age of the fetus. Beyond 34 weeks gestational age, the risks to the mother of remaining pregnant are usually greater than those of premature delivery of the fetus. At earlier gestational ages, however, betamethasone should be administered to promote fetal lung maturity, and the patient delivered accordingly. The patient's heart failure is managed similarly to other patients with heart failure using diuretics, digoxin, and vasodilators. Well over half of the patients with PPCM have excellent return to baseline of their cardiac activity within several months of delivery.

KEY POINTS

1. The changes in cardiac physiology during pregnancy can have an enormous impact on cardiac disease.
2. Common aspects of management include offering termination of pregnancy, medical stabilization, surgical or valvuloplasty repair if necessary, and consideration of the changes of pregnancy.
3. On labor and delivery, patients are commonly given prophylactic antibiotics, an early epidural, and an assisted vaginal delivery to minimize maternal stress and strain.
4. The most risky period of time for cardiac patients is during labor, delivery, and the puerperium.

■ MATERNAL RENAL DISEASE

Chronic renal disease can be divided into mild (Cr < 1.5), moderate (Cr from 1.5 to 2.8), and severe (Cr > 2.8), although other thresholds have been used. Renal blood flow and creatinine clearance increase during pregnancy in patients without renal disease, and this is also true initially in patients with renal disease. In fact, patients with mild renal disease will usually experience improvement in renal function throughout much of pregnancy. Moderate and severe patients, however, may experience decreasing renal function in the latter half of pregnancy that may persist postpartum in as many as half of pregnancies. Because of this, it is important to counsel these patients preconceptionally regarding the risks to them from pregnancy.

Patients with chronic renal disease have increased risk of preeclampsia, preterm delivery, and intrauterine growth restriction (IUGR) in addition to worsening renal disease. Because of this, they should be screened at least once per trimester with a 24-hour urine for creatinine clearance and protein. Patients who present in early pregnancy should be counseled regarding these risks and offered termination of pregnancy, particularly for the mother's health. Because of the risk to the fetus, antenatal fetal testing usually begins at 32 to 34 weeks gestation. For patients who have baseline proteinuria and hypertension, the diagnosis of preeclampsia can be difficult to make. In these patients, a baseline uric acid is assessed, and if normal at baseline can be used in the setting of worsening blood pressures to help diagnose preeclampsia. An increase in blood pressure of 30/15 above prepregnancy blood pressures can also be used.

KEY POINTS

1. Patients with mild renal disease suffer minimal effects, but may carry an increased risk of preeclampsia and IUGR, which is associated with the underlying diagnosis.
2. Patients with moderate or severe renal disease are at risk for preeclampsia and IUGR, as well as worsening renal disease during and after the pregnancy.
3. Careful monitoring of the patient's renal function and of fetal status are hallmarks of the management of these patients during pregnancy.

■ COAGULATION DISORDERS

Pregnancy is generally considered a "hypercoagulable" state. The pathogenesis of this state has not been elucidated, but several mechanisms have been proposed, including increased coagulation factors, endothelial damage, and venous stasis. The risk for superficial vein thrombosis (SVT), deep vein thrombosis (DVT), and pulmonary embolus (PE) is further increased postpartum, and pulmonary embolus remains one of the leading causes of maternal mortality.

Pathogenesis

No single cause of the hypercoagulability of pregnancy has been found, but there are several possible mechanisms hypothesized. The first is that there is an intrinsic increase in coagulability of the serum itself. In pregnancy, the production of clotting factors is increased and levels of all the clotting factors except XI and XIII are noted. Also noted in pregnancy is that the turnover time for fibrinogen is decreased and that there are increased levels of fibrinopeptide A, which is cleaved from fibrinogen to make fibrin. Additionally, there are increased levels of circulating fibrin monomer complexes. These levels increase further at the time of delivery and immediately postpartum. Finally, it has been hypothesized that the placenta synthesizes a factor that decreases fibrinolysis, but there is minimal evidence for this.

Another proposed source of hypercoagulability is increased exposure to subendothelial collagen secondary to increased endothelial damage during pregnancy, although no mechanism has been proposed. It has also been hypothesized that endothelial damage in the venous system during parturition increases the amount of thrombogenesis postpartum. This seems feasible, particularly as the etiology of pelvic vein thrombosis, but it does not account for the hypercoagulability throughout pregnancy.

Venous stasis may also account for some of the increase in venous thromboses during and after pregnancy. There are two principal causes for venous stasis in pregnancy. The first is decreased venous tone during pregnancy, which may be related to the smooth muscle relaxant properties of this high progesterone state. Second, the uterus, as it enlarges, compresses the inferior vena cava, the iliac, and pelvic veins. This compression, in particular, likely contributes to the increase in pelvic vein thromboses.

Superficial Vein Thrombosis (SVT)

Although **superficial vein thrombosis** is a painful complication of hypercoagulability, it is believed to be unlikely to lead to emboli. The diagnosis is usually obvious with a palpable, usually visible, venous cord that is quite tender, with local erythema and edema. Because of the low risk of emboli from SVT, it is not routinely treated other than symptomatically with warm compresses and analgesics. However, the patient should be informed of the signs and symptoms of DVTs and PEs because she may be at an increased risk for either.

Deep Vein Thrombosis (DVT)

Diagnosis of **deep vein thrombosis** is often made clinically with confirmation by Doppler studies or venography. The usual patient presents with unilateral lower extremity pain and swelling. On examination patients will often have edema, local erythema, tenderness, venous distension, and a palpable cord underlying the region of pain and tenderness. When clinical suspicion is high, the patient is usually sent for noninvasive lower extremity studies with the Doppler ultrasound for confirmation of a venous obstruction. Rarely, venography, the gold standard, will be used.

Treatment of DVT during pregnancy involves the use of heparin. Initially, the treatment is with IV heparin that is often continued with subcutaneous heparin throughout the remainder of the pregnancy and postpartum. Recently, low molecular weight heparin has been studied and found to be effective for both prophylaxis and treatment in pregnancy. Coumadin therapy is contraindicated in pregnancy secondary to evidence of fetal abnormalities caused by Coumadin. When given in the first trimester, it causes warfarin embryopathy that involves nasal hypoplasia and skeletal abnormalities. In addition, Coumadin appears to cause diffuse central nervous system (CNS) abnormalities, including optic atrophy, when given during pregnancy.

Pulmonary Embolus

Pulmonary embolus (PE) results when emboli from DVTs travel to the right side of the heart and then lodge in the pulmonary arterial system, leading to **pulmonary hypertension**, **hypoxia**, and, depending on the extent of the emboli, **right-sided heart failure** and **death**. Clinical suspicion of pulmonary embolus is raised whenever a patient presents with acute onset of shortness of breath, simultaneous onset of pleuritic chest pain, hemoptysis, and/or concomitant signs of DVT.

The diagnosis of PE usually involves the clinical picture correlated with a variety of diagnostic tests. A chest x-ray may be entirely normal. However, two common signs are the abrupt termination of a vessel as it is traced distally and an area of radiolucency in the area of the lung beyond the PE. An electrocardiogram may also be entirely normal. On occasion, however, it will show signs of right-heart strain with right-axis deviation, nonspecific ST changes, and peaked T-waves. A ventilation/perfusion scan is a radionuclide scan that first examines the perfusion of the lungs by detecting a radioisotope in the pulmonary circulation (Figure 11-1). An entirely normal perfusion scan rules out PE. However, if there is a defect in perfusion, a ventilation scan is performed. Mismatched defects in the ventilation and perfusion scans are suggestive of PE. Pulmonary angiography is the gold standard for diagnosis of PE. The pulmonary artery is catheterized and a radiopaque dye is injected. Diagnosis is made if there are intraluminal filling defects or if sharp vessel cutoffs are seen (Figure 11-2).

Treatment of mild PE is similar to treatment of DVT with IV heparin and, eventually, subcutaneous heparin therapy. In the postpartum period, Coumadin can be used as well. Massive PE leading to an unstable hypoxic patient is often treated with streptokinase for thrombolysis in addition to supportive measures. Patients are treated for a minimum of 6 months.

KEY POINTS

1. Pregnancy is a hypercoagulable state with increased clotting factors, endothelial damage, and venous stasis.
2. Pulmonary embolus is the leading cause of maternal death.
3. DVT and PE may be treated with heparin. Thrombolysis may be necessary for the unstable patient.

■ MATERNAL THYROID DISEASE IN PREGNANCY

Management of thyroid disease changes in pregnancy because of the V_D, increased circulating thyroid binding globulin, and sex hormone binding globulin (SHBG), which is secondary to estrogen stimulation of hepatic enzymes. Additionally, because metabolic demands increase in pregnancy, thyroid-stimulating hormone (TSH) and FT4 levels are commonly followed every 6 to 8 weeks.

Hyperthyroidism

The most common cause of hyperthyroidism is **Grave's disease**. Patients with medically managed Grave's disease can continue their **propylthiouracil (PTU)** or methimazole, which decrease production of the T4 moiety and in the case of PTU, block its peripheral conversion. Since Grave's disease is the result of thyroid-stimulating immunoglobulins (TSI), levels are checked and if elevated, the fetus is at risk of developing a fetal goiter. It is therefore important to follow these labs closely. In general, TSH should be kept between 0.5 and 5.0, but in pregnancy, it should be kept closer to 0.5 than 5.0.

Hypothyroidism

In patients with hypothyroidism, the most common etiology is **Hashimoto's thyroiditis**, and the second is

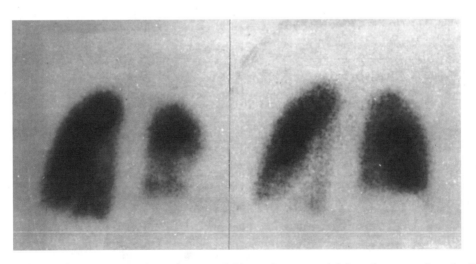

Figure 11-1 • In these posterior views, the perfusion lung scan (left) reveals segmental defects that are not "matched" in the normal ventilation scan (right). This is consistent with a high probability of pulmonary embolism.
(Reproduced with permission from Clark SL, et al. Critical Care Obstetrics. 2nd ed. Cambridge: Blackwell Science, 1991:162.)

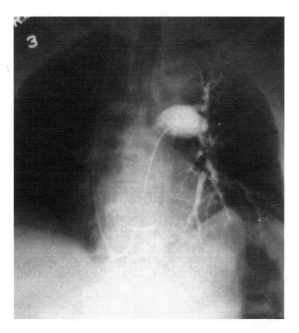

Figure 11-2 • Arteriogram of the left pulmonary artery showing filling defects and an unperfused segment of lung as demonstrated by the absence of contrast dye.
(Reproduced with permission from Clark SL, et al. Critical Care Obstetrics. 2nd ed. Cambridge: Blackwell Science, 1991:162.)

ablation of the thyroid after Grave's disease or cancer. The levels of TSH mentioned above should be kept low normal by increasing Synthroid supplementation throughout pregnancy and following the TSH level.

KEY POINTS

1. In pregnancy, there are particular changes to the thyroid system including increased V_D and metabolism.
2. In hyperthyroidism, TSIs should be screened for and, if elevated, fetal surveillance initiated to screen for fetal goiter and IUGR.
3. In hypothyroidism, increased Synthroid requirements are common.

■ SYSTEMIC LUPUS ERYTHEMATOSUS (SLE)

SLE and other associated collagen vascular disorders (CVD) such as Sjögren's syndrome, scleroderma, and antiphospholipid antibody syndrome can be particularly worrisome in pregnancy. There is particular concern in patients with concomitant hypertension or renal disease because these patients bear an even greater risk of developing preeclampsia, IUGR, and having preterm deliveries. The natural history of SLE in pregnancy tends to the one-third rule; that is one-third improve, one-third worsen, and one-third remain the unchanged. In general, it seems also that patients who are without flares immediately prior to pregnancy have a better course. Medications such as aspirin and corticosteroids are continued in pregnancy, whereas cyclophosphamide and methotrexate are not.

Early Pregnancy Complications

Patients with SLE and, in particular, antiphospholipid antibody syndrome, have a high risk of early pregnancy loss both in the first and second trimester. The pathophysiology of these losses is placental thrombosis. The high rate of second trimester losses is a hallmark of these diseases, and they will often show symmetric IUGR by 18 to 20 weeks gestation. Treatment and prophylaxis with low-dose aspirin, heparin, and corticosteroids have been tried with some improvement.

Later Pregnancy Complications

Just as in the early pregnancy losses, the placenta can become thrombosed in the third trimester as well, leading to IUGR and intrauterine fetal demise (IUFD). Because of this, frequent antenatal testing is performed, usually starting at week 32. Because of this risk of thrombosis, SQ heparin prophylaxis and low-dose aspirin have been used, both exhibiting some improvement. However, even on these agents, the risks are still quite higher than that of the baseline population. Patients are also at increased risk of developing preeclampsia.

Lupus Flares versus Preeclampsia

One of the most difficult differential diagnoses to sort out is that of a lupus flare versus preeclampsia in the pregnant lupus patient. Both diseases are likely mediated by circulating antigen-antibody complexes or tissue-specific antibodies that cause a vasculitis. The similarity between the two diseases is remarkable (Table 11-3). One method of differentiating

■ **TABLE 11-3**

Lupus Flare versus Severe Preeclampsia

Organ System	Lupus Complication	Severe Preeclampsia
Neuro	lupus cerebritis, seizures	seizures, visual changes
CV	hypertension	hypertension
Pulmonary	pulmonary edema	pulmonary edema
Renal	worsening renal disease	significant proteinuria, oliguria, renal failure
GI	hepatitis	liver dysfunction, ↑transaminases, hepatic edema
Heme	thrombocytopenia hemolytic anemia	thrombocytopenia, hemolytic anemia DIC

between the two is checking complement levels. Patients having a lupus flare will have reduced C3 and C4, whereas preeclamptics should have normal levels. Differentiating between the two conditions is important because the management for each highly differs. A lupus flare is managed with high-dose corticosteroids and, if unresponsive, cyclophosphamide. Worsening preeclampsia, on the other hand, is managed by delivery.

Neonatal Lupus

As with other maternal diseases, lupus can affect the fetus and neonate. There are two complications of interest. The first is a lupus syndrome related to maternal antigen-antibody complexes that have crossed the placenta and cause lupus in the neonate. These flares can be quite severe. The other complication seen is that of irreversible congenital heart block. SLE patients (and more commonly Sjögren's disease patients) can produce antibodies called anti-Ro (SSA) and anti-La (SSB) that are tissue-specific to the fetal cardiac conduction system. Anti-Ro seems much more likely to cause the congenital heart block that is seen in 1 : 20 patients with the antibody. Patients are screened for these antibodies at the first prenatal visit, and several interventions utilizing corticosteroids, plasmapheresis, and IVIG have been used. It is unclear whether any of these interventions improve outcomes.

KEY POINTS

1. Patients with SLE are at risk of developing complications throughout pregnancy.
2. Prophylaxis against pregnancy loss, preeclampsia, and IUGR has been tried with low-dose aspirin, heparin, and corticosteroids, all of which have some possible benefit.
3. Lupus flares and preeclampsia can be differentiated on the basis of complement levels.
4. Mothers with anti-Ro and anti-La antibodies are at risk of having a fetus with congenital heart block.

■ SUBSTANCE ABUSE IN PREGNANCY

Substance abuse in pregnancy contributes to maternal and fetal morbidity and mortality in both the antepartum and postpartum periods. The most commonly used substances are alcohol and cigarettes, both of which contribute to poor outcomes of pregnancy. The two most common illicit drugs used in pregnancy are cocaine and opiates, each of which has associated problems for the infant. Finally, even when infants are born with minimal effects from the intrapartum insult, substance abuse is an indicator for other social problems that may contribute to a poor environment for child rearing.

Alcohol

A constellation of abnormalities in the infants born to women who abuse alcohol during pregnancy have been included in the diagnosis of **fetal alcohol syndrome** (FAS). The syndrome has a spectrum of increasing severity in children of women who drink more heavily (2–5 drinks/day) during pregnancy.

FAS, which includes growth retardation, CNS effects, and abnormal facies, is estimated to occur in approximately 1:2000 live births. However, many milder cases may go unrecognized. Diagnosis is made by a history of alcohol abuse in the mother combined with the constellation of infant abnormalities. Other teratogenic effects of alcohol include almost every organ system. Cardiac defects are particularly associated with alcohol abuse.

Treatment

Several studies show that aggressive counseling programs for expectant mothers has led to a significant decrease in alcohol intake in greater than 50% of the participants. For patients who are at risk for alcohol withdrawal, barbiturates are often used for withdrawal symptoms because of the potential teratogenicity of benzodiazepines. Because alcoholics are at higher risk for nutritional deficiencies, special care should be taken to ensure adequate nutrition during pregnancy.

Caffeine

Caffeine is found in coffee (30–170 mg/cup), tea (10–100 mg/cup), and caffeinated soft drinks (30–60 mg/12 oz). It is the most commonly used drug during pregnancy, with almost 80% of all pregnant women being exposed in the first trimester. Studies on rats show teratogenicity at high levels of caffeine exposure. However, these studies have not been duplicated with humans. There does appear to be an increased risk of first- and second-trimester miscarriages with consumption of greater than 150 mg/day of caffeine. Patients should be advised of this risk and to reduce caffeine consumption during pregnancy to less than 150 mg/day.

Cigarettes

Cigarette smoking in pregnancy has been correlated with increased risk of spontaneous abortions, preterm births, abruptio placentae, and decreased birth weight. Further, infants exposed to cigarette smoking in the womb are at an increased risk for sudden infant death syndrome (SIDS) and respiratory illnesses of childhood. A dose-response effect has been noted for many of these outcomes. In the Ontario Perinatal Mortality Study, smokers were divided into less than 1 pack per day (PPD) and more than 1 PPD. A 20% increase in the risk of fetal death was found in those pregnancies in which patients smoked less than 1 PPD and a 35% increase in the more than 1 PPD group.

Treatment

Because of the demonstrated dose-response effect of smoking, patients should be counseled as to the increased risks for the fetus and advised at the very minimum to decrease cigarette use, although there is no demonstrated safe amount of smoking. Several studies show that smoking cessation programs targeting pregnant patients are more effective than those for nonpregnant patients. Further, primary care physicians of women of childbearing age should begin this counseling prior to pregnancy.

Cocaine

Cocaine use in pregnancy is correlated with abruptio placentae, IUGR and an increased risk for preterm labor and delivery. There has been a reported delivery of an infant with a massive cerebral infarction born to a woman who took a large dose of cocaine within 72 hours of delivery. The physiologic effects of cocaine, which causes vasoconstriction and hypertension, are consistent with this event, as well as the increased risk for abruption. Increasing amounts of evidence show that children who were exposed to cocaine in utero are at increased risk for CNS complications, including developmental delay.

Treatment

Patients who admit to cocaine use should be advised of its risks to themselves and their infants. Social services should be involved in prenatal care, and patients who continue to abuse the drug should be encouraged to enter a detoxification center.

Opiates

The two most common narcotics used in pregnancy are heroin and methadone. There are no known teratogenic effects of narcotics. In fact, there is likely to be more danger to fetuses from heroin withdrawal syndrome, including miscarriage, preterm delivery, and fetal death, than from chronic narcotic use. Patients using heroin in pregnancy should therefore be enrolled in methadone programs rather than advised to quit outright. Once infants are delivered, they will need careful monitoring and slow withdrawal from their narcotic addiction using tincture of opium. An aggressive effort should be made to taper their methadone postpartum.

KEY POINTS

1. Heavy alcohol abuse is correlated with FAS, which includes a constellation of growth restriction, CNS effects, and abnormal facies. Alcohol has also been correlated with other teratogenic effects, particularly cardiac defects.

2. Caffeine use greater than 150 mg/day has been correlated with an increased risk of spontaneous abortions.

3. Cigarette use during pregnancy has been correlated with growth restriction, abruptions, preterm delivery, and fetal death. Patients should be strongly encouraged to forgo use during pregnancy.

4. Cocaine use has been correlated with abruptio placentae and CNS effects in children. Patients should be advised to quit outright.

5. Narcotic abusers should be enrolled in methadone programs because the acute withdrawal effects of narcotics are more dangerous to the fetus than chronic use.

Postpartum Care and Complications

■ ROUTINE POSTPARTUM CARE

The puerperium, or postpartum period, is defined as the first 6 weeks after delivery. While still in the hospital, the patient often needs instruction about care of the neonate, breast-feeding, and her limitations, if any, during the ensuing weeks. In addition, the patient needs emotional support during the period of adjustment to the new member of the family and to her own physiologic changes.

Vaginal Deliveries

Routine medical issues in patients after vaginal delivery include pain control and perineal care. Usually, pain can be reduced with nonsteroidal anti-inflammatory drugs (NSAIDs) or acetaminophen. Low-dose narcotics are occasionally required for adequate patient comfort, particularly at the hour of sleep. For patients with vaginal deliveries that involved either episiotomies or lacerations, perineal care is particularly important. Ice packs around the clock can be quite beneficial for both pain and edema in the perineum and labia. When inspecting the perineum of a patient postpartum, it is important to ensure that the perineal repair is intact and that no hematomas have developed. It is also important to note whether the patient has hemorrhoids, which are common in pregnancy and postpartum, particularly after a long second stage of labor. These should resolve with time, but patients benefit symptomatically from over-the-counter hemorrhoidal medications, stool softeners, and ice packs.

Cesarean Section

Wound care and pain management are key issues in postcesarean care. Local wound care and observation for signs of wound infection or separation are part of routine care. Pain is usually managed with narcotics that can contribute to a postoperative ileus. Patients on narcotics should therefore also be on stool softeners and occasionally laxatives. NSAIDs should be used concomitantly for the cramping pain caused by uterine involution. Patients have usually received a first- or second-generation cephalosporin during the cesarean section as prophylaxis against infection. Although it is routine in many institutions to give additional doses, this has never been shown to further decrease the risk of infection.

Breast Care

All postpartum patients need breast care, regardless of whether or not they are nursing. Patients usually experience the onset of lactation, engorgement or "let down," approximately 24 to 72 hours postpartum. When this occurs, the breasts usually become uniformly warmer, firmer, and tender. Patients often complain of pain or warmth in the breasts and may experience a low-grade fever. For patients not breast-feeding, ice packs, a tight bra, analgesics, and anti-inflammatories are all useful. Patients who are breast-feeding obtain relief from the breast-feeding itself, although this can lead to its own difficulties, such as tenderness and erosions around the nipple.

Postpartum Contraception

Most patients are advised to have pelvic rest until the 6-week follow-up visit. However, many women resume sexual activity prior to this time. Thus, contraception is an important issue to address while patients are still in the hospital.

For patients interested in hormonal modes of contraception and who are breast-feeding, the progesterone-only minipill, Norplant, and Depo-Provera are first line recommended agents. Combination estrogen-progesterone OCPs have been shown to decrease milk production, so are usually recommended only to those patients who are not interested in breast-feeding. Progesterone-only contraceptives may decrease milk production as well, but this has not been shown to be clinically significant. They are therefore preferable to combination OCPs for patients who are dedicated to breast-feeding and interested in hormonal forms of birth control.

For patients interested in nonhormonal methods, condoms are particularly good because of the prophylaxis against sexually transmitted infections. The other barrier methods—the diaphragm and cervical cap—should be avoided until 6 weeks postpartum when the cervix has returned to its normal shape and size. Intrauterine devices (IUDs) may be inserted postpartum. However, these have a higher rate of extrusion in the immediate postpartum period because of the dilated cervix.

Discharge Instructions

Hospital stay after delivery is short, and while it has been mandated that insurance companies must cover up to 2 days after a vaginal delivery and 4 days after a cesarean delivery, many hospitals still discharge patients after 1 and 3 days respectively. After a vaginal delivery, the above issues of perineal care, contraception, and breast care are discussed with the patient. Further, a discussion regarding how common the postpartum "blues" can be as well as the availability of professionals to talk the patient through any problems as she transitions to home can be of help. Patients who have a cesarean delivery should be counseled regarding wound care and activity in addition to the above. With Pfannenstiel incisions that were stapled closed, the staples can be removed prior to discharge. Patients are often advised to avoid heavy lifting ("nothing heavier than your baby") and vigorous activities including driving. Before patients drive, it is recommended that they try to slam on the brakes as an experiment to be sure they are comfortable enough to drive.

> ### KEY POINTS
>
> 1. Two central issues in the immediate postpartum period, regardless of the mode of delivery, are pain management and wound care.
> 2. Condoms with a spermicidal foam or gel can be used by anyone postpartum.
> 3. Diaphragms and cervical caps need to be refitted at 6 weeks. IUDs are best placed at 6 weeks as well.
> 4. Depo-Provera, Norplant, or the progesterone-only minipill are the hormonal contraceptives of choice in the puerperium because they are less likely to decrease milk production in breast-feeding patients.
> 5. Discharge instructions should include both discussion of medical issues such as contraception and wound care. Instructions on social issues, such as the transition to home with the newborn, how to deal with some of the changes related to the delivery, and care of the baby are also needed.

■ POSTPARTUM COMPLICATIONS

The primary complications that arise postpartum include postpartum hemorrhage, endomyometritis, mastitis, and postpartum depression (Table 12-1). Postpartum hemorrhage usually occurs during the first 24 hours, while the patient is still in the hospital. However, it can also occur in patients with retained products of conception (POCs) for up to several weeks postpartum. Endomyometritis and mastitis usually occur 1 to 2 weeks after delivery. Postpartum depression can occur at any time during the puerperium and beyond and is probably grossly underdiagnosed.

Postpartum Hemorrhage

Postpartum hemorrhage is defined as blood loss exceeding 500 mL in a vaginal delivery and greater than 1000 mL in a cesarean section. If the hemorrhage occurs within the first 24 hours, it is deemed early postpartum hemorrhage; after 24 hours, it is considered late or delayed postpartum hemorrhage. Common causes of postpartum bleeding include uterine atony, retained POCs, placenta accreta, cervical lacerations, and vaginal lacerations (Table 12-2 and Table 12-3). While the cause of the hemorrhage is being investigated, the patient is simultaneously started on fluid resuscitation and preparations are

■ TABLE 12-1

Complications of Vaginal and Cesarean Deliveries

	Vaginal Delivery	Cesarean Section
Common complications	Postpartum hemorrhage	Postpartum hemorrhage
	Vaginal hematoma	Surgical blood loss
	Cervical laceration	Wound infection
	Retained POCs	Endomyometritis
	Mastitis	Mastitis
	Postpartum depression	Postpartum depression
Rare complications	Endomyometritis	Wound separation
	Episiotomy infections	Wound dehiscence
	Episiotomy breakdown	

■ TABLE 12-2

Risk factors for Postpartum Hemorrhage

Prior Postpartum Hemorrhage

Abnormal placentation
  Placenta previa
  Placenta accreta
  Hydatidiform mole

Trauma during labor and delivery
  Episiotomy
  Complicated vaginal delivery
  Low- or midforceps delivery
  Sulcal or sidewall laceration
  Uterine rupture
  Cesarean section or hysterectomy
  Cervical laceration

Uterine atony
  Uterine inversion
  Overdistended uterus
    Macrosomic fetus
    Multiple gestation
    Polyhydramnios
  Exhausted myometrium
    Rapid labor
    Prolonged labor
    Oxytocin or prostaglandin stimulation
    Chorioamnionitis

Coagulation defects—intensify other causes
  Placental abruption
  Prolonged retention of dead fetus
  Amnionic fluid embolism
  Severe intravascular hemolysis
  Severe preeclampsia and eclampsia
  Congenital coagulopathies
  Anticoagulant treatment

■ TABLE 12-3

Etiology of Postpartum Hemorrhage in Vaginal and Cesarean Deliveries

Vaginal Delivery	Cesarean Section
Vaginal lacerations	Uterine atony
Cervical lacerations	Surgical blood loss
Uterine atony	Placenta accreta
Placenta accreta	Uterine rupture
Vaginal hematoma	
Retained POCs	
Uterine inversion	
Uterine rupture	

made for blood transfusions. With blood loss greater than 2–3 liters, patients may develop a consumptive coagulopathy and require coagulation factors and platelets. In rare cases, if patients become hypovolemic and hypotensive, Sheehan's syndrome, or pituitary infarction, may occur. These patients present either with the absence of lactation secondary to the absence of prolactin or failure to restart menstruation secondary to the absence of gonadotropins. Each of the etiologies of postpartum hemorrhage is discussed sequentially; the obstetrician often has to consider and/or attempt to treat several diagnoses simultaneously.

Vaginal Lacerations and Hematomas

Vaginal lacerations with uncontrolled bleeding should be considered in the case of postpartum hemorrhage. Initially after a delivery, the perineum, labia, periurethral area, and deeper aspects of the vagina are examined for lacerations. These should be repaired at that time. However, deep sulcal tears or vaginal lacerations behind the cervix may be quite difficult to visualize without careful retraction. Occasionally, these lacerations will involve arteries and arterioles and lead to a significant postpartum hemorrhage. Adequate anesthesia, an experienced obstetrician, and assistance with retraction are all necessary to perform an adequate exploration and repair of these lacerations.

Occasionally, the trauma of delivery will injure a blood vessel without disrupting the epithelium above it. This leads to the development of a hematoma. If a patient has a larger than expected drop in hematocrit, an examination should be performed to rule out a vaginal wall hematoma. If one is discovered, it can be managed expectantly unless it is tense or expanding, in which case it should be opened, the bleeding vessel ligated, and the vaginal wall closed. Rarely, a patient will develop a retroperitoneal hematoma that can lead to a large blood loss into this space. Patients usually complain of back pain and there will be a large drop in hematocrit. Diagnosis is made via ultrasound or CT. These hematomas can also be managed expectantly. However, if the patient becomes unstable, surgical exploration and ligation of the disrupted vessels may be required.

Cervical Lacerations

Cervical lacerations can cause a brisk postpartum hemorrhage. Commonly, they are a result of rapid dilation of the cervix during the stage 1 of labor or of stage 2 labor beginning without complete dilation of the cervix. If a patient is bleeding at the level of the cervix or above, a careful exploration of the cervix should be performed. The patient should have adequate anesthesia via epidural, spinal, or pudendal block. The walls of the vagina are retracted so the cervix can be well visualized. When the anterior lip of the cervix is seen, it is grasped with a ring forcep. Then, another ring forcep can be used to grasp beyond the first and in this fashion the cervix should be "walked" around its entirety so that no lacerations, particularly on the posterior aspect, are missed. If any lacerations are seen, they are usually repaired with either interrupted or running absorbable sutures.

Uterine Atony

Uterine atony is the leading cause of postpartum hemorrhage. Patients are at a higher risk for uterine atony if they have chorioamnionitis, exposure to magnesium sulfate, multiple gestations, macrosomic fetus, a history of atony with any prior pregnancies, or if they are multiparous, particularly a grand multip (more than five deliveries). Uterine abnormalities or fibroids may also interfere with uterine contractions and lead to atony and increased bleeding. The diagnosis of atony is made by palpation of the uterus, which is soft, enlarged, and boggy. Occasionally the uterine fundus is well contracted, but the lower uterine segment, which has less contractile tissue, will be less so.

Atony is initially treated with IV oxytocin (Pitocin), which is usually given prophylactically as well. While the oxytocin is being administered, strong uterine massage should be performed to assist the uterus in contracting down. If atony continues, the next step is methylergonovine (Methergine), which is contraindicated in hypertensive patients. If the uterus is still atonic, the next step is to give prostin ($PGF_{2\alpha}$), which is contraindicated in asthmatics. The prostaglandin is thought to be more effective if injected directly into the uterine musculature, either transabdominally or transcervically, although this has not been demonstrated in studies. If atony continues despite maximal medical management, the patient is brought to the OR for a **dilation and curettage** (D&C) to rule out possible retained POCs. Patients with uterine atony unresponsive to these conservative measures, but bleeding at a rate that can tolerate some watchful waiting, may benefit from occlusion of pelvic vessels (uterine artery embolization) by interventional radiology to prevent the necessity of a hysterectomy. If this is unsuccessful, exploratory laparotomy with ligation of pelvic vessels and possible hysterectomy is required.

Retained POCs

Careful inspection of the placenta should always be performed. However, with vaginal delivery, it can often be difficult to determine whether a small piece of the placenta has been left behind in the uterus. Usually the retained fetal membranes or placental tissue pass in the lochia. However, they occasionally lead to endomyometritis and postpartum hemorrhage. If the suspicion is high for retained POCs, the uterus should be explored either manually if the cervix has not contracted down or by D&C. If hemorrhage continues once it has been ascertained that there are no further POCs via exploration, placenta accreta should be suspected.

Accreta

Placenta accreta, increta, and percreta are discussed briefly in Chapter 5 with antepartum hemorrhage. These conditions are the result of abnormal attachment of placental tissue to the uterus that may invade into or beyond the uterine myometrium, leading to incomplete separation of the placenta postpartum and postpartum hemorrhage. Risk factors for developing placenta accreta include placenta previa and prior uterine surgery, including cesarean delivery and myomectomy. Often the third stage will have been longer than usual and the placenta may have delivered in fragments. Accreta involves bleeding that is unresponsive to uterine massage and contractile agents such as oxytocin, ergonovines, and prostaglandins. Patients with accreta are brought to the operating room for surgical management via exploratory laparotomy.

Uterine Rupture

Uterine rupture is estimated to occur in 0.5% to 1.0% of patients with prior uterine scars and about 1:15,000–20,000 women with an unscarred uterus. It is an intrapartum complication but may occur with bleeding postpartum. It is rare for rupture to occur in a nulliparous patient. Risk factors include previous uterine surgery, breech extraction, obstructed labor, and high parity. Symptoms usually include abdominal pain and a "popping" sensation intra-abdominally. Treatment involves laparotomy and repair of the ruptured uterus. If hemorrhage cannot be controlled, hysterectomy may be indicated.

Uterine Inversion

Uterine inversion may occur in 1:2500 deliveries. Risk factors include fundal implantation of the placenta, uterine atony, placenta accreta, and excessive traction on the cord during third stage. Diagnosis is made by witnessing the fundus of the uterus attached to the placenta on placental delivery. Uterine inversion can be an obstetric emergency if hemorrhage occurs. Additionally, patients often experience an intense vasovagal response from the inversion and may require stabilization with the aid of an anesthesiologist before manual replacement of the uterus can be attempted, which should be the first step in treatment (Figure 12-1). Uterine relaxants such as nitroglycerin may be given to aid replacement. If this is unsuccessful, laparotomy is required to surgically replace the uterus.

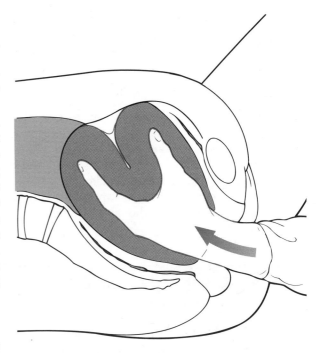

Figure 12-1 • Manual replacement of an inverted uterus.

Operative Management of Postpartum Hemorrhage

In the case of vaginal delivery, the management of postpartum hemorrhage is as described above. A differential diagnosis is created and a quick physical exam is performed to establish the likely etiology. If vaginal and cervical lacerations have been ruled out and the patient is unresponsive to uterotonic agents and massage, the patient should be moved to an operating room and a D&C performed. If this fails to stop the bleeding, a laparotomy is performed.

On entering the abdomen, the surgeon should note whether there is blood in the abdomen, which would indicate a uterine rupture. Unless the patient is unstable and coagulopathic secondary to excessive blood loss, the first surgical procedure is usually bilateral O'Leary sutures to tie off the uterine arteries. The second is ligation of the hypogastric, or internal iliac, arteries. If uterine atony is the cause of hemorrhage, B-Lynch sutures can be placed in an attempt to compress the uterus and achieve hemostasis. A uterine incision must first be made, through which a suture is looped around the uterus and used to tamp it back into place. If these measures fail to provide hemostasis, often the patient requires a puerperal hysterectomy (known as cesarean hysterectomy if that has been the mode of delivery).

If the patient has been delivered via cesarean section and there is evidence of accreta, the first step is usually to place hemostatic sutures in the placental bed. If these fail, or the patient has no focal site of bleeding, O'Leary sutures can be placed next with the uterus still open to watch the bleeding. If this fails, often the next step is to close the uterus with or without packing it and proceed to hypogastric artery ligation. If this fails, hysterectomy is the definitive procedure.

If a patient is not bleeding too briskly, with either vaginal or cesarean delivery, packing the uterus and obtaining an interventional radiology consult for uterine artery embolization is possible. This is reserved for those patients who are truly stable and desire future fertility.

KEY POINTS

1. Postpartum hemorrhage is an obstetric emergency.
2. Causes include uterine atony, uterine rupture, uterine inversion, retained POCs, placenta accreta, and cervical or vaginal lacerations.
3. Treatment may require use of blood products including fresh frozen plasma, cryoprecipitate, and platelets in patients who develop a consumptive coagulopathy.
4. Surgical management ranges from D&C to exploratory laparotomy, uterine artery ligation, hypogastric artery ligation, and, if these fail, hysterectomy.
5. In patients for whom there is enough time, an alternative to exploratory laparotomy is uterine artery embolization by interventional radiology.

Endomyometritis

Endomyometritis is a polymicrobial infection of the uterine lining that often invades the underlying wall. It is most commonly seen after cesarean sections but can be seen with vaginal deliveries as well, particularly if manual removal of the placenta was required. It is increased in patients with meconium, chorioamnionitis, and prolonged rupture of membranes.

Diagnosis is made in the setting of fever, elevated white blood count, and uterine tenderness, with a higher suspicion after cesarean sections. Endomyometritis commonly occurs 5 to 10 days after delivery but should still be suspected when all other sources of infection have been ruled out for several weeks after delivery. Because retained POCs can be the etiology of infection, an ultrasound is often obtained to examine the intrauterine contents.

Endomyometritis is usually treated with broad-spectrum intravenous antibiotics, or "triple" antibiotics. If retained POCs are suspected, a D&C is performed. Because the postpartum uterus is at greater risk for perforation, great care should be taken during dilation and a blunt rather than sharp curette should be used. Antibiotics are continued until the patient is afebrile for 48 hours, uterine pain and tenderness are absent, and the white blood cell count normalizes.

KEY POINTS

1. Endomyometritis is more common in patients with cesarean section than vaginal delivery, although patients with manual removal of the placenta are also at increased risk.
2. Diagnosis is clinical with fever, elevated white blood cell count, and uterine tenderness.
3. Treatment is with broad-spectrum antibiotics and D&C for retained POCs.

Mastitis

Mastitis is a regional infection of the breast, commonly caused by the patient's skin flora or the oral flora of breast-feeding infants. The organisms enter an erosion or cracked nipple and proliferate, leading to infection. Lactating women will often have warm, diffusely tender, and firm breasts, particularly at the time of engorgement or milk let-down. This should be differentiated from focal tenderness, erythema, and differences in temperature from one region of the breast to another, which are classic signs of mastitis. The diagnosis can be made with physical examination, a fever, and an elevated white blood count. Mastitis can be complicated by formation of an abscess, which then requires treatment by incision and drainage (I&D).

Mastitis can be treated with oral antibiotics. Dicloxacillin is commonly used. Patients should also continue to breast-feed, which prevents intraductal accumulation of infected material. Patients who are not breast-feeding should breast pump in the acute phase of the infection. Patients who are unresponsive to oral antibiotics are admitted for intravenous antibiotics until they remain afebrile for 48 hours.

Postpartum Depression

Many patients have the postpartum "blues" with mood swings and changes in appetite and sleep, if not frank postpartum depression. The pathophysiology of depression is poorly understood, but may be due to the rapid changes in estrogen, progesterone, and prolactin in postpartum patients. Greater than 50% of postpartum patients experience postpartum blues, whereas postpartum depression complicates greater than 5% of pregnancies. While these events are common, they are seen in higher rates in patients with a history of depression or other mental illness as well as in patients with poor support networks.

Diagnosis

Most patients have normal changes in appetite, energy level, and sleep patterns in the initial postpartum period that do not necessarily progress to frank depression. However, patients who experience low energy level, anorexia, insomnia, hypersomnolence, extreme sadness, and other depressive symptoms for greater than a few weeks may have postpartum depression. These patients often feel incapable of caring for their infants. Occasionally, depressed patients have suicidal ideation, which is a much clearer marker for depression and merits close observation.

Therapy and Prognosis

In patients with transient postpartum depression, symptoms usually pass on their own with support and encouragement. However, these patients can occasionally progress to a more severe postpartum depression or psychosis. In these situations, the caregiver needs to determine whether the patient is having suicidal or homicidal ideation. A social worker and professional counselor should be involved, as should the immediate family and any other individuals who are close to the patient and can provide support. Antidepressant medications are commonly used. While an episode of postpartum "blues" may resolve quite readily, depression and psychosis should be treated with medications. The SSRIs have been used for postpartum depression with good efficacy and appear to be safe for breast-feeding mothers. Most patients without a history of depression or other mental illness improve, usually to their prepregnant state.

Benign Disorders of the Lower Genital Tract

■ BENIGN LESIONS OF THE VULVA AND VAGINA

Many benign lesions and conditions of the vulva and vagina are infectious in nature; these are discussed in Chapter 16. However, noninfectious lesions—nonneoplastic epithelial disorders, cysts, and benign tumors—are also found; these conditions are described in this chapter.

■ CONGENITAL ANOMALIES

A variety of congenital defects occur in the external genitalia and vagina that can be associated with concomitant anomalies in the upper reproductive tract. Included are labial fusion, imperforate hymen, transverse vaginal septum, as well as partial and complete vaginal agenesis.

Labial Fusion

Labial fusion is associated with excess androgens. Most commonly, the etiology is the result of exogenous androgens but may also be due to an enzymatic error leading to increased androgen production. The most common form of enzymatic deficiency is 21-hydroxylase deficiency (Chapter 23) leading to **congenital adrenal hyperplasia**. This may be phenotypically demonstrated in the neonate with **ambiguous genitalia**, and hyperandrogenism with salt wasting, hypotension, hyperkalemia, and hypoglycemia. The neonates often present in adrenal crisis with salt-wasting seen approximately 75% of the time. This autosomal recessive trait occurs in roughly 1 : 40,000–50,000 pregnancies. The diagnosis is made

by **elevated 17α-hydroxyprogesterone** or urine 17-ketosteroid with decreased serum cortisol.

Treatment of this defect is with **cortisol**, which is not being produced by the adrenal cortex. The exogenous cortisol then negatively feeds back on the pituitary to decrease the release of adrenocorticotropic hormone (ACTH), thus inhibiting the stimulation of the adrenal gland that is shunting all steroid precursors into androgens. If salt-wasting is documented, a mineralocorticoid—usually fludrocortisone acetate—is also given. The labial fusion and other ambiguous genitalia often require **reconstructive surgery**.

Imperforate Hymen

The hymen is at the junction between the sinovaginal bulbs and the urogenital sinus. Congenital abnormalities of the hymen include imperforate hymen, microperforations, and septations (Figure 13-1). An imperforate hymen occurs when an opening does not develop in the hymen during the organogenesis of the reproductive tract. The result is an obstruction to the outflow tract of the reproductive system. It is often diagnosed at puberty with **primary amenorrhea** in the setting of **cyclic pelvic pain**. Patients may also experience both cyclic and persistent abdominal pain as the menstrual flow accumulates and, eventually, an increase in lower abdominal girth. On physical examination there is often hematocolpos; that is, a buildup of blood behind the hymen. Before puberty, there may be hydrocolpos or mucocolpos, which are buildups of secretions behind the hymen similar to that seen with a transverse vaginal septum. Treatment of imperforate hymen is with **surgical correction**.

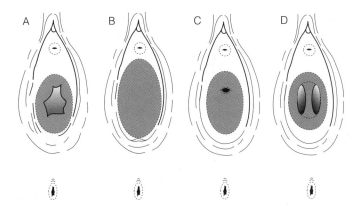

Figure 13-1 • Congenital abnormalities of the hymen. A: Normal. B: Imperforate. C: Microperforate. D: Septate.

Transverse Vaginal Septum

The vagina is formed as the müllerian system from above joins the sinovaginal bulb at the müllerian tubercle. The müllerian tubercle must be canalized for a normal vagina to form. If this does not occur, this tissue may be left as a transverse vaginal septum that lies roughly at the junction between the lower two-thirds and upper one-third of the vagina (Figure 13-2). This occurs in approximately 1:75,000 females. Similar to imperforate hymen, diagnosis is usually made at the time of puberty with primary amenorrhea accompanied by menstrual symptoms. The transverse vaginal septum differs from the imperforate hymen in that it is usually thicker and a normal hymen can be seen proximal to it in the vagina. Surgical correction is the only form of treatment.

Vaginal Atresia

Vaginal atresia is often confused with imperforate hymen or transverse vaginal septum. It occurs when the urogenital sinus fails to contribute the lower portion of the vagina. Instead, the absent lower vagina is replaced by fibrous tissue. It presents during adolescence with primary amenorrhea and cyclic pelvic pain. Physical examination reveals the absence of an introitus and the presence of a vaginal bulge. Pelvic imaging may show a large hematocolpos. Surgical correction can be achieved with a vaginal pull-through procedure.

Vaginal Agenesis

Vaginal agenesis may occur in **Mayer-Rokitansky-Kuster-Hauser (MRKH) syndrome** or testicular feminization. MRKH syndrome is characterized by the

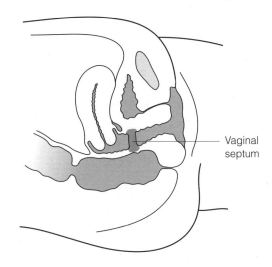

Vaginal septum

Figure 13-2 • Tranverse vaginal septum.

congenital absence or hypoplasia of the proximal vagina, cervix, uterus, and fallopian tubes. Ten percent of these patients have a normal uterus with functioning endometrium. Patients may or may not have a rudimentary pouch of a vagina developed from the sinovaginal bulb. In motivated patients, a vagina can be created using serial dilation of the perineal body, but this often takes months to years. If this fails, a neovagina can be created surgically using a split-thickness skin graft from the buttocks or a segment of the GI tract. Either way, once the vagina is created, continued dilation with dilators or intercourse is necessary to keep it open.

Testicular feminization syndrome occurs in 46,XY individuals who have an insensitivity to testosterone. Patients may have the beginning of a vagina as in MRKH, but will have undescended gonads rather than the normal ovaries of the 46,XX MRKH patient. The process of creating a vagina is similar to that for MRKH patients. In addition, patients with testicular feminization should have the undescended gonads surgically removed because they are prone to the development of seminomas. In addition, a social services consult is often appropriate and helpful.

■ NON-NEOPLASTIC EPITHELIAL DISORDERS OF THE VULVA AND VAGINA

Benign lesions of the skin, and mucosa of the vulva and vagina come under this broad category. Also included are the following disorders: vulvar dermatoses, lichen sclerosus, lichen planus, squamous hyperplasia, and vaginal adenosis. These disorders range from hypertrophic to atrophic lesions and must be differentiated from vulvar and vaginal carcinoma.

Pathogenesis

There are two types of **vulvar dermatoses**, also known as **vulvar eczema**: (1) an endogenous/atopic form, identical to classic eczema; and (2) an exogenous form that is secondary to external factors. In the **atopic/endogenous form**, an unknown immune mechanism is thought to alter immune regulation and results in atopic phenomenon such as eczema and asthma. Roughly 50% of patients with endogenous vulvar eczema have a personal or family history of asthma as well.

 Exogenous vulvar eczema is generally a contact dermatitis that 80% of the time is immediate and secondary to an irritant, and 20% of the time is chronic and secondary to an allergen. Because the stratum corneum of the vulva is not a very effective barrier the vulvar skin is highly susceptible to irritants compared to other parts of the body.

Seborrheic dermatitis is secondary to chronic inflammation in areas rich in sebaceous glands (scalp, face, axilla, groin, and upper trunk). The etiology is unknown, but it maybe secondary to a skin saprophyte called *Malassezia furfur*.

Although recognized on the vulva of females of all age groups, **lichen sclerosus** assumes major significance in postmenopausal women where it is associated with a 5% to 15% risk of cancer. The etiology is unknown, but several mechanisms have been proposed including genetic, immunologic, hormonal, and infectious.

Lichen planus is an atrophic inflammatory condition that results in chronic eruption of shiny, violaceous papules with white striae on the flexor surfaces, mucous membranes, and vulva. Lichen planus can cause vaginal synechiae/adhesions and can even develop into an erosive desquamative vaginitis. Lichen planus generally occurs in women age 30 to 60 and has two forms: drug-induced and spontaneous. Lichen planus can be diagnosed clinically and via biopsy. It is treated with topical steroids.

Squamous cell hyperplasia results from chronic scratching and rubbing. Patients often complain of vulvar itching with localized thickening of the vulvar skin. The involved area may range in color from white to gray secondary to edema. Lichen simplex chronicus is similar but involves reactive changes to chronic scratching and rubbing, rather than hyperkeratotic changes.

Vaginal adenosis is a benign lesion of the vaginal mucosa involving red grandular spots and patches. It typically and most frequently involves the upper third of the vagina and the anterior vaginal wall. Adenosis is found in 30% to 90% of women who have been exposed to diethylstilbestrol (DES) in utero. This epithelium usually contains various cell types, resembling müllerian structures such as the endocervix, endometrium, and fallopian tubes. Vaginal adenocarcinomas arise from the tuboendometrial cells, biopsy should therefore always be performed when vaginal adenosis is suspected not only to make the diagnosis, but also to rule out carcinoma.

Clinical Manifestations

History

Patients with benign lesions of the vulva and vagina present with a variety of complaints including vulvar itching, irritation, and burning. They may also report dysuria, dyspareunia, vulvodynia, and feel that the skin of their vulva is tender, bumpy, or thickened.

Physical Examination

These disorders range in appearance from erythematous plagues to hyperkeratotic white plagues. The lesions often involve excoriated areas secondary to scratching. Lichen planus typically is manifested by shiny, flat, violaceous papules, whereas lichen sclerosus typically appears in conjunction with atrophic changes such as thinning of the labia majora and minora (Figure 13-3). In lichen sclerosus fissures are often present as is fusion of the labia and white, wrinkly thinning of the perineum in a "keyhole" appearance around the anus. Occasionally petechiae and/or ecchymoses are present as a result of trauma from scratching. Vaginal adenosis presents as red grandular spots and patches and can be palpated submucosally, but occasionally can be seen on the surface.

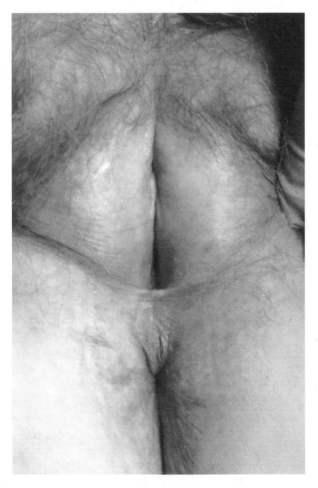

Figure 13-3 • A late case of lichen sclerosus. Note the thin, white, atrophic epithelium and labial fusion.
(Reproduced with permission from Champion RH. Textbook of Dermatology. 5th ed. Oxford: Blackwell Science, 1992:2852.)

Diagnostic Evaluation

Diagnosis is made histologically; therefore, all vulvar lesions should be **biopsied** unless your suspicion for vulvar dermatitis is high, the woman is premenopausal, and response to the treatment is immediate. Indications for definite biopsy include ulceration, unifocal lesions, suspicion of lichen sclerosus or other epithelial lesions, and unidentified lesions. Vaginal lesions can be biopsied and evaluated via **colposcopy**.

Differential Diagnosis

The differential diagnosis of non-neoplastic lesions of the vulva and vagina include disorders such as Behçet's syndrome, Crohn's disease, erythema multiforme, bullous pemphigoid, and plasma cell vulvitis. The differential also includes carcinomas such as squamous cell, basal cell, melanoma, sarcoma, and Paget's disease. Biopsies should therefore be performed and clinical correlations made.

Treatment

The histologic diagnosis is the basis for treatment. For all of these lesions, **healthy vulvar and vaginal hygiene** practices are of utmost importance. Patients should avoid tight-fitting clothes; pantyhose; pantyliners; scented soaps and detergents; bubble baths; washcloths; feminine sprays, douches, and powders. Patients should wear loose-fitting cotton underwear and loose-fitting clothing. They should use unscented detergents and soaps such as Neutrogena or Dove, and take morning and evening tub baths without additives.

High potency **topical steroids** such as clobetasol can be used to treat lichen sclerosus or planus, and low- to medium-potency steroids should be used for mild cases of dermatoses. The duration of use ranges from twice a day for 2 to 4 weeks for dermatoses, to daily for 6 to 12 weeks for lichen sclerosus. In most cases, patients benefit from a maintenance dose of one to three times per week to avoid recurrence. For lesions that respond poorly to topical steroids, intralesional steroids can be used.

No role has been found for the use of **topical estrogens** in the treatment of these disorders; however, estrogen is an effective treatment for postmenopausal vulvovaginal atrophy, and hormone replacement therapy (HRT) should be considered in women with changes secondary to estrogen deficiency, but *not* for lichen sclerosus.

Surgery generally plays a limited role in treatment of these disorders, except for in the case of postinflammatory sequelae such as adhesions and introital stenosis. Surgery is often necessary in the case of lichen planus when vaginal synechiae are involved.

KEY POINTS

1. Vulvar itching and lesions can be secondary to atopic skin disorders like eczema; irritants/allergens, and atrophic changes.
2. Lesions often become hypertrophic secondary to chronic irritation.
3. Diagnosis is made by palpation, colposcopy, and biopsy. Cancer should always be excluded by biopsy.
4. Treatment involves hygiene practices, avoidance of irritants, topical steroids, and intralesional steroids.

■ BENIGN CYSTS AND TUMORS OF THE VULVA AND VAGINA

A variety of cysts and tumors can arise on the vulva and vagina. Cysts can originate from occlusion of pilosebaceous ducts, sebaceous ducts, and apocrine sweat glands. Treatment of benign cystic and solid tumors is only needed if the lesions become symptomatic or infected.

Epidermal Inclusion Cysts

Epidermal inclusion cysts are **the most common tumor found on the vulva**. These cysts usually result from occlusion of a pilosebaceous duct or a blocked hair follicle. They are lined with squamous epithelium and contain tissue that would normally be exfoliated. These solitary lesions are normally small and asymptomatic; however, if these become superinfected and develop into abscesses, incision and drainage or complete excision is the treatment.

Sebaceous Cysts

When the duct of a sebaceous gland becomes blocked, a sebaceous cyst forms. The normally secreted sebum accumulates in this cyst. Cysts are often multiple and asymptomatic. As with any cyst, these can become superinfected with local flora and require treatment with incision and drainage (I&D).

Apocrine Sweat Gland Cysts

These sweat glands are found throughout the mons pubis and labia majora. They can become occluded and form cysts. **Fox-Fordyce disease** is a pruritic microcystic disease that results from occlusion of these sweat glands. As in the axillary region, if these cysts become infected and form multiple abscesses, **hidradenitis suppurativa** can result. Excision or incision and drainage are the treatments of choice. If an overlying cellulitis is present, antibiotics are often used as well.

Skene Gland Cysts

Skene glands, or paraurethral glands, are located next to the urethra meatus (Figure 13-4). Chronic inflammation of Skene glands can cause obstruction of the ducts and result in cystic dilation of the glands.

Benign Solid Tumors

There are many benign solid tumors of the vulva and the vagina. Some of the most common include

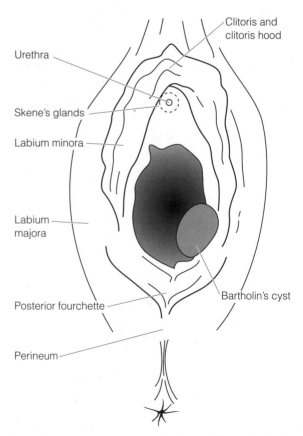

Figure 13-4 • Gross appearance of a Bartholin cyst of the vulva.

lipomas, hermangiomas and urethral caruncles. **Lipomas** are soft pedunculated or sessile tumors composed of mature fat cells and fibrous strands. These tumors do not require removal unless they become large and symptomatic. **Hemangiomas** are elevated soft red tumors most commonly found in infants. These tumors may grow rapidly and often ulcerate or bleed secondary to trauma. Most subsequently undergo spontaneous involution over several years. **Urethral caruncles** are small, red, fleshy tumors found at the distal urethral meatus. These occur almost exclusively in postmenopausal women as a result of vulvovaginal atrophy. This results in formation of an ectropion at the posterior urethral wall. These lesions are usually asymptomatic and no treatment is required. When bloody spotting results, a short course of systemic or topical estrogens is appropriate.

KEY POINTS

1. A variety of cysts from occlusion of ducts can arise on the vulva.
2. A solitary cyst is most likely epidermal in origin. These are the most common cysts found on the vulva.
3. A collection of cysts that are asymptomatic are most likely sebaceous cysts.
4. A collection of pruritic cysts is likely Fox-Fordyce disease, which is caused by occlusion of apocrine sweat glands.
5. Hidradenitis suppurativa is the result of abscess formation from superinfection of apocrine sweat glands and cysts.
6. Infection of any of these cysts is treated with I&D.
7. Lipomas, hermangiomas, and urethral caruncles are the most common benign solid tumors of the vulva and vagina.

Bartholin's Duct Cyst and Abscess

Bartholin's glands are located bilaterally at approximately 4 o'clock and 8 o'clock on the labia majora (see Figure 13-4). They are mucus-secreting glands with ducts that open just external to the hymenal ring. Obstruction of these ducts leads to an enlarged **Bartholin's cyst**. If the cyst remains small (1–2 cm) and is not causing any symptoms, it can be left untreated and will often resolve on its own or with sitz baths. However, some cysts can become quite large and cause pressure symptoms such as local pain,

dyspareunia, and difficulty walking. When a Bartholin duct cyst first presents in a woman over age 40, a biopsy should be performed to rule out the rare possibility of **Bartholin's gland carcinoma**.

If these cysts do not resolve, they can become infected and lead to a **Bartholin's gland abscesses**. These abscesses range in size and can be quite large, causing exquisite pain and tenderness and associated cellulitis. Bartholin's abscesses or symptomatic cysts should be treated like any other abscess: by drainage. However, simple incision and drainage can often lead to recurrence; therefore, one of two methods can be used.

1. Commonly performed in the emergent setting or in the office, this method involves making a small incision (5 mm) to drain and irrigate the abscess. Then a **Word catheter** with a balloon tip is placed inside the remaining cyst and inflated to fill the space. The balloon is left in place for 4 to 6 weeks, being serially reduced in size, while epithelialization of the cyst and tract occurs (Figure 13-5A, B).
2. **Marsupialization** is usually done for recurrent Bartholin's cysts or abscesses. The entire abscess or cyst is incised and the resulting space is sewn open (Figure 13-6). Epithelialization can then occur and there is no closed space where recurrent abscesses can form.

With either treatment, warm sitz baths several times per day are recommended both for pain relief and to decrease healing time. Adjunct antibiotic therapy is only recommended when the drainage is cultured for *Neisseria gonorrhoeae*, which occurs approximately 10% of the time. Concomitant cellulitis or an abscess that seems refractory to simple

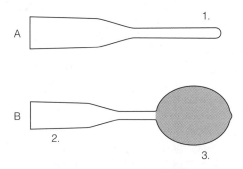

Figure 13-5 • Word catheter before inflation (A) and after inflation (B). 1. The balloon-tipped end is placed into the incision site on the Bartholin's cyst. 2. A small-gauge needle is inserted into the opposite end and 2–4 mL of water is injected. 3. The inflated balloon remains inside the cyst for 4 to 6 weeks until an epithelialized tract is formed to prevent blockage of the duct to recur.

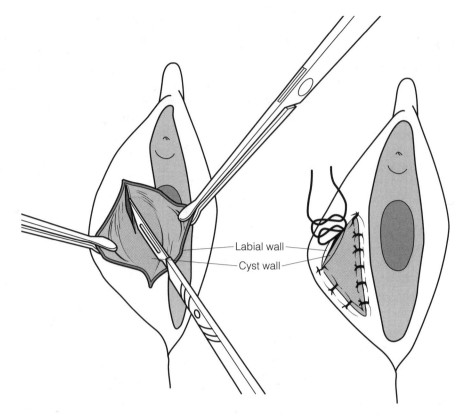

Figure 13-6 • Incision, drainage, and marsupialization of a Bartholin's abscess.

surgical treatment should also be treated with antibiotics that cover skin flora, primarily *Staphylococcus aureus*.

KEY POINTS

1. Bartholin's cysts and abscesses are located at 4 o'clock and 8 o'clock on the labia majora.
2. When uninfected, Bartholin's cysts are often asymptomatic and resolve on their own.
3. When a Bartholin's cyst first appears in a woman age 40+, the cyst should be biopsied to rule out the rare possibility of Bartholin's glands carcinoma.
4. Bartholin's abscesses can be treated like other abscesses with I&D but tend to recur unless appropriate drainage is provided with a Word catheter or marsupialization.
5. Antibiotic therapy is only recommended for abscesses with positive cultures for *N. gonorrhoeae* or concomitant cellulites (most commonly from *S. aureus* and skin flora).

■ BENIGN CERVICAL LESIONS

Congenital Anomalies

Isolated congenital anomalies of the cervix are rare. In case of a uterine didelphys with a double vagina, a double cervix (bicollis) may be found, but this does not arise in isolation. However, women who were exposed in utero to DES have some abnormality of the cervix approximately 25% of the time. These benign abnormalities include cervical collars, cervical hoods, cock's comb appearance, hypoplastic cervix, and pseudopolyps. Clear cell adenocarcinoma occurs in less than 0.1% of these patients but is a malignant process that can lead to untimely death.

Cervical Cysts

Most cervical cysts are dilated retention cysts called **nabothian cysts**. These are caused by blockage of an endocervical gland and usually expand to no more than 1 cm in diameter. Nabothian cysts are more commonly found in menstruating women; are usually asymptomatic, discovered on routine gynecologic examination, and require no treatment.

Cervical cysts can also be **mesonephric cysts**. These are remnants of the mesonephric (wolffian) ducts that can become cystic. These cysts differ from nabothian cysts in that they tend to lie deeper in the cervical stroma and on the external surface of the cervix.

Finally, in rare instances, **endometriosis** can implant on or near the cervix. These cysts tend to be red or purple in color and often the patient will have associated symptoms of endometriosis.

Cervical Polyps

True cervical polyps are benign growths that may be pedunculated or broad based; these can arise anywhere on the cervix and are often asymptomatic. Cervical polyps that do produce symptoms tend to be associated with intermenstrual or postcoital bleeding rather than pain of any kind, unless they are actually obstructing the cervical canal. Although cervical polyps are not usually considered a premalignant condition, they are generally removed, particularly those protruding from the cervical os. One reason for removal is that it can be difficult to determine whether a pedunculated polyp is actually uterine in origin and thus could be premalignant. Removal is often an office procedure with pedunculated polyps; however, dilation and curettage (D&C), with or without hysteroscopy, may be required for broad-based polyps of the endocervix.

Cervical Fibroids

Leiomyomas (myomas or fibroids) are common benign tumors of the uterine corpus; but may also arise in the cervix. Leiomyomas can cause symptoms of intermenstrual bleeding similar to both uterine fibroids and cervical polyps. However, depending on their location and size, these can also cause dyspareunia and bladder or rectal pressure. Once the possibility of cervical cancer is ruled out, an asymptomatic cervical fibroid can be followed with routine gynecologic care. Symptomatic fibroids can be surgically removed but, depending on their location, hysterectomy rather than myomectomy may be required.

Cervical Stenosis

Cervical stenosis can be congenital, a product of scarring after surgical manipulation or radiotherapy of the cervix, or secondary to obstruction with neoplasm, polyp, or fibroid. If cervical stenosis is asymptomatic and merely found on examination, it may be left untreated. However, if egress from the uterus is blocked in a premenopausal woman, oligo/amenorrhea, dysmenorrhea, or an enlarged uterus may result. An obstructive lesion should be removed. If the stenosis is secondary to scarring, the cervix should be gently dilated to allow the intrauterine contents to flow more easily.

KEY POINTS

1. Congenital cervical anomalies are usually associated with abnormalities in the uterus.
2. Cervical polyps are rarely cancerous but should be removed if they are causing bleeding or obstruction of the cervical canal.
3. Fibroids of the cervix can be a problem in pregnancy and may lead to poor dilation of the cervix; nonpregnant patients may have problems with cervical stenosis due to external compression.

Benign Disorders of the Upper Genital Tract

ANATOMIC ANOMALIES OF THE UTERUS

Pathogenesis

The superior vagina, cervix, uterus, and fallopian tubes are formed by fusion of the **paramesonephric (müllerian) ducts**. Uterine anomalies arise during embryonic development, generally as a result of incomplete fusion of the ducts, incomplete development of one or both ducts, or degeneration of the ducts (müllerian agenesis). These anomalies (Table 14-1) can vary in scope and severity from the presence of simple septa or bicornuate uterus to complete duplication of the entire female reproductive system (Figure 14-1). Of the disorders not related to drugs, the most common condition is the **septate uterus** due to malfusion of the paramesonephric ducts. Many anatomic uterine abnormalities may also be associated with **urinary tract anomalies** and **inguinal hernias**.

Epidemiology

Anatomic anomalies of the uterus are extremely rare. Several years ago, the incidence was estimated to be 0.02% of the female population. If estimated today, this percentage would most likely be somewhat higher due to the increased incidence of müllerian anomalies in women who were exposed in utero to diethylstilbestrol (DES) from 1940 to 1971.

Clinical Manifestations

History

Some uterine anomalies are asymptomatic and may never be discovered, whereas others may not be rec-

ognized until the onset of menarche or attempts at childbearing. Some symptoms associated with anomalies of the uterus include dysmenorrhea, dyspareunia, cyclic pelvic pain, and infertility.

Uterine septums are primarily composed of collagen fibers and lack an adequate blood supply to facilitate placentation and maintain a growing pregnancy. Thus, 25% of women with uterine septums may suffer from recurrent first-trimester pregnancy loss. A true **bicornuate uterus**, however, is more commonly complicated by the limited size of the uterine horn rather than by blood supply. As such, bicornuate uteri are associated with second-trimester abortion, preterm labor and delivery, and malpresentation.

Diagnostic Evaluation

The primary investigative tools for uterine abnormalities are pelvic ultrasound, CT, MRI, sonohystogram, hysterosalpingogram, hysteroscopy, and laparoscopy.

Treatment

Many uterine anomalies require no treatment. However, when the defect causes significant symptoms or interferes with reproduction, treatment options should be explored. Uterine septa can be excised with operative hysteroscopy. The ability to support a pregnancy with a bicornuate uterus has also been achieved with unification procedures.

TABLE 14-1

Classification of Müllerian Anomalies

Class I. Segmented müllerian agenesis or hypoplasia
A. Vaginal
B. Cervical
C. Fundal
D. Tubal
E. Combined

Class II. Unicornuate uterus
A. With a rudimentary horn
   1. With a communicating endometrial cavity
   2. With a noncommunicating cavity
   3. With no cavity
B. Without any rudimentary horn

Class III. Uterus didelphis

Class IV. Bicornuate uterus
A. Complete to the internal os
B. Partial
C. Arcuate

Class V. Septate uterus
A. With a complete septum
B. With an incomplete septum

Class VI. Uterus with internal luminal changes

KEY POINTS

1. Anatomic anomalies of the uterus are extremely rare. The most common condition unrelated to drug use is the septate uterus.
2. Anatomic anomalies of the uterus result from problems in the fusion of the paramesonephric (müllerian) ducts.
3. These anomalies may also be associated with urinary tract anomalies and inguinal hernias.
4. If present, symptoms include amenorrhea, dysmenorrhea, dyspareunia, cyclic pelvic pain, infertility, recurrent pregnancy loss, and premature labor.
5. Anomalies are diagnosed using physical exam, pelvic ultrasound, CT, MRI, hysterosalpingogram, hysteroscopy, and laparoscopy.
6. If implantation occurs on or near a uterine septum, the result may be recurrent early pregnancy loss due to decreased vascular supply of the septum.
7. Bicornuate uteri are associated with complications resulting from a small uterine cavity including second-trimester pregnancy loss, malpresentation, and premature labor and delivery.
8. Both septated uteri and bicornuate uteri can be treated surgically if symptomatic.

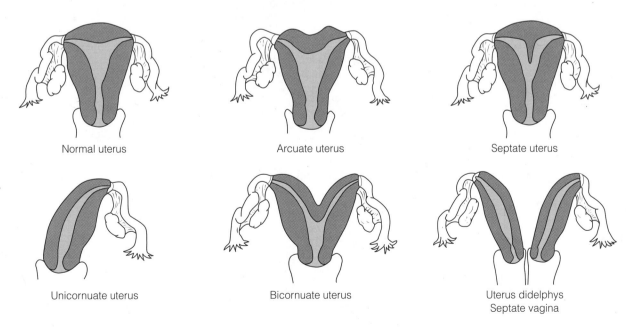

Normal uterus · Arcuate uterus · Septate uterus · Unicornuate uterus · Bicornuate uterus · Uterus didelphys Septate vagina

Figure 14-1 • Examples of anatomic anomalies of the uterus.

■ UTERINE LEIOMYOMA

Uterine leiomyomas, also called fibroids or uterine myomas, are local proliferation of smooth muscle cells of the uterus. Fibroids typically occur in women of childbearing age and then regress during menopause. These benign tumors constitute the most common indication for surgery for women in the United States. Approximately one-third of all hysterectomies performed are for uterine fibroids. Most fibroids, however, cause no major symptoms and require no treatment. Generally, fibroids only become problematic when their location results in heavy or irregular bleeding or infertility. Fibroids may also be identified when they become large enough to cause a mass effect on other pelvic structures resulting in pelvic pain and pressure, urinary frequency, or constipation.

Pathogenesis

The cause of uterine leiomyomas is unclear. Fibroids are **monoclonal** with each tumor resulting from propagation of a single muscle cell. Proposed etiologies include development from smooth muscle cells of the uterus or the uterine arteries, from metaplastic transformation of connective tissue cells, and from persistent embryonic rest cells. Recent studies have identified a small number of genes that mutate in fibroid tissue but not in normal myometrial cells.

Fibroids are hormonally responsive to estrogen. These can grow quickly and to huge proportions during pregnancy or when exposed to exogenous estrogens. During menopause, the tumors usually stop growing and may atrophy in response to naturally lower endogenous estrogen levels.

Uterine fibroids are classified by their location in the uterus (Figure 14-2). The typical classification includes **submucosal** (beneath the endometrium), **intramural** (in the muscular wall of the uterus), and **subserosal** (beneath the uterine serosa). Intramural leiomyomas are the most common type. Both submucosal and subserosal fibroids may become pedunculated. A **parasitic leiomyoma** is a pedunculated fibroid that becomes attached to the pelvic viscera or omentum and develops its own blood supply.

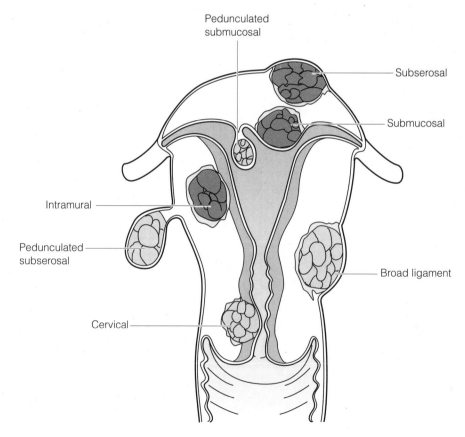

Figure 14-2 • Common locations of uterine fibroids.

Fibroids have a "**pseudocapsule**" of compressed smooth muscle cells that contain very few blood vessels and lymphatic vessels. As leiomyomas enlarge, they can outgrow their blood supply, infarct, and degenerate causing pain. Types of degenerative changes include **hyaline**, **cystic**, **red (hemorrhagic)**, **calcific**, and **sarcomatous**. During pregnancy, the growth and degeneration of fibroids can lead to infarction and hemorrhaging (red degeneration) within the tumors in 10% of pregnancies.

It is unclear whether fibroids have any malignant potential. Studies once suggested that malignant degeneration of a preexisting fibroid to a leiomyosarcoma is extremely rare; perhaps only 1 : 1000 cases. It is now believed that these cases may actually represent new neoplasias rather than the degeneration of an existing fibroid.

Epidemiology

It is estimated that 20% to 30% of all American women and 40% of African American women will develop leiomyoma by age 40.

Risk Factors

Women most at risk for uterine fibroids are those who are African American, nonsmokers, perimenopausal, or obese. The incidence of leiomyomas is three to nine times higher in black women in the United States compared to white, Asian, and Hispanic women. There is no known reason for this.

Clinical Manifestations

History

Most women with fibroids (50% to 65%) have no clinical symptoms. Of those who do (Table 14-2), abnormal uterine bleeding is by far the most common symptom, generally occurring in submucosal fibroids impinging on the endometrial cavity. Bleeding typically occurs as increasingly heavy periods of longer duration (menorrhagia). Blood loss from fibroids can lead to chronic iron-deficiency anemia, weakness, and dizziness.

In general, pelvic pain is not usually part of the symptom complex unless vascular compromise is present. This is most common in subserous pedunculated fibroids. Patients may, however, experience secondary dysmenorrhea with menses, particularly

TABLE 14-2
Clinical Symptoms of Uterine Leiomyomas
Bleeding
Longer, heavier periods
Endometrial ulceration
Pressure
Pelvic pressure and bloating
Constipation and rectal pressure
Urinary frequency or retention
Pain
Secondary dysmenorrhea
Acute infarct (especially in pregnancy)
Dyspareunia
Reproductive difficulties
Infertility (failed implantation/spontaneous abortion)
Intrauterine growth restriction
Increased cesarean sections
Increased malpresentation

when menorrhagia or metromenorrhagia are present. Pressure-related symptoms (pelvic pressure, fullness, or heaviness) vary depending on the number and location of leiomyomas. If a fibroid impinges on nearby structures, patients may complain of constipation, urinary frequency, or even urinary retention as the space within the pelvis becomes more crowded.

Uterine myomas are also associated with an increased incidence of infertility but are solely responsible for infertility in only 2% to 10% of cases. Fibroids may distort the endocervical canal, fallopian tubes, or endometrial cavity, thus interfering with conception or implantation and sometimes causing spontaneous abortion. The vast majority of women with fibroids, however, are able to conceive. Because fibroids have the potential for excessive growth during pregnancy, they may contribute to intrauterine growth restriction, malpresentation, premature labor, or dystocia. They may also block the presenting part, necessitating cesarean section.

Physical Examination

Depending on their location and size, uterine leiomyomas can sometimes be palpated on bimanual pelvic examination or on abdominal examination. Bimanual examination often reveals a nontender irregularly enlarged uterus with "lumpy-bumpy" or cobblestone protrusions that feel firm or solid on palpation.

Diagnostic Evaluation

The differential diagnosis for uterine leiomyoma depends on the patient's symptoms (Table 14-3). Because most women with leiomyomas are asymptomatic, the diagnosis is sometimes made only as an incidental finding on a pathology specimen.

Pelvic ultrasound is the most common means of diagnosis. Fibroids can be seen as areas of hypoechogenicity among normal myometrial material. MRI, hysterosalpingography (HSG), saline infusion sonography (sonohystogram), and hysteroscopy are additional tools for imaging the location and size of uterine fibroids.

Treatment

Most cases of uterine fibroids do not require therapy, and expectant management is appropriate. However, the diagnosis of leiomyoma must be unequivocal. Other pelvic masses should be ruled out, and the patient with actively growing fibroids should be followed every 6 months to monitor the size and growth.

When leiomyomas result in severe pain, infertility, urinary tract symptoms, or show evidence of postmenopausal growth, treatment should be considered. The choice of treatment depends on the patient's age, pregnancy status, desire for future pregnancies, and on the size and location of the fibroids.

Medical therapies for leiomyomas, including medroxyprogesterone (Provera), danazol, and gonadotropin-releasing hormone (GnRH) agonists (nafarelin acetate, Depot Lupron), have been found to shrink fibroids by **decreasing circulating estrogen** levels. Unfortunately, the tumors usually resume growth after medications are discontinued. For women nearing menopause, these treatments may be used as a temporizing measure until their own endogenous estrogens decrease naturally.

Uterine artery embolization (UAE) is being used with greater frequency as a less-invasive approach of treating symptomatic fibroids. The procedure is usually preformed by an interventional radiologist who catheterizes the femoral artery in order to inject permanent pledgettes into the uterine artery. The goal is to decrease the blood supply to the fibroid thereby causing degeneration and necrosis. Because the therapy is not specific to a given fibroid, the blood supply to the uterus and/or ovaries can be compromised. UAE should not be used in women who are planning to become pregnant after the procedure.

The indications for surgical intervention for fibroids are listed in Table 14-4. A **myomectomy** is the surgical resection of one or more fibroids from the uterine wall. Myomectomy is usually reserved for patients with symptomatic fibroids who wish to preserve their fertility. Myomectomies can be performed hysteroscopically, laparoscopically, or abdominally. The primary disadvantage of myomectomy is that fibroids recur in 50% of patients and adhesions frequently form that may further complicate pain and infertility.

Hysterectomy is the definitive treatment for leiomyomas. Vaginal hysterectomy can be performed for small myomas and total abdominal hysterectomy for large or multiple myomas. If the ovaries are diseased or if the blood supply has been damaged, then

---

TABLE 14-3

Differential Diagnosis of Uterine Fibroids*

Abnormal bleeding
Endometrial polyps
Endometrial hyperplasia
Endometrial cancer
Adenomyosis
Exogenous uterine bleeding

Pelvic mass or uterine enlargement
Pregnancy
Adenomyosis
Ovarian cysts
Ovarian neoplasm
Tubo-ovarian abscess
Leiomyosarcoma

Note: *Any of these conditions can coexist with fibroids.

TABLE 14-4

Indications for Surgical Intervention for Uterine Leiomyomas

Abnormal uterine bleeding, causing anemia

Severe pelvic pain or secondary amenorrhea

Size >12 weeks gestation obscuring evaluation of adnexae

Urinary frequency or retention

Growth after menopause

Infertility

Rapid increase in size

Source: *Adapted from Hacker N, and Moore JG. Essentials of Obstetrics and Gynecology. Philadelphia: WB Saunders, 1998:415.*

oophorectomy should be performed as well. Otherwise, the ovaries should be preserved in women under age 45. Surgical intervention should be avoided during pregnancy, although myomectomy or hysterectomy may be necessary after delivery.

Follow-Up

When hysterectomy is not indicated for a patient with leiomyomas, careful follow-up should take place to monitor the size and location of the tumors. At no time should a myoma go untreated if it obscures the evaluation of the adnexae. Rapid growth of a tumor in postmenopausal women may be a sign of leiomyosarcoma and should be investigated immediately. Postmenopausal estrogens and premenopausal oral contraceptives at low doses do not appear to pose a risk to the patient.

KEY POINTS

1. Fibroids are benign, estrogen-sensitive, smooth muscle tumors of unclear etiology found in 20% to 30% of reproductive-age women.
2. Fibroid incidence is three to nine times higher in black women compared to white, Asian, and Hispanic women. Risk is also increased in obese, nonsmoking, and perimenopausal women.
3. Fibroids may be submucosal, intramural, or subserosal and can grow to great size, especially during pregnancy.
4. Fibroids frequently result in degenerative changes, especially during pregnancy, but rarely if ever result in malignant degeneration (1:1000 cases).
5. Fibroids are asymptomatic in 50% to 65% of patients; when symptomatic, these can cause heavy bleeding (most common), pressure, pain, and infertility.
6. Fibroids are typically diagnosed by history, pelvic/abdominal examination, pelvic ultrasound, HSG, and/or hysteroscopy.
7. In most cases, no treatment is necessary.
8. Fibroids can be treated temporarily with Provera, danazol, or GnRH analogs to decrease estrogen and shrink the tumors, or myomectomy to resect the tumors when future fertility is desired.
9. Fibroids are treated definitively by hysterectomy in the case of severe pain, when large or multiple, when causing urinary symptoms, and when evidencing postmenopausal or rapid growth.

■ ENDOMETRIAL HYPERPLASIA

Pathogenesis

Endometrial proliferation is a normal part of the menstrual cycle that occurs during the follicular- or estrogen-dominant phase of the cycle. **Simple proliferation** is an overabundance of histologically normal endometrium. However, when the endometrium is exposed to continuous endogenous or exogenous estrogen in the absence of progesterone, simple endometrial proliferation can advance to endometrial hyperplasia. **Endometrial hyperplasia** is the abnormal proliferation of glandular and stromal elements of the endometrium resulting in histologic alterations in its cellular architecture and/or cytologic atypia. These lesions do not necessarily involve the entire endometrium, but rather may develop focally among normal endometrium. These lesions do not automatically advance to carcinoma if left untreated but they can occur simultaneously with endometrial carcinoma.

The histologic variations of endometrial hyperplasia are outlined in Table 14-5. When only **architectural changes** are present, the hyperplasia is known as either simple or complex. When **cytologic atypia** is present along with architectural changes, then it is said to be either *atypical* simple or *atypical* complex hyperplasia.

1. **Simple hyperplasia** is the simplest form of hyperplasia. It represents an abnormal proliferation of both the stromal and glandular endometrial elements. Less than 1% of these lesions progress to carcinoma.
2. **Complex hyperplasia** consists of abnormal proliferation of the glandular endometrial elements without proliferation of the stromal elements. In these lesions, the glands are crowded in a back-to-back fashion and are of varying shapes and sizes, *but no cytologic atypia* is present. Approximately 3% of these lesions progress to carcinoma if left untreated.

In addition to the architectural changes seen in simple and complex hyperplasia, **cytologic atypia** may be found in more severe forms of endometrial hyperplasia. These cytologic changes include large nuclei with lost polarity, increased nuclear-to-cytoplasmic ratios, prominent nuclei, and irregular clumped chromatin. In these cases, the hyperplasia is further divided into *atypical* simple hyperplasia and *atypical* complex hyperplasia.

■ **TABLE 14-5**

Classification of Endometrial Hyperplasia and Progression to Endometrial Cancer

Architectural Type	Cytologic Atypia	Progression to Endometrial Cancer (in %)
Simple hyperplasia	Absent	1
Complex hyperplasia	Absent	3
Atypical simple hyperplasia	Present	8
Atypical complex hyperplasia	Present	29

3. **Atypical simple hyperplasia** involves cellular atypia and mitotic figures in addition to glandular crowding and complexity. These lesions progress to carcinoma in about 8% of cases if untreated.
4. **Atypical complex hyperplasia** is the most severe form of endometrial hyperplasia. It progresses to carcinoma in approximately 29% of untreated cases.

Epidemiology

Endometrial hyperplasia typically occurs in the menopausal or perimenopausal woman, but may also occur in the years immediately after menarche if ovulation is infrequent.

Risk Factors

Patients at risk for endometrial hyperplasia, like those at risk for endometrial carcinoma, are at risk due to **unopposed estrogen exposure** (Table 14-6). This includes women with obesity, nulliparity, late menopause, and exogenous estrogen use without progesterone. Chronic anovulation, polycystic ovarian syndrome, and estrogen-producing tumors such as granulosa-theca cell tumors also put women at increased risk for endometrial hyperplasia.

Clinical Manifestations

History

Patients with endometrial hyperplasia typically present with irregular or excessive uterine bleeding. Uterine bleeding in a postmenopausal woman should raise high suspicion of endometrial hyperplasia or carcinoma.

Physical Examination

Occasionally, the uterus will be enlarged in endometrial hyperplasia. This is attributed to both the increase in the mass of the endometrium and to the

■ **TABLE 14-6**

Risk Factors for Endometrial Hyperplasia

Obesity

Nulliparity

Late menopause (> age 55)

Exogenous estrogen use without progesterone

Chronic anovulation

Diabetes mellitus

Tamoxifen use

growth of the myometrium in response to continuous estrogen stimulation.

Diagnostic Evaluation

The diagnosis of endometrial hyperplasia is made pathologically by endometrial biopsy. Although dilation and curettage (D&C) was once the gold standard for sampling the endometrium, modern endometrial biopsies enjoy a 90% to 95% accuracy rate and have thus become the method of choice for evaluation of endometrial hyperplasia. However, when an office biopsy cannot be obtained due to insufficient tissue, patient discomfort, or cervical stenosis, then D&C of the uterus is required to rule out endometrial hyperplasia and carcinoma, except in women under age 30. D&C is also recommended in patients who have atypical complex hyperplasia on biopsy because approximately 29% of those patients will have a coexistent endometrial carcinoma.

Treatment

The treatment of endometrial hyperplasia depends on the histologic variant of the disease and on the age of the patient. Simple, complex, atypical simple, and atypical complex hyperplasia can all be treated medically with **progestin therapy**. Typically, medroxy-progesterone (Depo Provera) or oral progesterone

(Provera or Megace) is used in doses that will inhibit and eventually reverse the endometrial hyperplasia. The progestin is usually administered for 3 months; then a repeat endometrial biopsy is performed to evaluate the regression of disease. The progestin therapy may be repeated if residual disease is found on repeat biopsy.

Patients without cytologic atypia (i.e., those with simple or complex hyperplasia) may be managed with D&C with or without hysteroscopy. These patients should also be reevaluated with endometrial sampling every 3 to 6 months.

Atypical complex hyperplasia is often treated surgically by hysterectomy given the significant (29%) risk of developing endometrial cancer and because most women with the disorder are either perimenopausal or postmenopausal. In younger patients with atypical complex hyperplasia and chronic anovulation who wish to preserve fertility, endometrial curettage, longer-term progestin management, and ovulation induction may assist patients in becoming pregnant.

KEY POINTS

1. Endometrial hyperplasia represents a broad spectrum of abnormal proliferation of the endometrium accompanied by architectural abnormalities and/or cytologic atypia.
2. It is caused by prolonged exposure to exogenous or endogenous estrogen in the absence of progesterone.
3. It includes risk factors for unopposed estrogen exposure such as obesity, nulliparity, chronic anovulation, late menopause, and unopposed estrogen use.
4. Endometrial hyperplasia is classified as simple or complex if only architectural alterations exist or as atypical simple or atypical complex if cytologic atypia is also present.
5. Risk of malignant transformation is 1% in simple hyperplasia, 3% in complex hyperplasia, 8% in atypical simple hyperplasia, and 29% in atypical complex hyperplasia.
6. Endometrial hyperplasia is diagnosed pathologically by endometrial biopsy or D&C.
7. It is usually treated medically with progestin therapy for 3 months, followed by resampling of the endometrium.
8. It can also be treated surgically with hysterectomy if symptoms persist and if future childbearing is not desired.

■ OVARIAN CYSTS

Pathogenesis

In general, ovarian masses can be divided into functional cysts and neoplastic growths. Benign and malignant neoplasms of the ovary are discussed in detail in Chapter 30. **Functional cysts** of the ovaries result from normal physiologic functioning of the ovaries and are divided into follicular cysts and corpus luteum cysts.

Follicular cysts—the most common functional cysts—arise after failure of a follicle to rupture during follicular maturation and may vary in size from 3–8 cm. Follicular cysts are classically asymptomatic and usually unilateral. Large follicular cysts can cause a tender palpable ovarian mass and can lead to ovarian torsion. Most follicular cysts disappear spontaneously within 60 days.

Corpus luteum cysts are common functional cysts that occur during the luteal phase of the menstrual cycle. Most corpus luteum cysts are formed when the corpus luteum becomes enlarged (>3 cm) and hemorrhagic (corpus hemorrhagicum), or fails to regress after 14 days. These cysts can cause a delay in menstruation and dull lower quadrant pain. Patients with a ruptured corpus luteum cyst can present with acute pain and signs of hemoperitoneum late in the luteal phase.

Theca lutein cysts are small bilateral cysts filled with clear, straw-colored fluid. These ovarian cysts result from stimulation by abnormally high β-human chorionic gonadotropin (e.g., from a molar pregnancy, choriocarcinoma, or clomiphene therapy).

Epidemiology

Seventy-five percent of ovarian masses in women of reproductive age are **functional cysts** and 25% are **nonfunctional neoplasms**. Although functional ovarian cysts can be found in females of any age, they most commonly occur between puberty and menopause. Women who smoke have a twofold increase for functional cysts.

Clinical Manifestations

History

Patients with functional cysts present with a variety of symptoms depending on the type of cyst. Follicular cysts tend to be asymptomatic and only occasionally cause menstrual disturbances such as prolonged intermenstrual intervals or short cycles. Larger follicular cysts can cause aching pelvic pain, dyspareunia, and can lead to ovarian torsion. Corpus luteum cysts may cause local pelvic pain and either amenorrhea or delayed menses. Acute abdominal pain may result from a hemorrhagic corpus luteum cyst, a torsed ovary, or from a ruptured follicular cyst.

Physical Examination

The findings on bimanual pelvic examination varies with the type of cyst. Follicular cysts tend to be less than 8 cm and simple or unilocular in structure. Lutein cysts are generally larger than follicular cysts and often feel more firm or solid on palpation. A torsed or ruptured cyst will cause pain on palpation, acute abdominal pain, and rebound tenderness.

Diagnostic Evaluation

After a thorough history and physical, the primary diagnostic tool for the work-up of ovarian cyst is the **pelvic ultrasound**. This study evaluates the structure of the growth as more cystic or solid in nature to guide further work-up and treatment. A CA-125 level is often obtained from patients who are at high risk for ovarian cancer; it is not, however, a diagnostic or screening test per the American College of Obstetrics and Gynecology (ACOG) guidelines.

The differential diagnoses for ovarian cysts include ectopic pregnancy, pelvic inflammatory disease, torsed adnexa, tubo-ovarian abscess, endometriosis, fibroids, and ovarian neoplasms.

Treatment

Treatment of ovarian cysts depends on the age of the patient and the characteristics of the cyst. Table 14-7 outlines the management options using these criteria. In general, a palpable ovary or adnexal mass in a premenarchal or postmenopausal patient is suggestive of an ovarian neoplasm rather than a func-

tional cyst and exploratory laparotomy is in order. Likewise, reproductive-age women with cysts larger than 8 cm that persist for longer than 60 days or are solid or complex on ultrasound probably do not have a functional cyst. These lesions should be closely investigated with diagnostic laparoscopy or laparotomy.

For patients of reproductive age with cysts less than 6 cm in size, observation with a follow-up ultrasound is the appropriate action. Most follicular cysts should resolve spontaneously within 60 days. As another alternative, patients are sometimes started on **oral contraceptives** during this observation period to suppress gonadotropin stimulation of the cyst and to prevent future cyst formation. Cysts that do not resolve within 60 days—despite observation and gonadotropin suppression—require evaluation with a pelvic ultrasound and possible laparoscopy or laparotomy.

KEY POINTS

1. Functional cysts result from normal physiologic functioning of the ovaries.
2. Follicular cysts result from unruptured follicles. These are usually asymptomatic unless torsion occurs. Management includes observation for 6 to 8 weeks with or without oral contraceptives, followed by pelvic ultrasound.
3. Corpus luteum cysts result from an enlarged and/or hemorrhagic corpus luteum. These may cause a missed period or dull lower quadrant pain. Corpus luteum cysts should resolve spontaneously or may be suppressed with oral contraceptives if recurrent.
4. Any palpable ovary or adnexal mass in a premenarchal or postmenopausal patient is suggestive of ovarian neoplasm and should be investigated with exploratory laparoscopy or laparotomy.

■ TABLE 14-7

Management of a Cystic Adnexal Mass

Age	Size of Cyst (cm)	Management
Premenarchal	>2	Exploratory laparotomy
Reproductive	<6	Observe for 6 to 8 weeks then repeat ultrasound
	6–8	Observe if unilocular; explore if multilocular or solid on ultrasound
	>8	Exploratory laparoscopy/laparotomy for ovarian cystectomy
Postmenopausal	Palpable	Exploratory laparoscopy/laparotomy for ovarian oophorectomy

Endometriosis and Adenomyosis

◼ ENDOMETRIOSIS

Pathogenesis

Endometriosis is the presence of endometrial tissue (glands and stroma) outside the endometrial cavity. Endometrial tissue can be found anywhere in the body but the most common sites are the ovary and the pelvic peritoneum. Endometriosis in the ovary appears as a cystic collection known as an **endometrioma**. Other common sites include the most dependent parts of the pelvis including the uterosacral ligaments, the anterior and posterior cul-de-sacs, and the posterior uterus and broad ligaments (Figure 15-1). Although not commonly found, endometriosis has been identified in the lung and brain.

There are three main theories about the etiology of endometriosis. The Halban theory proposes that endometrial tissue is transported via the **lymphatic system** to various sites in the pelvis, where it grows ectopically. Meyer proposes that multipotential cells in peritoneal tissue undergo **metaplastic transformation** into functional endometrial tissue. Finally, Sampson suggests that endometrial tissue is transported through the fallopian tubes during **retrograde menstruation**, resulting in intraabdominal pelvic implants.

Endometrial implants cause symptoms by disrupting normal tissue, forming adhesions and fibrosis, and causing severe inflammation. Interestingly, the severity of symptoms does not necessarily correlate with the amount of endometriosis. Women with widely disseminated endometriosis or a large endometrioma may experience little pain, whereas women with minimal disease in the cul-de-sac may suffer severe pain.

Epidemiology

The incidence of endometriosis is estimated to be between 10% and 15%. Because **surgical confirmation is necessary** for the diagnosis of endometriosis, the true prevalence if the disease is unknown. It is found almost exclusively in women of reproductive age, and is the single most common reason for hospitalization of women in this age group. Approximately 20% of women with chronic pelvic pain and 30% to 40% of women with infertility have endometriosis.

Risk Factors

Women with **first-degree relatives** (mother or sisters) with endometriosis are seven times more likely to develop the disorder than women without this risk factor. A relationship has also been demonstrated between endometriosis and some autoimmune disorders (e.g., lupus). For unclear reasons, endometriosis is identified less often in black women.

Clinical Manifestations

History

The hallmark of endometriosis is **cyclic pelvic pain** beginning 1 or 2 days before the onset of menses and lasting the first few days of the cycle. Women with chronic endometriosis and teenagers with endometriosis may not demonstrate this classic pain pattern. Other symptoms associated with endometriosis are dysmenorrhea, dyspareunia, abnormal bleeding, and infertility. Endometriosis is one of the most common diagnoses in the evaluation of infertility.

Symptoms of endometriosis vary depending on

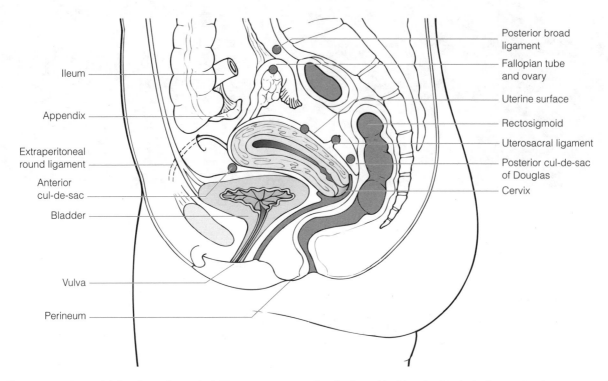

Ileum

Appendix

Extraperitoneal round ligament

Anterior cul-de-sac

Bladder

Vulva

Perineum

Posterior broad ligament

Fallopian tube and ovary

Uterine surface

Rectosigmoid

Uterosacral ligament

Posterior cul-de-sac of Douglas

Cervix

Figure 15-1 • Potential sites for endometriosis. The most common sites (indicated by blue dots) include the ovaries, the uterosacral ligaments, the anterior and posterior cul de sacs, and the posterior uterus and posterior broad ligaments.

the area involved. Dysmenorrhea usually begins in the third decade, worsens with age, and should be considered in women who develop dysmenorrhea after years of pain-free cycles. Dyspareunia is usually associated with deep penetration that can aggravate endometriae lesions in the cul-de-sac or on the uterosacral ligaments.

Endometriosis is also a cause of **infertility**. Although the exact mechanism is unclear, endometriosis is thought to distort the pelvic architecture, interfere with tubal mobility, and cause tubal obstruction from dense adhesions.

Physical Examination

The physical findings associated with early endometriosis may be subtle or nonexistent. To maximize the likelihood of physical findings, the physical exam should be performed during early menses when implants are likely to be largest and most tender. When more disseminated disease is present, the physician may find **uterosacral nodularity** on rectovaginal examination or a **fixed** or **retroverted uterus**. When the ovary is involved, a tender, fixed **adnexal mass** may be palpable on bimanual examination.

Diagnostic Evaluation

The only way to definitively diagnose endometriosis is through **direct visualization** with laparoscopy or laparotomy. Peritoneal biopsy is not necessary but is helpful in confirming the diagnosis of endometriosis. Endometrial implants may appear as rust-colored to dark brown "powder burns" or raised, blue-colored "mulberry" or "raspberry" lesions. The areas may be surrounded by reactive fibrosis that can lead to dense adhesions in extensive disease. The ovary itself can develop large cystic collections of endometriosis filled with thick, dark, old blood known as **endometriomas** or "**chocolate cysts**."

Once the diagnosis of endometriosis is confirmed, the anatomic location and extent of the disease can be used to properly classify the operative findings. The American Fertility Society's revised classification schema is reproduced in Table 15-1. Although not commonly used, this classification method uses a point system to stage endometriosis based on the location, diameter, and depth of lesions and density of adhesions.

■ TABLE 15-1

Classification of Endometriosis

American Society for Reproductive Medicine Revised Classification of Endometriosis

Patient's name _____   Date _____

Stage I   (minimal) —1–5
Stage II   (mild)   —6–15   Laparoscopy _____ Laparotomy _____ Photography _____
Stage III (moderate)—16–40   Recommended treatment _____
Stage IV   (severe)   —>40   _____
Total _____   Prognosis _____

Peritoneum	Endometriosis	<1 cm	1–3 cm	>3 cm
	Superficial	1	2	4
	Deep	2	4	6
Ovary	R Superficial	1	2	4
	Deep	4	16	20
	L Superficial	1	2	4
	Deep	4	16	20

	Posterior Cul-de-sac Obliteration	Partial		Complete
		4		40

	Adhesions	<1/3 Enclosure	1/3–2/3 Enclosure	>2/3 Enclosure
Ovary	R Filmy	1	2	4
	Dense	4	8	16
	L Filmy	1	2	4
	Dense	4	8	16
Tube	R Filmy	1	2	4
	Dense	4*	8*	16
	L Filmy	1	2	4
	Dense	4*	8*	16

*If the fimbriated end of the fallopian tube is completely enclosed, change the point assignment to 16.
Denote appearance of superficial implant types as red [(R), red, red-pink, flamelike, vesicular blobs, clear vesicles], white [(W), opacifications, peritoneal defects, yellow-brown], or black [(B) black, hemosiderin deposits, blue]. Denote percent of total described as R___%, W___%, and B___%. Total should equal 100%.

Differential Diagnosis

The differential diagnosis for endometriosis includes chronic pelvic inflammatory disease, recurrent acute salpingitis, adenomyosis, fibroids, adhesions, hemorrhagic corpus luteum, ectopic pregnancy, and ovarian neoplasms.

Treatment

The treatment choice for patients with endometriosis depends on the extent and location of disease, the severity of symptoms, and the patient's desire for future fertility. Expectant management may be used in patients with minimal or nonexistent symptoms and in patients actively attempting to conceive. For other patients, both surgical and medical options are available.

Medical treatment for endometriosis is aimed at suppression and atrophy of the endometrial tissue. Although medical therapies can be quite effective, these are temporizing measures rather than permanent treatments because the endometrial implants and symptoms often recur following cessation of treatment.

Current medical regimens for the treatment of endometriosis include NSAIDS, either continuous or cyclic administration of oral contraceptives, and use of Provera (medroxyprogesterone). These treatments induce a state of "**pseudopregnancy**" by suppressing both ovulation and menstruation and thereby avoid the cyclic pelvic pain and dysmenorrhea. This therapy is believed best for patients with milder endometriosis who are not currently seeking to conceive.

Patients can also be placed in a reversible state of "**pseudomenopause**" with the use of danazol (Danocrine), an androgen derivative, or gonadotropin-releasing hormone (GnRH) agonists such as leuprolide acetate (Lupron) and nafarelin (Synarel). Both classes of drugs suppress follicle-stimulating hormones (FSHs) and luteinizing hormones (LHs). As a result, the ovaries do not produce estrogen, which would normally stimulate endometrial implants. Existing endometrial implants atrophy, and new implants are prevented.

However, these effects are temporary, and the endometriosis usually eventually recurs after cessation of therapy. The drawback to danazol is that patients may experience some **androgen-related, anabolic side effects** including acne, oily skin, weight gain, edema, hirsutism, and deepening of the voice. Likewise, headache, vasomotor flushing, sweating, and atrophic vaginitis may result from **estrogen deficiency** caused by GnRH agonists such as Lupron. Moreover, these treatments can be costly and often have limited insurance coverage.

Because endogenous estrogen levels are decreased by GnRH agonists, the side effects of these medications are similar to those seen during menopause including hot flashes and loss of bone density. Therefore, the use of these medications is generally limited to 6 months. However, newer treatment regimens known as "**add back therapy**" minimize bone loss by adding a small dose of estrogen to the GnRH agonist. With add back therapy, the patient receives the benefits of the GnRH agonist but bone loss is minimized by the small added dose of estrogen.

Surgical treatment for endometriosis can be classified as either conservative or definitive.

1. **Conservative surgical therapy** typically involves ablation or excision of visible endometriosis during laparoscopy while preserving the reproductive organs to allow for future fertility. For patients with infertility, the potential for conception after conservative surgical treatment depends on the extent of the disease (Table 15-2). For patients with pain, pain control can be optimized by the use of medical therapy after conservative treatment with surgery.
2. **Definitive surgical therapy** includes total abdominal hysterectomy and bilateral salpingo-oophorectomy (TAHBSO), lysis of adhesions, and removal of endometriosis lesions. This therapy is reserved for cases in which childbearing is complete and for women with severe disease or symptoms that are refractory to conservative medical or surgical treatment.

KEY POINTS

1. Endometriosis is the presence of endometrial tissue outside the endometrial cavity, most often in the ovary or pelvic peritoneum.
2. It is estimated to occur in 10% to 15% of women of reproductive age.
3. The hallmark of endometriosis is cyclic pelvic pain. Symptoms (dysmenorrhea, dyspareunia, abnormal bleeding, and infertility) may not correlate with extent of disease.
4. Complications of endometriosis include intra-abdominal inflammation and bleeding that can cause scarring and adhesion formation. These can cause of infertility and small bowel obstructions.
5. Direct visualization with diagnostic laparoscopy or laparotomy is the only way to definitively diagnose endometriosis.
6. Endometriosis can be treated medically (NSAIDs, OCPs, danazol, GnRH agonists) to reduce pain, but these methods are used mainly as temporizing agents.
7. Endometriosis can be treated surgically with conservative therapy to ablate implants and adhesions thereby preserving the potential for future fertility.
8. Endometriosis can be treated definitively with surgery, including TAHBSO, lysis of adhesions, and removal of endometriosis lesions.

TABLE 15-2		
Conception Rates after Ablation of Endometrial Implants		
Extent of Disease	**Stage of Disease**	**Conception Rates (in %)**
Mild	1 & 2	75
Moderate	3	50–60
Severe	4	30–40

■ ADENOMYOSIS

Pathogenesis

Adenomyosis is an extension of endometrial tissue into the uterine myometrium. In the past, adenomyosis was referred to as endometriosis interna. This terminology is no longer used because adenomyosis and endometriosis are two distinct and different clinical entities (Table 15-3).

The cause of adenomyosis is not known. The current theory is that high levels of estrogen stimulate hyperplasia of the basalis layer of the endometrium. For unknown reasons, the barrier between the endometrium and myometrium is broken and the endometrial cells can then invade the myometrium. Because this disease occurs most frequently in parous women, it is thought that endomyometritis may be the first insult to the endometrial-myometrial barrier and eventually predisposes the myometrium to subsequent invasion.

Adenomyosis causes the uterus to become diffusely enlarged and globular due to **hypertrophy** and **hyperplasia** of the myometrium adjacent to the ectopic endometrial tissue. The disease is usually most extensive in the posterior uterine wall. Because the endometrial tissue in adenomyosis extends from the **basalis layer** of the endometrium, it does not undergo the proliferative and secretory changes traditionally induced by cyclic ovarian hormone production. Unlike uterine fibroids, individual areas of adenomyosis are not encapsulated.

Adenomyosis may also present as a well-circumscribed, isolated region known as an **adenomyoma**. Adenomyomas contain smooth muscle cells as well as endometrial glands and stroma. These nodular growths may be located in the myometrium or extend into the endometrial cavity as a polyp.

Epidemiology

The incidence of adenomyosis is 15%. The disease generally develops in parous women in their late 30s or early 40s. It occurs very infrequently in nulliparous women.

Risk Factors

Adenomyosis, endometriosis, and uterine fibroids frequently coexist. About 15% to 20% of patients with adenomyosis also have **endometriosis**, and 50% to 60% of patients with adenomyosis also have **uterine fibroids**.

Clinical Manifestations

History

Thirty percent of patients with adenomyosis are **asymptomatic** or have symptoms minor enough that medical attention is not sought. Symptomatic adenomyosis occurs most often in parous women between age 35 and 50. When symptoms do occur, the most common are secondary dysmenorrhea (30%), menorrhagia (50%), or both (20%). Patients typically present with increasingly excessively heavy or prolonged menstrual bleeding (menorrhagia). They may also complain of increasingly severe dysmenorrhea that may begin up to 1 week before menses and last until cessation of bleeding. Other patients may only experience pressure on the bladder or rectum due to an enlarged uterus.

Physical Examination

The pelvic examination of a patient with adenomyosis may reveal a diffusely enlarged globular uterus. The uterus may be two to three times normal size but is usually <14 cm. The consistency of the uterus is typically softer than the firmer, rubbery uterus containing fibroids. The adenomyomatous uterus may be mildly tender just before or during menses but should have normal mobility and no associated adnexal pathology.

Diagnostic Evaluation

Adenomyosis is a clinical diagnosis and imaging studies—although helpful—are not cost effective. When used, however, MRI is the most accurate imaging tool for identifying adenomyosis. However, because the cost of MRI can be prohibitive, pelvic ultrasound is usually the initial imaging modality.

■ TABLE 15-3

Terminology of Endometriosis	
Adenomyosis	An extension of endometrial tissue into the uterine myometrium leading to menorrhagia or metromenorrhagia. The uterus becomes soft, globular. The definitive treatment is hysterectomy.
Adenomyoma	A well-circumscribed collection of endometrial tissue within the uterine wall. They may also contain smooth muscle cells and are not encapsulated. Adenomyomas can also extend into the endometrial cavity in the form of a polyp.
Endometriosis	The presence of endometrial cells outside the endometrium. The hallmark of the disorder is cyclic pelvic pain. These estrogen-sensitive lesions can be treated with NSAIDs, OCPs, progestins, GnRH agonists, or surgery.
Endometrioma	A cystic collection of endometrial cells on the ovary; also known as "chocolate cysts."
Leiomyoma	Local proliferations of smooth muscle cells within the uterus, often surrounded by a psuedocapsule. Also known as fibroids, these benign growths may be located on the intramural, subsurosal, or submucosal portion of the uterus.

MRI is then used if adenomyosis is suggested by pelvic ultrasound. Ultimately, hysterectomy is the only definitive means of diagnosing adenomyosis.

Differential Diagnosis

The differential diagnosis for adenomyosis includes disease processes resulting in uterine enlargement, menorrhagia, and/or dysmenorrhea including uterine fibroids, polyps, menstrual disorders, endometrial hyperplasia, endometrial cancer, pregnancy, and adnexal masses.

Treatment

The treatment for adenomyosis depends on the severity of the dysmenorrhea and menorrhagia. Women with minimal symptoms or those near menopause may be managed with analgesics alone. Nonsteroidal anti-inflammatory drugs (NSAIDs), oral contraceptive pills (OCPs), and menstrual suppression with progestins or continuous OCPs have also been found to be helpful.

Hysterectomy is the only definitive treatment for adenomyosis. It is particularly important to distinguish adenomyosis from uterine fibroids. If adenomyosis is mistaken for uterine fibroids, a surgeon attempting a myomectomy may find only diffuse adenomyosis and perform a hysterectomy instead. Endometrial biopsy should be performed to rule out concomitant endometrial carcinoma before a hysterectomy is performed for adenomyosis.

KEY POINTS

1. Adenomyosis is the extension of endometrial tissue into the myometrium, making the uterus symmetrically enlarged and globular.
2. It occurs in 15% of women, most of whom are parous and in their late 30s or early 40s.
3. Fifteen percent of women with adenomyosis also have endometriosis and 50% will also have uterine fibroids.
4. Patients typically present with increasing secondary dysmenorrhea and/or menorrhagia; 30% of patients are asymptomatic.
5. Patients presenting with dyspareunia, dyschezia, and metrorrhagia have an increased probability of having adenomyosis.
6. Minimal symptoms may be treated with analgesics, NSAIDs, OCPs, or progestins.
7. Hysterectomy is the only definitive treatment for adenomyosis.

Infections of the Lower Female Reproductive Tract

■ URINARY TRACT INFECTIONS

One of the most common infections of the lower genitourinary tract treated by clinicians is the common **urinary tract infection** (UTI). Women commonly present with symptoms of urethritis (discomfort or pain at the urethral meatus or a burning sensation throughout the urethra with micturition) or cystitis (pain in the midline suprapubic region, and/or frequent urination). UTIs are most common in sexually active women, and increased in women with diabetes mellitus and sickle-cell disease. They are diagnosed at a rate of about 1% per year in adult women, although the true rate of occurrence is most likely higher. The rates are higher in women than men secondary to the shorter length of the urethra and its proximity to the vagina and rectum.

Diagnosis

When a woman presents with dysuria and urinary frequency, the diagnosis of UTI should lead the differential. The urine can be sent for urinalysis and sediment. A high prevalence of leukocytes or leukocyte esterase in the absence of a vaginal infection is indicative of a UTI. If the sediment has a high bacterial count without the presence of inflammatory cells, this is most likely contamination. To distinguish contamination from true infection, the urinalysis and sediment can be repeated with urine collected via catheterization. Patients are often diagnosed and treated for UTI in the setting of a positive urinalysis with concomitant symptoms of dysuria and urinary frequency once **pyelonephritis** is ruled out by checking for costovertebral angle tenderness (CVAT). The

diagnosis can be confirmed with a urine culture. The common organisms that cause UTIs include bacteria that colonize the GI tract such as *E. coli* and *S. saprophyticus*. Other common organisms that cause UTIs are *P. mirabilis*, *K. pneumoniae*, and *Enterococcus*. If the urine culture is negative, the diagnosis should be reconsidered. In patients with symptoms consistent with urethritis, organisms such as *C. trachomatis* and *N. gonorrhoeae* should be considered and screened for using a midstream collection. Another etiology of urethritis is herpes simplex virus (HSV) infection. In patients with symptoms of cystitis, but a negative culture, the diagnosis of interstitial cystitis should be entertained.

Treatment

Most uncomplicated UTIs can be treated with oral antibiotics. It is important to both begin treatment on initial diagnosis as well as follow-up culture sensitivities to be certain the pathologic organisms are covered. Initial treatment is often begun with ampicillin, trimethoprim-sulfamethoxazole, macrodantin, or cephalexin. However, the local sensitivities of common organisms should be known. For example, the rates of ampicillin-resistant *E. coli* can vary between 5% to 35% in different hospitals. More aggressive treatment of UTIs may use fluoroquinolones such as ciprofloxacin. Patients with symptoms consistent with pyelonephritis are usually admitted and treated in hospital with IV antibiotics. Outpatient management has been studied and is used increasingly in reliable patients without other medical issues.

THE EXTERNAL ANOGENITAL REGION

Various infectious diseases affect the external genitalia. In the female patient, the entire perianal area and mons should be considered in addition to the vulva. The skin overlying these areas is subject to the same infections that can occur anywhere on the epidermis, but the exposure and environment differ and must be considered when discussing these infections. There are also a variety of focal and systemic processes that can cause lesions or symptoms in this region. Anogenital lesions are usually categorized as ulcerative or nonulcerative, and common symptoms include pain and itching.

VULVITIS

The most common cause of vulvitis, and usually of vulvar pruritus, is **candidiasis**. It is also a common cause of vaginitis and is discussed in greater detail later in this chapter. A candidal vulvitis usually presents with vulvar erythema, pruritus, and small satellite lesions. If the vulvitis does not respond to the usual treatment with topical or systemic antifungals, symptoms may be due to other causes such as allergic reaction, chemical or fabric irritants, and vulvar dystrophies. Malignancy should always be ruled out in the setting of chronic vulvar irritation.

ULCERATED LESIONS

Many primary vulvar ulcers are caused by sexually transmitted diseases (STDs) (Table 16-1) such as **herpes, syphilis, chancroid**, and **lymphogranuloma venereum**. However, even with a diagnosis of an infectious process, these lesions can be associated with malignant processes as well.

There are conditions other than infections that can lead to vulvar ulcerations. Crohn's disease can have linear "knife cut" vulvar ulcers as its first manifestation, preceding gastrointestinal or other systemic manifestations by months to years. Behçet's disease leads to tender and highly destructive vulvar lesions that often cause fenestrations in the labia and extensive scarring.

Syphilis

The spirochete *Treponema pallidum* causes the chronic systemic infection of **syphilis**. It is transmitted primarily through sexual contact. The incidence of primary and secondary syphilis in the United States increased through the 1980s until 1990, when the CDC noted a peak of 50,578 reported cases followed by a sharp decline to 8550 cases reported in 1997 and only 5979 cases reported in 2000. During this time, there was a concomitant decrease in latent syphilis as well, although at a slower rate of decline. Currently, the incidence is decreasing in both het-

TABLE 16-1

Infectious Causes of Ulcerated Lesions

	Syphilis	Herpes	Chancroid	LGV
Incubation period	7–14 days	2–10 days	4–7 days	3–12 days
Primary lesion	Papule	Vesicle	Papule/pustule	Papule/vesicle
Number of lesions	Single	Multiple	1–3, occasionally more	Single
Size	5–15 mm	1–3 mm	2–20 mm	2–10 mm
Painful	No	Yes	Yes	No
Diagnostic test	Dark-field microscopy RPR/MHA-TP/FTA-ABS	Viral culture	Gram's stain with "school of fish" appearance	Complement fixation
Treatment	Penicillin	Acyclovir	Ceftriaxone or azithromycin	Doxycycline

erosexual men and women with a decline among the gay population as well, likely secondary to increased safe sexual practices directed at decreasing human immunodeficiency virus (HIV) transmission.

T. pallidum most likely enters the body through minute abrasions in the skin or mucosal surface and replicates locally. Initial lesions therefore commonly occur on the vulva, vagina, cervix, anus, nipples, or lips. The initial lesion that characterizes the primary stage is a painless, red, round, firm ulcer approximately 1 cm in size with raised edges known as a **chancre** (Figure 16-1). It develops approximately 3 weeks after inoculation and is usually associated with concomitant regional adenopathy. Material expressed from the chancre usually reveals motile spirochetes under dark-field microscopy.

The secondary stage of syphilis occurs as *T. pallidum* disseminates. Between 1 and 3 months after the primary stage resolves, the secondary stage appears as a maculopapular rash and/or moist papules on the skin or mucous membranes. Classically, the rash appears on the palms of the hands or soles of the feet. The dermatologic manifestations of secondary syphilis is why syphilis is known as the "great imitator." There may be other organ system involvement with meningitis, nephritis, or hepatitis.

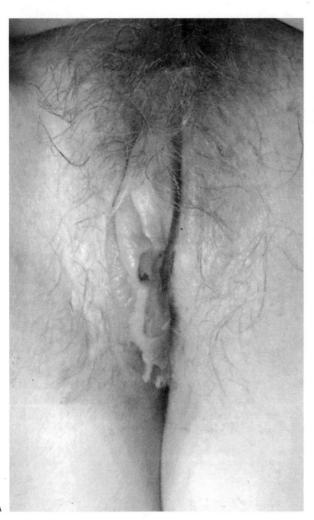
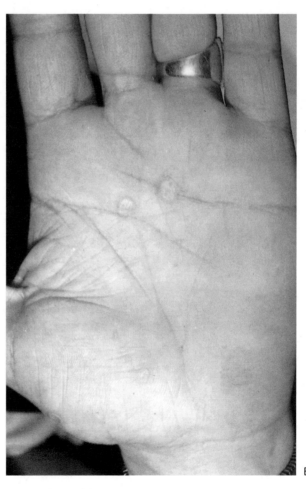

A

B

Figure 16-1 • A: Slightly indurated primary chancre of 2-days' duration that was neither painful nor tender. It points to the need for a high index of suspicion concerning all genital lesions. Dark-filled microscopy prevents diagnostic error and embarrassment. B: Papulosquamous secondary syphilis involving the palm. C: Typical coppery-red papules in secondary syphilis. D: Healing gumma. Delay in diagnosis is suggested by widespread pigmentation and scarring. Response to treatment was slow and the final scarring led to permanent edema of the foot, sometimes called "paradoxical healing."
(Reproduced with permission from Champion RH. Textbook of Dermatology. 5th ed. Oxford: Blackwell Science, 1992:2852.)

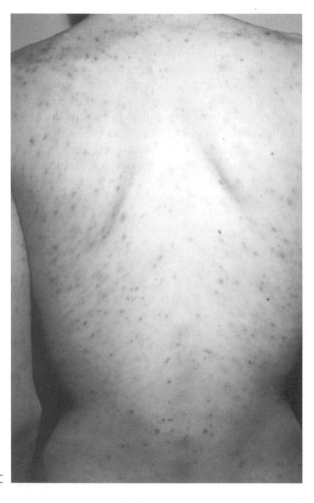

C

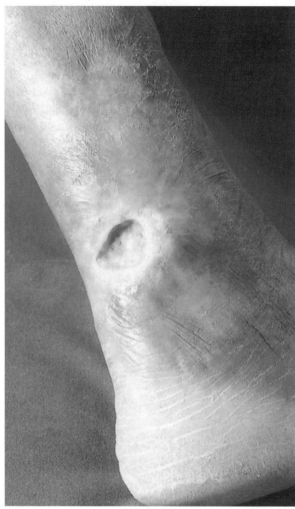

D

Figure 16-1 • *Continued.*

All lesions resolve spontaneously, and this stage can be entirely asymptomatic. After resolution of this stage, the infection enters a latent phase that can last for years.

Tertiary syphilis is quite uncommon today but is characterized by granulomas (gummas) of the skin and bones; cardiovascular syphilis with aortitis; and neurosyphilis with meningovascular disease, paresis, and tabes dorsalis.

Diagnosis

T. pallidum is commonly screened for via a nonspecific antibody test. Either the rapid plasmin reagin (RPR) or the Venereal Disease Research Laboratory (VDRL) test can be used as a screening test. The diagnosis is confirmed with more specific testing: either the microhemagglutination assay for antibod-

ies to *T. pallidum* (MHATP) or the fluorescent treponemal antibody-absorption (FTAABS) technique. False-positive results in these latter two tests occur less than 1% of the time. Primary, secondary, tertiary, and neurosyphilis can be diagnosed by the presenting signs and symptoms described above. However, patients who are asymptomatic with a positive titer are considered to be in early (less than 1 year) or late latency.

Treatment

Penicillin is still the drug of choice when treating syphilis. Early syphilis can be treated with benzathine penicillin G, 2.4 million units intramuscularly one time. For syphilis of more than 1-year's duration, the same dose can be given weekly for 3 weeks. Alternative regimens to penicillin include IV ceftriaxone given QOD for 10 days, and tetracycline 500 mg orally QID or doxycycline 100 mg orally BID for two to four weeks.

Neurosyphilis is a more serious infection and requires aqueous crystalline penicillin G, 2–4 million units intravenously every 4 hours for 10 to 14 days, followed by three weekly doses of benzathine penicillin. There is no recommended treatment alternative for neurosyphilis. Patients with a penicillin allergy will therefore require desensitization. Treatment success can be verified by following RPR or VDRL titers, which should decline fourfold in 3 to 6 months.

Of note, two to eight hours after administering treatment for syphilis, patients may experience malaise, fever, headache, pharyngitis, and/or rash. This is the Jarisch-Herxheimer reaction that was initially recognized in the treatment of neurosyphilis, but can be seen with any syphilitic treatment, most commonly with secondary syphilis. This reaction is not considered a drug reaction, but related to the treatment of syphilis, and can be seen with the treatment of other spirochetes as well, such as Lyme disease.

KEY POINTS

1. A painless chancre is the initial lesion of syphilis.
2. Syphilis is screened for with the RPR and VDRL tests and confirmed with either the MHATP or FTAABS.
3. Benzathine penicillin is the drug of choice for treating syphilis. Neurosyphilis requires intravenous penicillin.
4. Patients being treated for syphilis may experience the Jarisch-Herxheimer reaction, seen most commonly in treatment of secondary syphilis.

Genital Herpes

HSV infections are quite common in the perioral and genital regions. Although only about 5% of women report a history of genital herpes infection, as many as 25% to 30% test antibody positive. Although some women have the classic "severe" presentation of genital herpes with painful genital ulcers, many women have a mild initial presentation or are entirely asymptomatic. Because of the asymptomatic nature of many initial presentations it is difficult to get an estimate on the true incidence of disease;

however, there has been a steady increase in patient visits to a physician for herpes over the past two decades, with approximately 200,000 office visits in 2000. In those individuals with a history of genital herpes, the causative organism is shown to be HSV-2 in approximately 63% and HSV-1 in the remaining 37% of cases. Initial infections usually begin with flu-like symptoms including malaise, myalgias, nausea, diarrhea, and fever. Vulvar burning and pruritus precede the multiple vesicles that appear next and usually remain intact for 24 to 36 hours before evolving into painful genital ulcers (Figure 16-2). These ulcers can require a mean of 10 to 22 days to heal. After this initial herpes outbreak, recurrent episodes can occur as frequently as one to six times per year. Because of the possibility of frequent recurrence and the devastating consequences of neonatal herpes, pregnant women should have vaginal examinations around the time of delivery. Those with lesions should be delivered via cesarean section.

Diagnosis

Diagnosis is made clinically with an examination of the vesicles and ulcers in conjunction with a sexual history. A **Tzanck smear** can be made from one of the lesions and examined for multinucleated giant cells with a characteristic appearance. Viral cultures are used as the gold standard for diagnosis, and specific antibody titers may be used to determine whether the patient has a primary infection as well as the serotype of the causative organism.

Treatment

Although many palliative treatments have evolved over the years such as sitz baths for comfort and analgesics to reduce the pain, there is no "cure" for

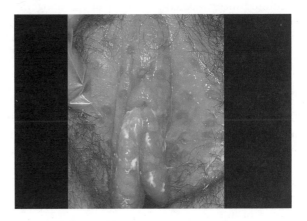

Figure 16-2 • Genital herpes.

herpes. For a **primary infection**, acyclovir 200 mg five times per day or 400 mg TID can reduce the length of infection and the length of time a patient has viral shedding. With severe HSV infections, such as those that occur in immunocompromised patients, intravenous acyclovir should be used at a dose of 5 mg/kg every 8 hours. For individuals with frequent recurrences, prophylactic or suppression therapy of 400 mg orally QD can be used. Alternate antiviral medications such as valacyclovir are also used, particularly if there is a concern for resistance in patients who have been on acyclovir suppression.

KEY POINTS

1. Genital herpes infections are caused by HSV-2 63% of the time; the remaining 37% are caused by HSV-1.
2. Herpes classically appears as multiple vesicles that develop into painful ulcers.
3. Treatment is usually palliative, although acyclovir can reduce the length of primary infection and suppressive therapy may decrease the number of recurrences.

Chancroid

Chancroid is caused by **Haemophilus ducreyi**. Globally, it is a common STD, although the incidence in North America has declined steadily since 1987, with just 78 reported cases in 2000. Reported cases are likely to grossly underestimate true incidence since *H. ducreyi* is difficult to culture. Males are affected more than females by ratios of 3:1 to 25:1.

Chancroid appears as a painful, demarcated, nonindurated ulcer located anywhere in the anogenital region. There is often concomitant painful inguinal lymphadenopathy. Usually, just a single ulcer is present, but multiple ulcers and occasionally extragenital infections have been known to occur.

Diagnosis

Diagnosis is a problem because *H. ducreyi* is difficult to culture. Often, transporting the culture swab in Amies or Stuart transport media or chocolate agar can aid in the culture. Direct Gram's stains have not been a consistent method of diagnosis. The diagnosis is therefore often made clinically by ruling out other sources of infection.

Treatment

Treatment regimens include ceftriaxone 250 mg intramuscularly once, azithromycin 1 g orally once, or erythromycin 500 mg QID for 7 days. Alternative regimens include ciprofloxacin 500 mg orally BID for 3 days or Bactrim DS 1 tablet orally BID for 7 days. As with most other STDs, sexual partners should be treated as well.

KEY POINTS

1. Chancroid manifests as a painful genital ulcer and, usually, concomitant lymphadenopathy.
2. Chancroid is difficult to diagnose and neither cultures nor Gram's stains have been particularly consistent.
3. Treatment regimens can include a variety of antibiotics; the simplest are single doses of PO azithromycin or IM ceftriaxone.

Lymphogranuloma Venereum

The L-serotypes of *Chlamydia trachomatis* can cause the systemic disease **lymphogranuloma venereum** (LGV). The primary stage of this illness is often a local lesion that may be either a papule or a shallow ulcer, and is often painless, transient, and can go unnoticed. The secondary stage (inguinal syndrome) is characterized by painful inflammation and enlargement of the inguinal nodes. Systemic manifestations include fever, headaches, malaise, and anorexia. The tertiary stage (anogenital syndrome) of this disease is characterized by proctocolitis, rectal stricture, rectovaginal fistula, and elephantiasis. Initially, an anal pruritus will develop with a concomitant mucous rectal discharge.

Treatment

Treatment of LGV is with doxycycline, 100 mg orally BID for 21 days. With persistent illness, the antibiotic regimen can be repeated. If the external genitalia and rectum are disfigured and scarred, surgical measures may be required.

■ NONULCERATIVE LESIONS

One of the most common nonulcerative lesions is the condyloma (Figure 16-3). **Condyloma acuminata** are

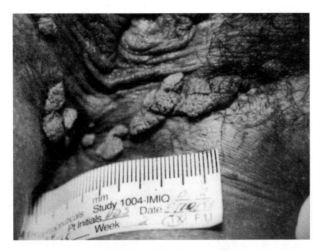

Figure 16-3 • Extensive external condylomata acuminata. These fleshy, exophytic growths are covered with small, papillary surface projections. Some of the lesions are pedunculated; others are sessile.
(Reproduced with permission from Blackwell RE. Women's Medicine. Blackwell Science, 1996:317.)

"warty" lesions that occur anywhere in the anogenital region and are considered a STD. Other nonulcerative lesions include **molluscum contagiosum**, caused by a pox virus; and lesions caused by **Phthirus pubis**, the crab louse, and **Sarcoptes scabiei**, the itch mite.

Finally, when considering nonulcerative lesions, folliculitis should always be included in the differential diagnosis because the skin in the pubic region has hair follicles. In rare cases, folliculitis can lead to larger lesions such as boils, carbuncles, and abscesses. The usual source of these infections is skin flora, primarily *Staphylococcus aureus*. Factors contributing to these lesions in the anogenital region include tight undergarments, sanitary pads, poor hygiene, diabetes, and immunosuppression.

Human Papillomavirus

The most clinically evident results of infection with human papillomavirus (HPV) are **condyloma acuminata** or **genital warts**. The annual incidence of genital warts is estimated to be over 1:1000. However, of more significance in terms of morbidity and mortality, HPV is associated with cervical cancer and other squamous cell malignancies of the female and male reproductive tracts. It is estimated that the incidence of HPV has been increasing in the United States, with an estimated prevalence between 20% to 45%. It is clearly a STD with 60% to 80% of partners being affected.

Although genital warts often occur throughout the lower reproductive tract, patients usually present with anogenital lesions that they have identified or that have become pruritic or caused bleeding. Condyloma acuminata are most commonly caused by serotypes 6 and 11, whereas cervical cancer is more often associated with serotypes 16, 18, and 31.

Diagnosis

Diagnosis of condyloma acuminata is usually made via clinical examination. The wart has a raised papillomatous or spiked surface. Initially, the lesions are small, 1–5 mm diameter lesions, but these can evolve into larger pedunculated lesions and eventually into cauliflower-like growths, particularly in immunocompromised patients. In addition to the vulva, perineal body, and anogenital region, these lesions can also arise in the anal canal, on the walls of the vagina, and on the cervix. When uncertain of diagnosis or for lesions that are unresponsive to therapy, a biopsy of the lesion can be made for definitive diagnosis.

Treatment

Treatment of the lesions includes local excision, cryotherapy, topical trichloroacetic acid, topical 25% podophyllin, and 5-fluorouracil cream (Efudex 5%). The medical treatments are usually repeated weekly by the clinician until all lesions are gone. For motivated patients with uncomplicated condyloma that can be reached, both imiquimod (Aldara) and podofilox (Condylox) can be used. Imiquimod is used three times per week and needs to be washed off after 6 to 10 hours, whereas podofilox is applied BID for 3 days and left in place. These patients can self-treat and follow-up with clinicians every 3 to 4 weeks until the lesions have resolved. For larger condylomas or those unresponsive to medical treatment, the CO_2 laser may be used to vaporize the lesion. Regardless of treatment modality, a recurrence rate of approximately 20% is seen in all patients.

KEY POINTS

1. HPV causes condylomata but, more seriously, is correlated with cervical cancer.
2. Genital warts are usually diagnosed by appearance but can be confirmed with biopsy.
3. Treatment is usually with cryotherapy or topical medications; larger lesions are usually excised or vaporized with the CO_2 laser.

Molluscum Contagiosum

Molluscum contagiosum is caused by a pox virus that is spread via close contact with an infected person or via autoinoculation. The lesion is a small, 1–5 mm, domed papule with an umbilicated center (Figure 16-4). Also known as "water warts," these lesions contain a waxy material that reveals intracytoplasmic molluscum bodies under microscopic examination when stained with Wright's stain or Giemsa stain. Molluscum lesions can occur anywhere on the skin except on the palms of the hands and soles of the feet. These lesions are often asymptomatic and generally resolve on their own. These can be removed via local excision and/or treatment of the nodule base with trichloroacetic acid or cryotherapy.

Phthirus pubis and *Sarcoptes scabiei*

The nonulcerative lesions caused by **Phthirus pubis**, the crab louse; and **Sarcoptes scabiei**, the itch mite, are similar. Signs and symptoms of these two infections include pruritis, irritated skin, vesicles, and burrows. The primary difference is that lesions from *P. pubis*, or **pediculosis**, are usually confined to the pubic hair, whereas **scabies** may spread throughout the entire body. Thus, when treating with lindane (Kwell) shampoo, pediculosis can be cured with application to specific areas, whereas it is more effective to treat scabies by using lindane lotion over the entire body.

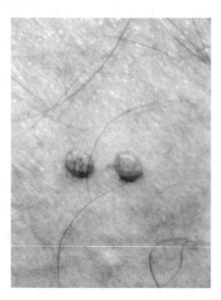

Figure 16-4 • Two typical molluscum lesions, one of which shows a mosaic appearance.

■ VAGINAL INFECTIONS

Symptoms related to vaginal infections are the leading cause of visits to a gynecologist. The vagina provides a warm, moist environment that can be colonized by various organisms. When anything upsets the balance of microflora in the vagina such as antibiotics, diet, systemic illness, or the introduction of a pathogen, overgrowth of one variety of organism can lead to symptoms including itching, pain, discharge, burning, and odor. Common organisms that cause symptoms with overgrowth include *Candida* (Figure 16-5) and *Gardnerella*; the most common pathogenic protozoan is *Trichomonas*. These can each be easily diagnosed and treated quite effectively with antimicrobials. However, any chronic vaginitis with pruritis, pain, bleeding, and/or ulcerated lesions that do not respond to drug therapy should be investigated to rule out malignancy.

Bacterial Vaginosis

The vagina is commonly colonized with multiple bacteria, predominantly *Lactobacillus* sp. that generally maintain the vaginal pH below 4. **Bacterial vaginosis** (BV) can develop when there is a shift in the predominant bacterial species in the vagina. Although bacterial vaginosis is likely to be polymicrobial, one of the most common organisms present in culture is *Gardnerella vaginalis*. BV is quite common and is the leading cause of vaginitis, with prevalence rates of 5% of college populations and as high as 60% in STD clinics. Risk factors include lower

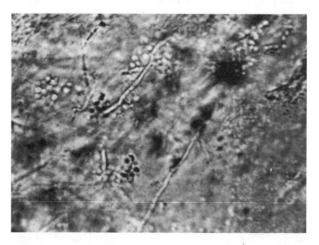

Figure 16-5 • *Candida albicans*, KOH mount of skin scraping. (Reproduced with permission from Crissey JT. Manual of Medical Mycology. Boston: Blackwell Science, 1995:90.)

socioeconomic status, IUD usage, multiple sexual partners, and smoking. BV is particularly concerning during pregnancy, where it has been associated with preterm birth.

Diagnosis

Many patients with BV may be asymptomatic or have an isolated increase in vaginal discharge. However, symptomatic patients complain of a profuse nonirritating discharge, often with a malodorous "fishy" amine odor. Diagnosis is made most commonly with microscopic examination of a wet prep of a vaginal swab that has an elevated pH of 5–6 and reveals clue cells (Figure 16-6). These are vaginal epithelial cells that are diffusely covered with bacteria. The amine odor of bacterial vaginosis can be enhanced by adding KOH to a vaginal prep (**the whiff test**), and this is considered pathognomonic.

Vaginal cultures can also be performed and may often reveal G. vaginalis, Bacteroides and other anaerobes. However, the clinical diagnosis is usually made from vaginal preps.

Treatment

Treatment of BV is usually with either metronidazole 500 mg orally BID for 7 days or clindamycin 300 mg TID for 7 days. Both antibiotics are also available in gel or cream and can be used topically. It has been found that using 375 mg instead of 500 mg of metronidazole is as effective, and has fewer GI side effects. A 2 g single dose therapy has been studied. However, it is less than 75% effective in BV when compared to 85% to 90% cure rates for the week-long treatment. Patients need to be reminded of metronidazole's antabuse effect when taken with alcohol.

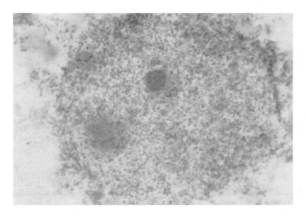

Figure 16-6 • Bacterial vaginosis.

KEY POINTS

1. Bacterial vaginosis is polymicrobial but usually attributed to *Gardnerella*.
2. The discharge is usually thin, yellow, and has a characteristic "fishy" amine odor; the whiff test exaggerates this odor with KOH.
3. Formal diagnosis is made by visualizing clue cells on wet prep.
4. First-line treatment is metronidazole (Flagyl) for a 7-day course.

Yeast Infections

Candidiasis probably causes 30% of the vaginitis that leads women to be seen by a gynecologist. Many more of these infections are treated by women using over-the-counter (OTC) preparations. Candidiasis is caused by *Candida albicans* in 80% to 90% of all cases, with the remaining cases caused by other candidal species. Predisposing factors for candidal overgrowth include the use of broad-spectrum antibiotics, diabetes mellitus, and decreased cellular immunity as seen in AIDS patients or those on immunosuppressive therapies. Yeast infections are also associated with intercourse and may increase during the late luteal phase of the menstrual cycle.

Diagnosis

Typical symptoms of genital candidiasis include vulvar and vaginal pruritus, burning, dysuria, dyspareunia, and vaginal discharge. On physical examination there is vulvar edema and erythema with a scant vaginal discharge. Only approximately 20% of patients display the characteristic white plaques adherent to the vaginal mucosa or the cottage cheese–like discharge. Diagnosis is usually made by microscopic examination of a KOH prep of the vaginal discharge that reveals characteristic branching hyphae and spores as well as a vaginal pH of 4–5. Although the KOH preparation is estimated to have a sensitivity of 25% to 80%, the Gram's stain is almost 100% sensitive for yeast infections. The most sensitive test is culture on Sabouraud's agar. Clinically, treatment is often instituted on the basis of clinical signs and symptoms.

Treatment

Treatment includes any of the azole agents via topical applications, typically Monistat-7 as an OTC preparation or terazole cream by prescription. Nystatin suppositories or powder may prove to be effective as well. Other local therapies include boric acid capsules 600 mg every day for 2 weeks or the application of 1% aqueous solution of gentian violet. More recently, fluconazole (Diflucan) 150 mg orally once has been shown to be as effective as any of the local treatments. For chronic recurring candidal infections, ketoconazole 400 mg orally every day for 1 to 2 weeks has been shown to be effective.

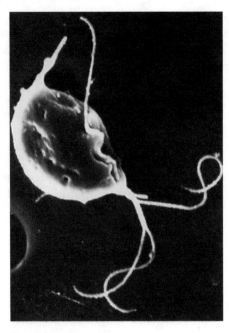

Figure 16-7 • Scanning electron micrograph of *Trichomonal vaginalis*. The undulating membrane and flagella of *Trichomonas* are its characteristic features.
(Reproduced with permission from Cox FEG, ed. Modern Parasitology: A Textbook of Parasitology. 2nd ed. Oxford: Blackwell Science, 1993:9.)

KEY POINTS

1. As with vulvitis, the number one cause of vaginitis is *Candida*.
2. Diagnosis is often made with a wet prep (trich and BV) or KOH prep (yeast).
3. In the absence of microscopic evidence, symptoms and type of discharge should dictate the treatment.

Trichomonas vaginalis

Trichomonas vaginalis is a unicellular, anaerobic flagellated protozoan that can cause vaginitis. It inhabits the lower genitourinary tracts of women and men, and there are approximately 3 million cases diagnosed annually in the United States. The disease is sexually transmitted, with 75% of sexual partners possessing positive cultures.

Diagnosis

The signs and symptoms of *T. vaginalis* include a profuse discharge with an unpleasant odor. The discharge may be yellow, gray, or green in coloration and may be frothy in appearance. Vaginal pH is in the 6–7 range. Vulvar erythema, edema, and pruritus can also be noted. The characteristic erythematous, punctate epithelial papillae, or "strawberry" appearance of the cervix is apparent in only 10% of cases. Symptoms are usually worse immediately after menses because of the transient increase in vaginal pH at that time.

Diagnosis of *Trichomonas* is made via microscopic examination of wet preps of vaginal swabs. The protozoan is slightly larger than a white blood cell with three to five flagella. Often, active movement of the flagella and propulsion of the organism can be seen (Figure 16-7). The diagnosis can be confirmed when necessary with culture, but this is not commonly used.

Treatment

The mainstay of treatment for *T. vaginalis* infections is metronidazole (Flagyl) 2 g orally in a single dose. As opposed to BV, this regimen has been found to be as effective as the more traditional 250 mg orally TID for 7 days. An alternative treatment to metronidazole is clotrimazole cream topically for 7 days. However, it is unclear whether this regimen is particularly effective. Because of the high rate of concomitant infections in sexual partners, both partners should be treated to prevent reinfection.

KEY POINTS

1. Seventy-five percent of sexual partners of those with *Trichomonas* will also be colonized and should be presumptively treated.
2. Diagnosis is made via wet prep, but is usually presumed with a profuse, malodorous, gray-green, frothy discharge.
3. Treatment is metronidazole 2 g orally one time.

■ INFECTIONS OF THE CERVIX

The organisms that most commonly cause cervicitis and infections of the upper reproductive tract differ from those that most commonly cause infections of the lower reproductive tract. **Neisseria gonorrhoeae** and **Chlamydia trachomatis** are the two most common organisms that cause cervicitis and the only organisms shown to cause mucopurulent cervicitis. Clinically, cervicitis is diagnosed as cervical motion tenderness in the absence of other signs of pelvic inflammatory disease (PID).

Other organisms can cause infections of the cervix including HSV, HPV, mycoplasma hominis, and ureaplasma ureolyticum. HSV causes either herpes lesions or a white plaque that resembles cervical cancer. Infection with HPV leads to condyloma and is thought to be an etiology of cervical cancer. Neither mycoplasma nor ureoplasma has been shown to be correlated with active disease, but may cause nonmucopurulent cervicitis and bacterial vaginosis.

Neisseria gonorrhoeae

Despite a 50% decrease in incidence in the 1990s, gonococcal infections remain the second-leading reported STDs in the United States, with approximately 360,000 cases reported in 2000. Most cases occur in the 15- to 29-year-old age group. Among sexually active women, 15- to 19-year-olds have two times the incidence of 20- to 24-year-olds. However, the highest overall prevalence is in the 20- to 24-year-old age group because this group includes the highest percentage of sexually active individuals.

Multiple risk factors have been associated with gonococcal infections, including low socioeconomic status, urban residence, nonwhite and non-Asian ethnicity, early age of first sexual activity, illicit drug use, prostitution, being unmarried, and previous gonococcal infections. Condoms, diaphragms, and spermicides decrease the risk of transmission. There are also seasonal variations in the incidence of gonorrhea in the United States with a peak observed in late summer.

Transmission between the sexes is unequal, with male-to-female transmission estimated at 80% to 90% compared to an estimated 20% to 25% female-to male-transmission rate after a single sexual encounter. This difference in transmission is most likely related to the type of epithelium exposed in the different sexes. In males, the external surface of the penis is primarily keratinized epithelium, whereas females receive primary contact with mucosa of the vagina and the nonkeratinized epithelium of the cervix. Further, male ejaculation increases the amount of exposure time in women, which supports the use of condoms as an exceptional prophylactic measure against gonococcal transmission.

Gonococcus can infect the anal canal, the urethra, the oropharynx, and Bartholin glands, in addition to the more commonly reported cervicitis, PID, or tupoovarian abscess (TOA). Gonococcal exposure in neonates can cause conjunctivitis. As many as 1% of recognized gonococcal infections may proceed to a disseminated infection. This infection begins with fevers and erythematous macular skin lesions and proceeds to a tenosynovitis and septic arthritis.

Diagnosis

Identification of the causative organism, *N. gonorrhoeae*, a gram-negative diplococcus resembling paired kidney beans, is necessary for definitive diagnosis. Isolation using the modified Thayer-Martin chocolate agar has a sensitivity of 96% in endocervical cultures. Recently, many hospitals and health care facilities have begun using a gonococcal DNA probe similar to that used to diagnose *Chlamydia*.

Treatment

The recommended treatment is ceftriaxone 250 mg intramuscularly once. Therapy should be followed by a week-long course of doxycycline 100 mg orally BID or a 1 g dose of azithromycin to treat likely concomitant chlamydial infections. Ofloxacin may be used as a single agent to treat both organisms and, recently, a 2 g dose of azithromycin has been shown to be effective against gonorrhea.

KEY POINTS

1. *N. gonorrhoeae* causes a reported 2 million infections per year.
2. Common conditions caused include cervicitis, PID, TOA, and Bartholin abscess.
3. Diagnosis can be made with culture, Gram's stain, or DNA probe.
4. Treatment for uncomplicated infections is ceftriaxone 250 mg intramuscularly once.
5. Treatment for *N. gonorrhoeae* should always include doxycycline 100 mg orally BID for 1 week to treat likely concomitant chlamydial infections.

Chlamydia trachomatis

Chlamydia trachomatis is a pathogen that causes ocular, respiratory, and reproductive tract infections. In the United States, its transmission is primarily via sexual contact, although vertical transmission from a mother to a newborn is also seen. Interestingly, while there has been a decrease in reported gonococcal infections through the year 2000, reported chlamydial infections have increased to over 700,000. This is most likely secondary to the advent of a genetic probe that uses polymerase chain reaction (PCR) enhancement of the DNA for *C. trachomatis* (traditionally difficult to diagnose because they are obligate intracellular organisms and culture poorly) and aggressive screening programs of sexually active women. Prevalence is estimated at 3% to 5% in asymptomatic women, and 5% to 7% of pregnant women have had positive chlamydiazyme tests. Epidemiologically, *C. trachomatis* infections are parallel to those of *N. gonorrhoeae*, with higher rates seen among women age 15–29, with earlier age of first coitus, and greater number of sexual partners.

Another reason for the higher prevalence of chlamydial infections is that carriers of both sexes are often entirely asymptomatic. This is particularly unfortunate in women, in whom chronic infections may lead to scarring in the fallopian tubes that may result in infertility or increased risk of ectopic pregnancies. Common sites of infection include the endocervix, urethra, and rectum. Clinical manifestations of symptomatic chlamydial infections are often quite similar to those of *N. gonorrhoeae* and include symptoms of cervicitis, urethritis, and PID. As previously discussed, the L-serotypes of *C. trachomatis* can cause the systemic disease LGV.

Treatment

Treatment of choice for chlamydial infections is doxycycline 100 mg orally BID for 1 week or a one-time 1 g dose of azithromycin. Alternative regimens include tetracycline 500 mg orally QID or, for the pregnant patient, erythromycin 500 mg orally QID. For LGV, the treatment regimen should be extended to 3 weeks. When treating chlamydial infections, most physicians treat *N. gonorrhoeae* concomitantly with a single intramuscular injection of 250 mg ceftriaxone.

KEY POINTS

1. Chlamydial infections tend to coincide with gonococcal infections. However, the incidence of gonococcal infections has decreased, whereas the incidence of chlamydial infections has increased.
2. Many chlamydial infections are entirely asymptomatic.
3. Treatment is with doxycycline 100 mg BID; alternatively, a one-time 1 g dose of azithromycin can be used.
4. LGV is caused by the L-serotypes of *Chlamydia*.

Upper Female Reproductive Tract and Systemic Infections

■ THE UPPER FEMALE REPRODUCTIVE TRACT

The main reason why women—not men—experience upper reproductive tract, pelvic, and abdominal infections is the absence of a mucosal lining or epithelium between these spaces and the external body. Although defenses such as ciliary movement creating flow and cervical mucous exist, there is essentially an open tract between the vagina, the pelvis, and abdomen. This can lead to ascending infections of the uterus, fallopian tubes, adnexae, pelvis, and abdomen. This open ascending tract may also lead to the acquisition of toxic shock syndrome (TSS). Further, because the vaginal epithelium is easily abraded during intercourse, transmission of systemic infections such as human immunodeficiency virus (HIV) and hepatitis B and C is more common from men to women than the converse.

■ ENDOMETRITIS

Pathogenesis

Endometritis is an infection of the uterine endometrium; if the infection invades into the myometrium, it is known as **endomyometritis**. Endometritis and endomyometritis are usually preceded by instrumentation or disruption of the intrauterine cavity. It is seen most commonly after cesarean section, but also after vaginal deliveries, dilation and evacuation (D&E), dilation and curettage (D&C), and intrauterine device (IUD) placement. Nonpuerperal endometritis is not commonly recognized but is probably coexistent with 70% to 80% of

pelvic inflammatory disease (PID). Its etiology is related to ascent of infection from the cervix, which then proceeds to the fallopian tubes to cause acute salpingitis and, eventually, widespread PID. Diagnosis of endomyometritis is made in the clinical settings described above with a bimanual exam revealing uterine tenderness, fever, and elevated white blood cell (WBC) count.

Chronic endometritis is often asymptomatic but is clinically significant because it leads to other pelvic infections and, uncommonly, endomyometritis. It is often a polymicrobial infection with a variety of pathogens, including skin and gastrointestinal flora in addition to the usual flora colonizing the lower reproductive tract. It can be suspected in patients with chronic irregular bleeding, discharge, and pelvic pain. The diagnosis can be made in a nonpuerperal patient with endometrial biopsy showing plasma cells.

Treatment

Treatment of severe endomyometritis is usually clindamycin 900 mg intravenously (IV) every 8 hours and gentamicin loaded with 2 mg/kg IV and then maintained with 1.5 mg/kg IV every 8 hours. Less severe endometritis is often treated with a cephalosporin such as cefoxitin 2 g IV every 6 hours or cefotetan 2 g IV every 12 hours. Treatment course continues until the patient is asymptomatic and/or afebrile for 48 hours. Chronic endometritis is treated with a 3-week course of doxycycline 100 mg PO BID.

■ PELVIC INFLAMMATORY DISEASE (PID)

Acute salpingitis, or more generally **pelvic inflammatory disease** (PID), is the most common serious complication of sexually transmitted diseases (STDs). As many as 1 million cases are estimated to occur annually in the United States. The economic costs of initial treatment are estimated at greater than $3.5 billion, which is in addition to the treatment for the principal sequelae, including infertility and increased ectopic pregnancies. Infertility is estimated to occur in 20% of all PID patients, and the risk of ectopic pregnancy is increased as much as tenfold. Other sequelae, including chronic pelvic pain, dyspareunia, and pelvic adhesions, may also require surgical therapy, contributing to the economic costs and morbidity of this disease.

Among sexually active women, the incidence of this disease is higher in the 15- to 19-year-old age group (three times greater than in the 25- to 29-year-old age group). This may be attributed to higher-risk behavior of this age group. It may also be related to decreased immunity to STD agents in younger women, although the pathophysiology is unclear. Finally, the younger age group is less likely to have regular gynecological care or to seek medical attention until bacterial vaginosis or cervicitis has progressed to the more symptomatic PID (Figure 17-1).

Other risk factors for PID include nonwhite and non-Asian ethnicity, being unmarried, recent history of douching, and cigarette smoking. Barrier contraceptives have been shown to decrease the incidence of PID, whereas IUDs are considered a risk factor for PID.

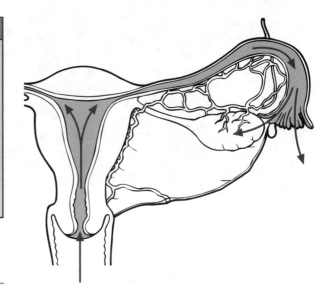

Figure 17-1 • Route of intra-abdominal spread of gonorrhea and other pathogenic bacteria.

Clinical Manifestations

The principal symptom of acute salpingitis is abdominal or pelvic/adnexal pain. The character of the pain can range (burning, cramping, stabbing) and can be unilateral or bilateral. Pain may also be absent in what has been deemed "silent" PID. Other associated symptoms include increased vaginal discharge, abnormal odor, abnormal bleeding, gastrointestinal disturbances, and urinary tract symptoms. Fever is a less common symptom, seen in only 20% of women with PID.

Diagnosis

Diagnosis is made clinically with an elevated WBC count, fever, pelvic pain, cervical motion tenderness, and adnexal tenderness. Cervical cultures are done to find a causative organism but, due to the disease's polymicrobial nature, should not dictate the treatment regimen. The definitive diagnosis is made via laparoscopy. In practice, this is usually performed only when appendicitis cannot be ruled out by clinical examination, although there are several small ongoing trials looking at the effectiveness of laparoscopy under local anesthesia for the diagnosis of PID. Ultrasonography is not useful in the diagnosis of uncomplicated PID. Occasionally, PID is complicated by **Fitzhugh-Curtis syndrome**. This is a perihepatitis from the ascending infection resulting in right upper quadrant pain and tenderness and liver function test (LFT) elevations.

The principal organisms suspected of causing PID are *N. gonorrhoeae* and *C. trachomatis*. However, cultures from the upper reproductive tract have shown that most PID is likely to be polymicrobial, including anaerobic organisms such as *Bacteroides* species and facultative bacteria such as *Gardnerella*, *Escherichia coli*, *H. influenzae*, and streptococci.

Treatment

Because of the high rate of ambulatory treatment failures and the seriousness of sequelae, patients are often hospitalized for treatment of PID, particularly those who are teenagers, unable to tolerate POs, pregnant, noncompliant, or who have been refractory to outpatient therapy. PID is usually treated with a broad-spectrum cephalosporin plus doxycycline because of its polymicrobial nature. A typical regimen is cefoxitin 2 g IV every 6 hours or cefotetan 2 g IV every 12 hours given until the patient is asymptomatic for 48 hours with a concomitant 10- to 14-day course of doxycycline 100 mg orally BID. In patients allergic to cephalosporins, IV clindamycin and gentamicin can be used. On an outpatient basis, ceftriaxone 500 mg IM every day or cefoxitin 2 g IM plus 1 g of probenecid orally along with oral doxycycline is used with close follow-up for resolution of symptoms. PID is rare in pregnant patients; because tetracyclines and fluoroquinolones are contraindicated in pregnancy, clindamycin and gentamicin is the treatment of choice within pregnancy.

KEY POINTS

1. There may be as many as 1 million cases of PID reported annually.
2. Twenty percent of patients with PID will become infertile.
3. PID can be diagnosed with uterine and adnexal tenderness, fever, elevated WBC count, and cultures or tests for gonorrhea and *Chlamydia*.
4. Because of the seriousness of this disease and its sequelae, patients are often hospitalized and treated with IV antibiotics.

■ TUBO-OVARIAN ABSCESS

Persistent PID can lead to the development of tubo-ovarian abscess (TOA) (Figure 17-2). Most so-called TOAs are actually tubo-ovarian complexes (TOC), the difference being that complexes are not walled off like the true abscess and are thus more responsive to antimicrobial therapy. Estimates of the progression from PID to TOA range from 3% to 16%; thus, any PID not responsive to therapy should be investigated further to rule out TOA.

Diagnosis

The diagnosis of TOA can be made clinically in the setting of PID and the appreciation of an adnexal or posterior cul-de-sac mass or fullness. WBC count is usually elevated with a left shift and the erythrocyte sedimentation rate (ESR) is often elevated as well. Cultures should include endocervical swabs and blood cultures to rule out sepsis. Culdocentesis that reveals gross pus is diagnostic but has been used less as imaging studies have been used more. Ultrasound diagnosis of pelvic abscess has increased as this modality has been refined. Pelvic computed tomography (CT) may be required, particularly in obese patients for whom ultrasound use is limited. Finally, laparoscopy can lead to a definitive diagnosis but is usually only used when the clinical picture is unclear.

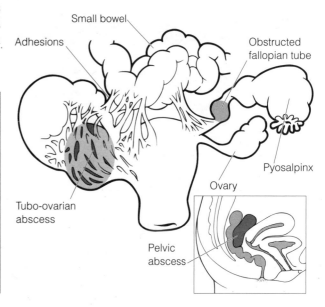

Figure 17-2 • Findings associated with chronic pelvic inflammatory disease, including tubo-ovarian abscess, adhesions, pyosalpinx, and an abscess located in the posterior cul-de-sac.

Treatment

Unless the abscess is ruptured, causing peritoneal signs, surgical treatment can be avoided and patients can be treated with antibiotics. The standard of care is to hospitalize any patient with a TOA/TOC and treat with broad-spectrum antibiotics. The first-line choice is often cefoxitin 2 g IV every 6 hours with doxycycline 100 mg IV/PO BID. If there is no response to this therapy, coverage can be expanded to triple antibiotic therapy such as ampicillin, gentamicin, and clindamycin or metronidazole. In patients allergic to penicillin, clindamycin and levofloxacin is an alternative regimen. The course of this disease can be followed by symptoms, clinical examination, temperature, WBC count, and, if these are equivocal, imaging studies. Typically, a repeat pelvic exam is performed after the patient has been afebrile for 48 hours to monitor for resolution of tenderness, after which time the patient can be converted to oral antibiotics to complete a 10- to 14-day course in anticipation of discharge from the hospital.

For more serious TOAs, either unresponsive to antibiotic therapy or with gross rupture, surgical intervention is necessary. Usually unilateral salpingo-oophorectomy is curative for the unilateral TOA. For bilateral TOAs, often a total abdominal hysterectomy and bilateral salpingo-oophorectomy (TAHBSO) may be necessary.

KEY POINTS

1. Chronic or acute PID can lead to TOAs or TOCs.
2. Diagnosis of TOA or TOC is most likely when there is an adnexal mass in the setting of PID symptoms. Confirmation is usually achieved with an imaging study such as pelvic ultrasound or CT.
3. Treatment includes hospitalization and IV antibiotics. For TOAs not responsive to antibiotics, adnexal surgery is the definitive cure.

■ TOXIC SHOCK SYNDROME (TSS)

TSS reached its peak in the United States in 1980 when the rate was 3 : 100,000 menstruating women. Since 1984, there have been fewer than 300 cases per year. Initially, TSS was correlated with high absorbency tampons and menstruation. Nonmenstrually related TSS has been associated with vaginal infections, vaginal delivery, cesarean section, postpartum endometritis, miscarriage, and laser treatment of condylomata.

Diagnosis

TSS is caused by colonization or infection with specific strains of *Staphylococcus aureus* that produce an epidermal toxin—toxic shock syndrome toxin-1 (TSST-1). This toxin and other staphylococcal toxins are likely to cause most of the symptoms of TSS. Symptoms include high fever (>102°F), erythematous rash, desquamation of the palms and soles 1 to 2 weeks after the acute illness, and hypotension. Gastrointestinal disturbances, myalgias, mucous membrane hyperemia, increased blood urea nitrogen (BUN) and creatinine, platelet count less than 100,000, and alteration in consciousness can also be seen. Blood cultures are often negative, possibly because the exotoxin is absorbed through the vaginal mucosa.

Treatment

Because of the seriousness of the disease (2% to 8% mortality rate), hospitalization is always indicated. For more severe cases in which patients are hemodynamically unstable, admission to an intensive care unit may be necessary. Of highest priority is treatment of hypotension with IV fluids and pressors if needed. Because this disease is caused by the exotoxin, treatment with IV antibiotics does not often shorten the length of the acute illness. However, it does decrease the risk of recurrence, which has been as high as 30% in women who continued to use high-absorbency tampons.

KEY POINTS

1. TSS peaked in 1984; currently, there are fewer than 300 cases per year in the United States.
2. Symptoms, which include fever, rash, and desquamation of palms and soles, are most likely caused by an *S. aureus* toxin, TSST-1.
3. Because of the seriousness of this illness, patients are hospitalized and treated with IV antibiotics and, if necessary, hemodynamic support.

HUMAN IMMUNODEFICIENCY VIRUS (HIV)

HIV is the causative agent of acquired immunodeficiency syndrome (AIDS). HIV is transmitted via sexual contact, via parenteral inoculation, and **vertically** from mothers to infants via a **transplacental route**, during birth from direct exposure, and via breast milk. As of June 2001, there had been about 800,000 cumulative cases of AIDS reported to the CDC, and it is estimated that there are 2 to 4 times that number of HIV carriers in the United States. Although women account for only 7% of AIDS cases in the United States, they are one segment of the population in which the incidence is currently rising. Worldwide, women represent a far more substantial proportion of those affected with HIV. In 2001, there were approximately 40 million patients with HIV, 3 million deaths due to HIV, and 1.1 million deaths directly attributed to HIV in women.

Infection with HIV—a retrovirus—leads to decreased cellular immunity because various cells carrying the CD4 antigen become infected, including helper T cells, B cells, monocytes, and macrophages. Initially, the infection is entirely asymptomatic, although the individual is a carrier of the disease; this stage can last from 5 to 7 years. This disease may appear initially with the AIDS-related complex, which includes lymphadenopathy, night sweats, malaise, diarrhea, weight loss, and unusual recurrent infections such as oral candidiasis, varicella-zoster, or herpes simplex. As the infection further decreases cellular immunity, full-blown AIDS develops with opportunistic infections such as *Pneumocystis carinii* pneumonia, toxoplasmosis, *Mycobacterium avium intracellulare*, cytomegalovirus, and various malignancies such as Kaposi's sarcoma and non-Hodgkin's lymphoma.

Diagnosis

The diagnosis of HIV infection is made initially via a screening test. Most commonly, the test is an enzyme-linked immunosorbent assay (ELISA) using HIV antigens, to which patient serum is added. A positive test results when antigen-antibody complexes form. This test does have false-positive results that, in low-risk populations, may occur more often than true positive results. Positive tests are therefore always confirmed by a Western blot. Another level of confirmation may be obtained if a viral load is sent and is positive. Viral loads are used to follow the progression of disease.

Treatment

There is no known cure for HIV or AIDS. The approach to this disease is prevention of transmission, prophylaxis of opportunistic infections, and prolonging the lives of infected patients by slowing progression of disease with antiretroviral agents. Great efforts are being directed toward prevention of HIV transmission by encouraging modification of risky behavior. Condoms are recommended for sexually active patients. IV drug users should avoid sharing needles and use clean needles. With improved screening methods, the risk of HIV infection from blood transfusion is currently estimated at less than 1 : 1,000,000.

Prophylaxis and treatment of the opportunistic infections in HIV-positive patients are discussed in *Blueprints Medicine*. Delaying the progress of the disease is accomplished primarily with nucleoside analogs and protease inhibitors. The nucleoside analogs—zidovudine (AZT), ddI, ddC, 3TC, and d4T—act to inhibit reverse transcriptase and interfere with viral replication. Protease inhibitors (indinavir, saquinavir, ritonavir) interfere with the synthesis of viral particles and have been effective in increasing CD4 counts and decreasing viral load. Because the action mechanisms of these two groups differ, a synergistic effect is seen with combination therapy known as **highly active antiretroviral therapy (HAART)**.

Beyond this simple review of HIV management, there are issues regarding HIV infection in women that deserve special emphasis. First, obstetric care of the HIV patient demands attention to both the ongoing care of the patient as well as the prevention of vertical transmission to the fetus. Second, the high incidence of invasive cervical cancer in this population requires more aggressive screening than in the general population.

Approximately 25% to 30% of infants born to untreated HIV-infected mothers become infected with HIV. Current evidence suggests that AZT administration during the antepartum (after the first trimester), intrapartum, and neonatal period can reduce the risk of maternal-fetal HIV transmission by two-thirds in women with mildly symptomatic HIV disease. There is also evidence that cesarean section prior to rupture of membranes can decrease the rate of transmission. More recent studies looking at triple therapy and protease inhibitors suggest that reducing viral load markedly reduces transmission. It is difficult to say whether cesarean section will actually make a difference in transmission rates in patients who have well-controlled disease with undetectable viral loads. In addition, there are many studies worldwide that are looking further at prevention of vertical transmission.

The high incidence of **invasive cervical cancer** in HIV-infected women is an important issue in gynecologic outpatient management. Studies confirm the synergistic association of HIV and human papillomavirus (HPV), the causative agent in squamous cell carcinoma of the cervix. The Centers for Disease Control and Prevention currently recommends routine Pap smears at initial evaluation and 6 months later. Thereafter, yearly evaluations are sufficient if results are negative unless there is documentation of previous HPV infection, squamous intraepithelial lesion, or symptomatic HIV disease, in which case the Pap smear should be repeated at 6-month intervals.

KEY POINTS

1. HIV is transmitted via sexual contact, sharing IV needles, and any activity where infected blood is introduced to a noninfected host.
2. HIV infection is screened for with the ELISA test and confirmed with a Western blot.
3. There is currently no cure for HIV infection so treatment focuses on antiretroviral agents such as nucleoside analogs and protease inhibitors and treatment of the multiple opportunistic infections.
4. Vertical transmission rates during pregnancy have been shown to decrease with antiretroviral treatment and by cesarean section, and are positively associated with viral load.

PATHOGENESIS

As shown in Figure 18-1, normal support of the pelvic organs is provided by a complex network of muscles (e.g., levator muscles), fascia (e.g., urogenital diaphragm, endopelvic fascia), and ligaments (e.g., uterosacral and cardinal ligaments). Damage to any one of these structures can potentially result in a weakening or loss of support to the pelvis and pelvic organs (Figure 18-2). Damage to the anterior vaginal wall can result in herniation of the bladder (**cystocele**) or urethra (**urethrocele**) into the vaginal vault. Injuries to the endopelvic fascia of the rectovaginal septum can result in herniation of the rectum (**rectocele**) or small bowel (**enterocele**) into the vaginal vault. And injury or stretching of the cardinal ligaments and other pelvic support structures can result in descensus, or prolapse, of the uterus (**uterine prolapse**). After hysterectomy, some women may experience prolapse of the vagina secondary to loss of support structures during surgery (**vaginal vault prolapse**).

Pelvic relaxation can cause pelvic pressure and pain, urinary incontinence, dyspareunia, and bowel and bladder dysfunction. Pelvic support can be compromised by birth trauma; chronic increases in intra-abdominal pressure from obesity, chronic cough, or heavy lifting; intrinsic weakness; and atrophic changes due to aging or estrogen deficiency.

Pelvic organ prolapse quantitative (POP-Q) refers to an objective, site-specific system for describing, quantifying, and staging pelvic support in women. It provides a standardized means for documenting, comparing, and communicating clinical findings of pelvic organ prolapse that focuses on the extent of prolapse and not on which organ part is presumed to be prolapsing within the defect (Figure 18-3). In order to quantitatively assess the degree of prolapse involved, POP-Q utilizes six points within the pelvis that are measured in relation to a fixed point of reference: the hymen (Figure 18-4). The POP-Q system is approved for the description of female pelvic organ prolapse by the International Continence Society, the American Urogynecologic Society, and the Society of Gynecologic Surgeons. POP-Q is not used uniformly by clinicians because it is quite complicated, but it is helpful in the research setting and in comparing patients' exams over time and among different examiners.

EPIDEMIOLOGY

The problem of pelvic relaxation is increased in postmenopausal women as tissues become less resilient and the accumulative stresses on the pelvis take effect. Black and Asian women have a much lower rate of uterine prolapse than do white women.

RISK FACTORS

The incidence of pelvic relaxation is increased for those patients who have chronically increased abdominal pressure due to chronic cough, straining, ascites, and large pelvic tumors. Obstructed labor and traumatic delivery are also risk factors for pelvic relaxation as are aging and menopause.

CLINICAL MANIFESTATIONS

History

The symptoms reported with pelvic relaxation vary depending on the structures involved and the degree

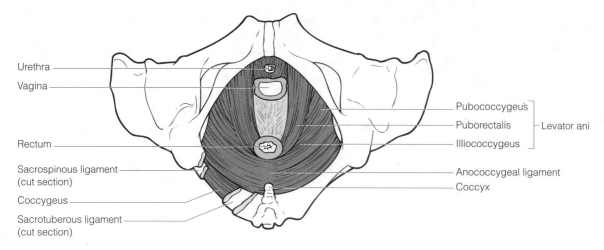

Urethra
Vagina
Rectum
Sacrospinous ligament (cut section)
Coccygeus
Sacrotuberous ligament (cut section)

Pubococcygeus
Puborectalis
Illiococcygeus
Levator ani
Anococcygeal ligament
Coccyx

Figure 18-1 • Normal structural support of the pelvis.

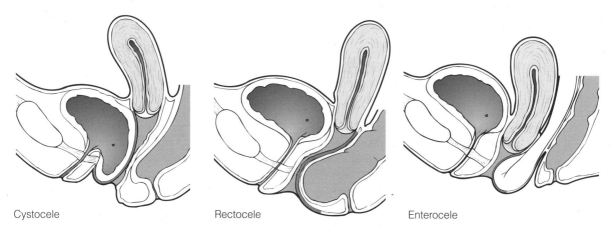

Cystocele

Rectocele

Enterocele

Figure 18-2 • Anatomic defects in pelvic relaxation.

of prolapse (Table 18-1). With small degrees of pelvic relaxation, patients are often asymptomatic. With more extensive relaxation, patients often complain of **pelvic pressure**, heaviness in the lower abdomen, or a **vaginal bulge** that may worsen at night or become aggravated by prolonged standing, vigorous activity, or lifting heavy objects. Urinary incontinence, frequency, urgency, and retention are other symptoms that may also be reported by patients with pelvic relaxation.

Physical Examination

Pelvic relaxation is best observed by separating the labia and viewing the vagina while the patient strains or coughs. **Urethroceles** and **cystoceles** may cause a downward movement of the anterior vaginal wall when the patient strains (Figure 18-5). Rectoceles

TABLE 18-1
Symptoms of Pelvic Relaxation
Pelvic pressure or heaviness
Backache
Dyspareunia
Urinary incontinence
Other urinary symptoms
Frequency
Hesitancy
Incomplete voiding
Recurrent infection
Rectal symptoms
Constipation
Painful defecation
Incomplete defecation

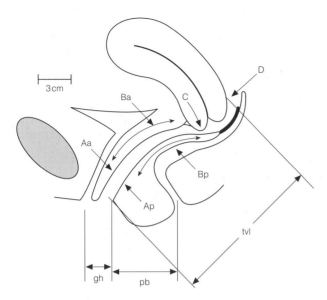

Figure 18-3 • Six sites (points Aa, Ba, C, D, Bp, Ap), genital hiatus (gh), perineal bodoy (pb), and total vaginal length (tvl) used for pelvic organ support quantitation.

Aa	Ba	C
gh	pb	tvl
Ap	Bp	D

Figure 18-4 • Three-by-three grid used to express the quantified pelvic organ prolapse (POP-Q) system. Aa = point A of the anterior wall; Ba = point B of the anterior wall; C = cervix or cuff; D = posterior fornix; gh = genital hiatus; pb = perineal body; tvl = total vaginal length; Ap = point A of the posterior wall; Bp = point B of the posterior wall.

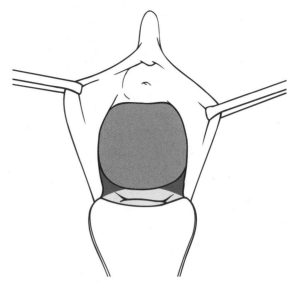

Figure 18-5 • Cystocele.

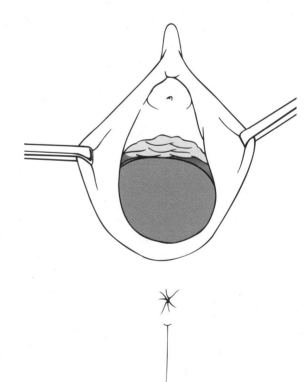

Figure 18-6 • Rectocele.

and enteroceles are best visualized by using a Sims speculum or the lower half of a Grave's speculum to provide better visualization of the anterior and posterior vaginal walls individually (Figure 18-6). A prolapsed uterus can also be viewed using either of these methods or by palpation.

The degree of pelvic relaxation is determined by the amount of descent of the structure. In **first-degree** pelvic relaxation, the structure is in the upper two-thirds of the vagina. In **second-degree** pelvic relaxation, the structure descends to the level of the introitus. In **third-degree** pelvic relaxation, the structure protrudes outside of the vagina.

DIAGNOSTIC EVALUATION

The diagnosis of pelvic relaxation depends primarily on the history and physical examination. Other tools that may be useful in the diagnosis of cystocele and urethrocele include urine cultures, cystoscopy, urethroscopy, and urodynamic studies, if indicated. When rectocele is suspected from a history of chronic constipation and difficulty passing stool, obstructive lesions should be ruled out using anoscopy or sigmoidoscopy. A barium enema study may also help to show a rectocele or enterocele but is not always essential to diagnosis.

DIFFERENTIAL DIAGNOSIS

Although rare, the differential diagnosis for cystocele and urethrocele includes urethral diverticula and Skene glands abscess. When a rectocele is suspected, obstructive lesions of the colon and rectum (lipomas, fibromas, sarcomas) should be investigated. Cervical elongation, prolapsed cervical polyp, and prolapsed cervical and endometrial tumors may be mistaken for uterine prolapse as can lower uterine segment fibroids.

TREATMENT

Regardless of the etiology, symptomatic pelvic relaxation is essentially a structural problem and therefore requires therapies that reinforce the lost support to the pelvis. These structural remedies may include hormonal therapies to maximize intrinsic pelvic support or exercises to strengthen the pelvic musculature (Kegel exercises). Likewise, mechanical support devices (pessaries) and surgical repair of the defect may also be utilized.

In postmenopausal women, **estrogen replacement** (systemic or vaginal) can be an important supplemental treatment, improving tissue tone and facilitating reversal of atrophic changes in the vaginal mucosa.

In motivated patients with mild symptoms, a first attempt at treatment may involve the use of **Kegel exercises** to strengthen the pelvic musculature. These exercises involve the tightening and releasing of the pubococcygeus muscles repeatedly throughout the day to strengthen the muscles and increase pelvic support.

Vaginal pessaries act as mechanical support devices to replace the lost structural integrity of the pelvis and to diffuse the forces of descent over a wider area. Pessaries are indicated for patients in whom surgery is contraindicated but whose symptoms are severe enough to require treatment. These are used in pregnant and postpartum women as well. These devices are placed in the vagina, positioned like a diaphragm, and serve to hold the pelvic organs in their normal position (Figure 18-7). The use of vaginal pessaries requires a highly motivated patient and close initial follow-up to avoid vaginal trauma and necrosis. Close follow-up also ensures proper placement and hygiene to minimize the risk of leukorrhea and infections.

Symptomatic patients who are not helped by nonoperative approaches may require **surgical correction**. In general, surgical repair for pelvic relaxation produces very good results. As outlined in Table 18-2, correction of cystoceles and rectoceles can be accomplished by **anterior** and **posterior colporrhaphy**, respectively. These procedures repair of the **fascial defect** through which the herniation occurred. With significant uterine prolapse, abdominal or vaginal **hysterectomy** may be indicated. **Vaginal vault prolapse** is corrected by suspension of the vaginal apex to various fixed points within the pelvis. The degree of success depends on the skill of the surgeon, the degree of pelvic relaxation, and the age, weight, and lifestyle of the patient.

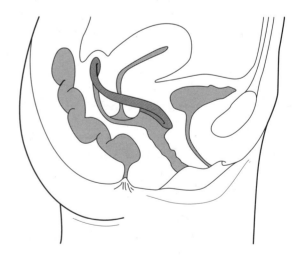

Figure 18-7 • Placement of a vaginal pessary to treat pelvic relaxation.

■ TABLE 18-2

Surgical Treatment of Genital Prolapse

Classification	Surgical Treatment
Cystocele	Anterior colporrhaphy Removal of excess anterior vaginal mucosa and plication of the endopelvic fascia to reelevate the bladder
Rectocele	Posterior colporrhaphy Similar to anterior colporrhaphy, except the rectal fascia is plicated posteriorly
Enterocele	Vaginal enterocele sac ligation Enterocele (hemia) sac is identified, ligated, and the vagina reinforced to prevent recurrence
Uterine prolapse	Vaginal hysterectomy and McCall culdoplasty Hysterectomy followed by plication of the uterosacral ligaments to prevent future vault prolapse

Vaginal vault prolapse (after hysterectomy)	Sacrospinous ligament suspension
	    Transvaginal suturing of the endopelvic fascia of the vaginal apex to the sacrospinous ligament
	Abdominal sacral colpopexy
	    Uses intervening mesh to attach the vaginal apex to the sacrum

KEY POINTS

1. Pelvic relaxation can result in prolapse of the bladder (cystocele), urethra (urethrocele), rectum (rectocele), small bowel (enterocele), uterus (uterine prolapse), or vagina (vaginal vault prolapse) into the vaginal vault.
2. Causes include birth trauma, chronic increases in intra-abdominal pressure, intrinsic weakness, and pelvic change due to aging.
3. Pelvic relaxation can result in pelvic pressure and pain, dyspareunia, bowel and bladder dysfunction, and urinary incontinence.
4. Pelvic relaxation is diagnosed primarily by history and physical examination, but may also require urine cultures, cystoscopy, urethroscopy, urinary dynamic studies, anoscopy, sigmoidoscopy, and barium enema as indicated.
5. Relaxation of the pelvic organs can be treated nonsurgically with Kegel exercises, vaginal pessaries and/or estrogen replacement. Surgical treatment options include a variety of supportive sling and suspension procedures, anterior and/or posterior colporrhaphy, and abdominal or vaginal hysterectomy.

Urinary Incontinence

■ EPIDEMIOLOGY

The involuntary loss of urine is common, affecting an estimated 25 million Americans of all ages. Nearly 50% of all women experience occasional urinary incontinence and 20% of women over age 75 are affected daily. Urinary incontinence is often a major reason for placing individuals in nursing homes with some 30% of nursing home residents suffering from urinary incontinence. The incidence of urinary incontinence increases with age and with increasing degrees of pelvic relaxation.

The four primary types of urinary incontinence are described in Table 19-1. **Stress incontinence** is characterized by urine loss with exertion or straining (coughing, laughing, exercising) and is typically caused by pelvic relaxation and displacement of the urethrovesical junction. This differs from **urge incontinence**, also known as detrusor instability, where urine leakage is due to involuntary and uninhibited bladder contractions. The cause is usually idiopathic but may be due to infection, bladder stones, urinary diverticula or neurologic disorders such as Alzheimer's, multiple sclerosis, or stroke.

Total incontinence is characterized by continuous urine leakage secondary to urinary fistulas. In the United States, almost all cases of total incontinence result from pelvic surgery or pelvic radiation. Finally, **overflow incontinence** may present with incomplete voiding, urinary retention, and overdistension of the bladder due to poor or absent bladder contractions. The causes of overflow incontinence vary widely from the use of certain medications to neurologic disorders and postoperative overdistension.

■ ANATOMY

Understanding the anatomy and physiology of the lower urinary tract and pelvic floor is crucial to understanding the mechanism behind each type of urinary incontinence (Figure 19-1). The bladder, or detrusor muscle, is a meshwork of smooth muscle layers ending in the **trigone** area at its base. The **internal sphincter** is at the junction of the bladder and the urethra. This is also known as the UVJ or **urethrovesical junction**. The urethra is made of smooth muscle. It is suspended by the pubourethral ligaments that originate at the lower pubic bone and extend to the middle third of the urethra to form the **external sphincter**.

Urinary continence at rest is possible because the **intraurethral pressure** exceeds the **intravesical pressure**. Continuous contraction of the internal sphincter is one of the primary mechanisms for maintaining continence at rest. The external sphincter provides about 50% of urethral resistance and is the second line of defense against incontinence. When the UVJ is in its proper position, any sudden increase in intra-abdominal pressure is transmitted equally to the bladder and proximal third of the urethra. Therefore, as long as the intraurethral pressure exceeds the intravesical pressure, continence is preserved.

In addition to the internal and external sphincters, continence is also maintained via the action of the **submucosal vasculature** of the urethra. When this vasculature complex fills with blood, the intraurethral pressure is increased thus preventing involuntary loss of urine (Figure 19-2). The filling mechanism of this system—known as **mucosal coaptation**—is estrogen sensitive, which explains why the estrogen-deficient postmenopausal state can lead to incontinence.

Neurologic control of the bladder and urethra is

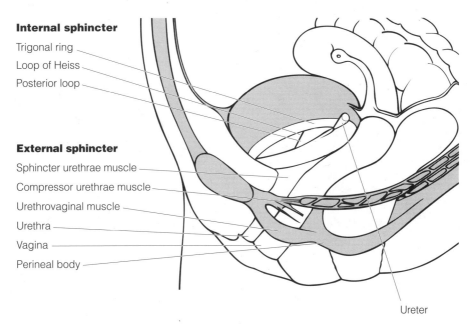

Internal sphincter
- Trigonal ring
- Loop of Heiss
- Posterior loop

External sphincter
- Sphincter urethrae muscle
- Compressor urethrae muscle
- Urethrovaginal muscle
- Urethra
- Vagina
- Perineal body

Ureter

Figure 19-1 • Anatomy of the lower urinary tract.

TABLE 19-1

Primary Types of Urinary Incontinence

Stress incontinence
Urine loss with exertion or straining (coughing, laughing, exercising) typically associated with pelvic relaxation and displacement of the urethrovesical junction.

Urge incontinence
Urine leakage due to involuntary and uninhibited bladder contractions known as detrusor instability.

Total incontinence
Continuous urine leakage due to urinary fistula resulting from pelvic surgery or pelvic radiation.

Overflow incontinence
Incontinence due to poor or absent bladder contractions that lead to urinary retention with overdistension of the bladder and overflow incontinence.

---

provided by both the **autonomic** (sympathetic and parasympathetic) and **somatic nervous systems** (Figure 19-3). The parasympathetic nervous system allows micturition to occur. Parasympathetic control of the bladder is supplied by the pelvic nerve derived from S2, S3, and S4 of the spinal cord. The sympathetic nervous system prevents micturition by contracting the bladder neck and internal sphinc-ter. Sympathetic control of the bladder is achieved via the hypogastric nerve originating from T10 to L2 of the spinal cord. Finally, the somatic nervous system aids in voluntary prevention of micturition by inner-vating the striated muscle of the external sphincter and pelvic floor through the pudendal nerve.

During micturition, the bladder releases its con-tents under voluntary control through a series of coordinated activities by the urethra and detrusor muscle. Stretch receptors in the bladder wall send a signal to the central nervous system (CNS) to begin voluntary voiding. This triggers inhibition of the sym-pathetic sacral and pudendal nerves thereby causing relaxation of the urethra, external sphincter, and levator ani muscles. This is closely followed by acti-vation of the parasympathetic pelvic nerve, resulting in contraction of the detrusor muscle, and micturi-tion begins.

■ PHYSICAL EXAMINATION

Care of all patients with urinary incontinence should begin with obtaining a thorough medical and surgi-cal history. The physical examination should include both internal and external pelvic examinations. Because the innervation of the lower urinary tract is closely associated with the innervation of the lower extremities and rectum, patients should receive a

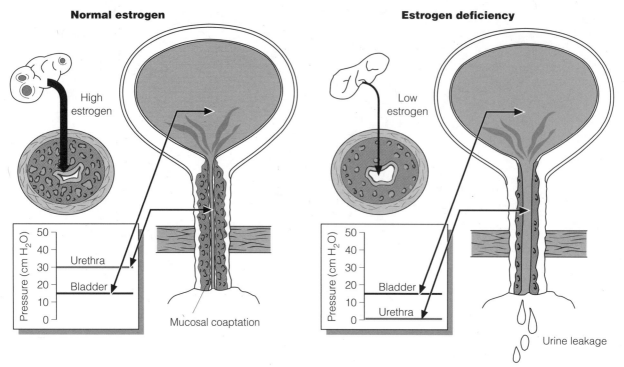

Normal estrogen

High estrogen

Pressure (cm H₂O)

Urethra

Bladder

Mucosal coaptation

Estrogen increases urethral resting pressure, making involuntary urine loss more difficult.

Figure 19-2 • Urethral mucosal coaptation.

Estrogen deficiency

Low estrogen

Pressure (cm H₂O)

Bladder

Urethra

Urine leakage

Estrogen deficiency decreases urethral resting pressure and facilitates urine leakage.

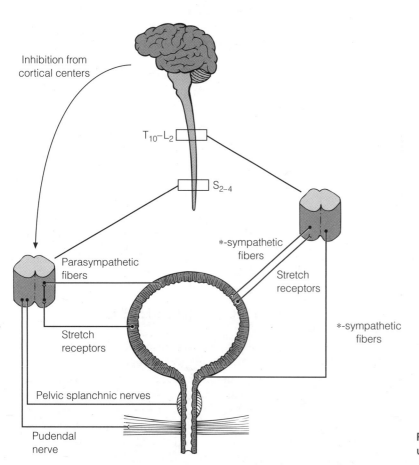

Inhibition from cortical centers

T_{10}–L_2

S_{2-4}

*-sympathetic fibers

Parasympathetic fibers

Stretch receptors

Stretch receptors

*-sympathetic fibers

Pelvic splanchnic nerves

Pudendal nerve

Figure 19-3 • Innervation of the lower urinary tract.

thorough neurologic examination. In particular, deep tendon reflexes, anal reflex, pelvic floor contractions, and the bulbocavernosus reflex (contraction after gentle tapping or squeezing of the clitoris) should be elicited.

■ DIAGNOSTIC EVALUATION

Fortunately, a variety of diagnostic tests are available for the evaluation of urinary incontinence. A **voiding diary** can be used to document the specific circumstances of the patient's voiding habits. A **urinalysis** and **urine culture** should be obtained to rule out infection as a cause of incontinence. The scope of this text precludes an exhaustive compilation of every diagnostic modality. The most common are the standing stress test, the cotton swab test, cystometrogram, and uroflowmetry.

A **standing stress test** is performed by having the patient with a full bladder stand over a towel or sheet with feet placed shoulder distance apart. The patient is asked to cough, and the physician observes to verify a loss of urine. Alternatively, the physician can ask the patient to cough while in the lithotomy position. Either method may be used to document stress incontinence. The stress test has low specificity and sensitivity.

The purpose of the **cotton swab test** is to diagnose a hypermobile bladder neck associated with genuine stress incontinence. The physician inserts a lubricated cotton swab into the urethra to the angle of the urethrovesical junction (Figure 19-4). When the patient strains as if urinating, the urethrovesical junction descends and the cotton swab moves. The change in cotton swab angle is normally less than 30° (Figure 19-4A), but will range from 30° to 60° with a hypermobile bladder neck (Figure 19-4B).

A **cystometrogram** can distinguish between genuine stress incontinence and detrusor instability. Pressure sensors are used to determine bladder and sphincter tone as the bladder is filled with fluid. Observations can be made about the bladder filling capacity, the presence or absence of a detrusor reflex, and the patient's ability to control or inhibit the strong desire to void.

Uroflowmetry measures the rate of urine flow through the urethra when a patient is asked to spontaneously void while sitting on a uroflow chair. This is particularly useful in patients complaining of hesitancy, incomplete bladder emptying, poor stream, and urinary retention.

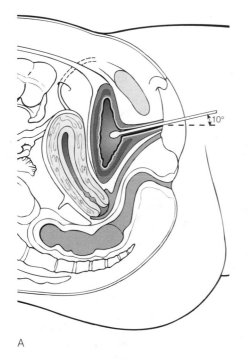

A

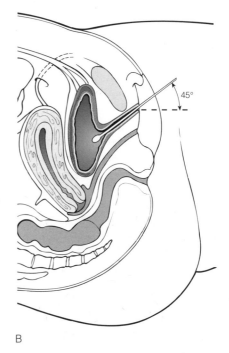

B

Figure 19-4 • A, B: Cotton swab test.

KEY POINTS

1. The incidence of urinary incontinence increases with age and with increasing degrees of pelvic relaxation.
2. The four primary types are stress incontinence, urge incontinence, total incontinence, and overflow incontinence.
3. Causes include pelvic relaxation, detrusor instability or insufficiency, and urinary fistulas.
4. Under normal circumstances, urinary incontinence is avoided due to the complex system of muscles, ligaments, sphincters, and nerves that keep the intraurethral pressure greater than the intravesical pressure.
5. Urinary incontinence can be diagnosed using the history and physical examination, urinalysis, urine culture, standing stress test, cotton swab test, cystometrography, and uroflowmetry as needed.

■ STRESS INCONTINENCE

Pathogenesis

Stress incontinence, also known as genuine stress incontinence and true stress incontinence, is the involuntary release of urine through the intact urethra in response to a sudden increase in **intra-abdominal pressure** such as coughing or exercise. In most cases, pelvic relaxation causes the bladder neck to become hypermobile so that increases in intra-abdominal pressure are no longer transmitted equally to the bladder and urethra. Instead, increases in intra-abdominal pressure are transmitted primarily to the bladder. Therefore, as intravesical pressures exceed intraurethral pressure, urinary stress incontinence occurs (Figure 19-5).

Risk Factors

The risk factors for urinary stress incontinence include factors that affect the normal transmission of intra-abdominal pressure, those that increase intravesical pressure, and those that decrease intraurethral pressure (Table 19-2). The three major risk factors for urinary stress incontinence include **pelvic relaxation** (affects transmission), chronically **increased intra-abdominal pressure** (increases intravesical pressure), and **menopause** (decreases intraurethral pressure due to coaptation). Other risk factors are outlined in Table 19-2.

TABLE 19-2

Risk Factors for Urinary Stress Incontinence

Conditions causing pelvic relaxation
Vaginal childbirth
Aging
Genetic factors

Conditions causing chronic increases in intra-abdominal pressure
Constipation
Chronic coughing from lung disease, smoking
Chronic heavy lifting
Obesity (does not cause incontinence, but worsens it)

Conditions that weaken the urethral closing mechanism
Estrogen deficiency
Scarring
Denervation
Medications

History

Patients with urinary stress incontinence may present with a sole complaint of involuntary loss of urine with coughing, laughing, sneezing, and straining. With more severe stress incontinence, urine leakage may occur with activities that cause even small increases in intra-abdominal pressure, such as walking or changing positions. Table 19-3 describes the grading system for stress incontinence. If pelvic relaxation is also involved, patients may report feeling a bulge, pressure, or pain in the vagina.

Diagnostic Evaluation

Table 19-4 lists the criteria for diagnosing urinary stress incontinence.

TABLE 19-3

Gradations of Urinary Stress Incontinence

Grade I	Incontinence only with severe stress such as coughing, sneezing, or jogging.
Grade II	Incontinence with moderate stress such as rapid moving or walking up and down stairs.
Grade III	Incontinence with mild stress such as standing. The patient is continent in the supine position.

Source: Adapted from Hacker N, Moore JG. Essentials of Obstetrics and Gynecology. Philadelphia: WB Saunders, 1998: 461.

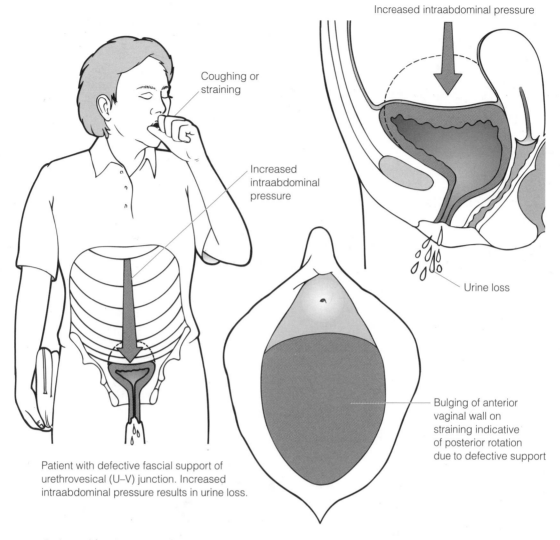

Increased intraabdominal pressure

Coughing or straining

Increased intraabdominal pressure

Urine loss

Patient with defective fascial support of urethrovesical (U–V) junction. Increased intraabdominal pressure results in urine loss.

Bulging of anterior vaginal wall on straining indicative of posterior rotation due to defective support

Figure 19-5 • Patient with urinary stress incontinence.

Treatment

The goal of stress incontinence treatment is to maximize pelvic support and to restore the anatomic position of the UVJ. This can be accomplished using a number of therapies.

Pelvic diaphragm exercises (**Kegel exercises**) result in an increase in resting and active muscle tone and thereby increase urethral closing pressure in cases of mild incontinence.

Pessaries and other intravaginal devices are used to physically elevate and support the bladder neck, which restores normal anatomic relationships. As a result, increases in intra-abdominal pressures are transmitted equally to the bladder and urethra and continence is maintained. Although pessaries are non-invasive, they preclude sexual intercourse and require close medical supervision to avoid infection of the vaginal mucosa or damage to the vaginal tissues.

A variety of **behavior modifications** have been useful in improving mild stress incontinence including biofeedback and bladder training.

Medical therapies including estrogen and **alpha-adrenergic agents** (phenylpropanolamine and pseudoephedrine) work to increase urethral sphincter tone and enhance urethral closure. Topical or systemic **estrogen** can be used to increase urethral tone by enhancing mucosal coaptation.

Surgery for genuine stress incontinence aims to restore normal anatomy by returning the hypermobile bladder neck to its original position. Disadvan-

TABLE 19-4

Criteria and Tools for Diagnosing Stress Incontinence

Normal urinalysis

Negative urine culture

Normal neurologic examination

Poor anatomic support (suggesting pelvic relaxation)
  Cotton swab test
  x-ray
  Urethroscopy

Demonstrable leakage with stress
  Stress test
  Pad test

Normal cystometrogram or urethrocystometry
  Normal residual urine volume
  Normal bladder capacity and sensation
  No involuntary detrusor contractions

Source: Adapted from DeCherney A, Pernoll M. Current Obstetric and Gynecologic Diagnosis and Treatment. Norwalk: Appleton & Lange, 1994:837.

tages of surgery include the risks of an invasive procedure and the risk of failure with resumption of symptoms over time. Several approaches have been employed with roughly equal success. These include the abdominal retropubic urethropexies (Marshall-Marchetti-Krantz and Burch procedures), paravaginal defect repair, vaginal needle suspensions (Pereyra, Stamey, and Raz procedures) and suburethral slings. Patients with intrinsic sphincter deficiency have been helped by periurethral collagen injections.

KEY POINTS

1. Stress incontinence is the involuntary loss of urine with physical activity (e.g., laughing, coughing, exercising).
2. It is usually due to pelvic relaxation (e.g., with aging or after childbirth) that results in a hypermobile bladder neck or from intrinsic sphincter deficiency.
3. Risk factors for stress urinary incontinence include pelvic relaxation, chronically increased intra-abdominal pressure (e.g., obesity, chronic cough), and estrogen deficiency in menopause.
4. Diagnostic evaluation includes a thorough history and physical, urine culture and analysis, standing stress test, cotton-swab test, and use of a voiding

diary. Urodynamics (cystometrogram, uroflowmetry) can be used as indicated.
5. Stress incontinence can be treated with pelvic exercises, medication to enhance urethral sphincter closure (estrogen, Propadrine), or surgery to restore the intra-abdominal position of the proximal urethra.

■ DETRUSOR INSTABILITY

Pathogenesis

Detrusor instability, also known as **urge incontinence**, is usually caused by involuntary and uninhibited detrusor contractions during the filling phase of bladder function. Under normal circumstances, these contractions should not occur.

Most detrusor instability is **idiopathic**. Some conditions known to cause involuntary bladder contractions include urinary tract infections (UTIs), bladder stones, bladder cancer, suburethral diverticula, and foreign bodies (Figure 19-6). Detrusor overactivity, or detrusor hyperreflexia, may also be due to neurologic disease such as stroke, Alzheimer's disease, Parkinson's disease, multiple sclerosis, and diabetes mellitus (Table 19-5).

TABLE 19-5

Common Causes of Urge Incontinence

Detrusor instability
UTIs
Urethral obstruction
Urethral compression (previous surgery)
Bladder stones
Bladder cancer
Suburethral diverticula
Foreign bodies

Detrusor hyperreflexia
Cerebrovascular accident
Alzheimer's disease
Parkinsonism
Multiple sclerosis
Diabetes
Peripheral neuropathies
Autonomic neuropathies
Cauda equina lesions

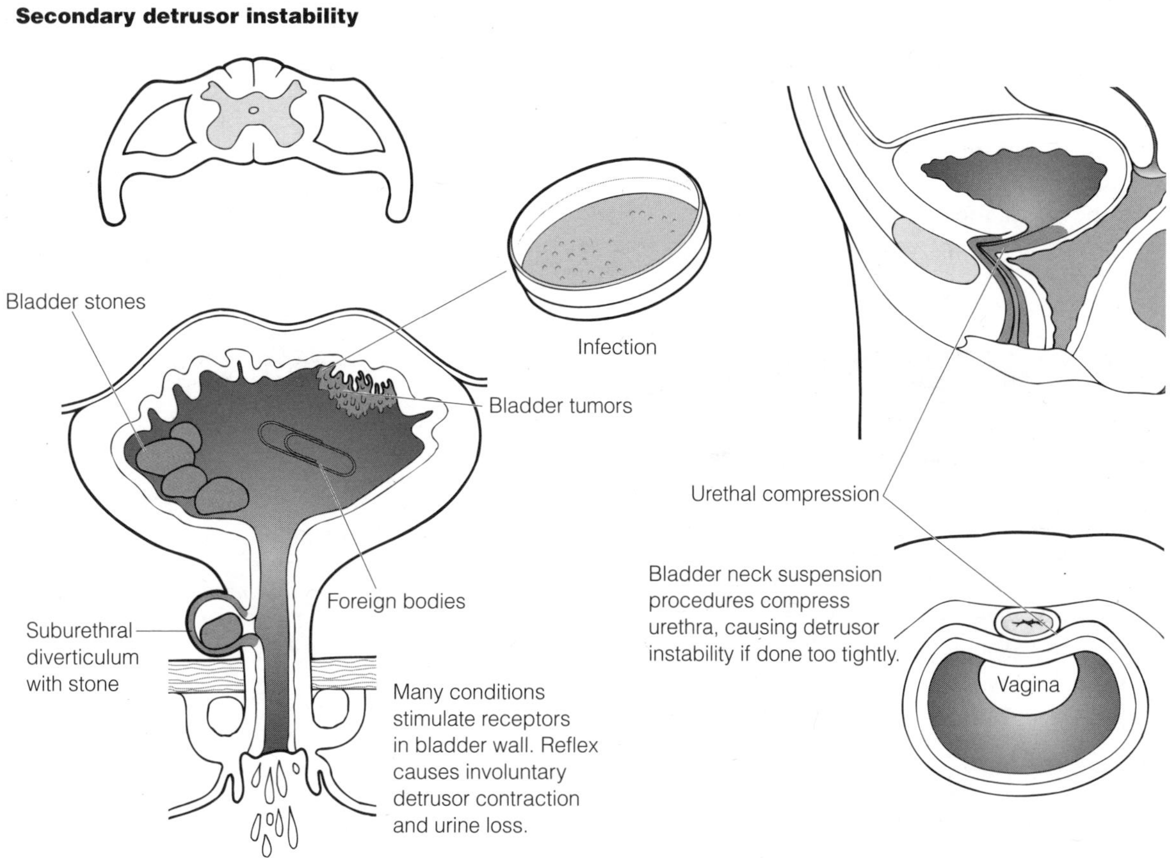

Secondary detrusor instability

Bladder stones

Infection

Bladder tumors

Urethal compression

Foreign bodies

Bladder neck suspension procedures compress urethra, causing detrusor instability if done too tightly.

Vagina

Suburethral diverticulum with stone

Many conditions stimulate receptors in bladder wall. Reflex causes involuntary detrusor contraction and urine loss.

Figure 19-6 • Causes of detrusor instability.

Epidemiology

In the general population, the incidence of detrusor instability is 10% to 15%.

Clinical Manifestations

History

Patients with urge incontinence usually present with a history of involuntary urine loss whether or not the bladder is full. Many women complain of not being able to reach the bathroom in time or of dribbling or leakage triggered by just seeing a bathroom.

Physical Examination

Detrusor instability presents with symptoms that suggest bladder overactivity, including urinary urgency, frequency (more than seven times a day), stress incontinence, and nocturia (more than one time per night). Given the wide differential for detrusor instability, patients should also be asked about neurologic symptoms, history of previous anti-incontinence surgery, and hematuria (suggestive of cancer, stones, or infection).

Treatment

The treatment of urge incontinence will depend on the etiology of disease. Bladder training, Kegel exercises, biofeedback, hypnosis, and psychotherapy are methods of **behavior modification** that have had moderate success in controlling urge incontinence. Bladder training begins by establishing a regular voiding schedule that is modified to gradually lengthen the intervals between voiding until the patient reestablishes cortical control over the voiding reflex.

Medical therapy for urge incontinence is designed to enhance urine storage and relax the bladder. Bladder contractions are caused by stimulation of the parasympathetic nervous system through the release of acetylcholine. Therefore, the most frequently used and most effective medications for urge incontinence are **anticholinergics** (e.g., Pro-Banthine, oxybutynin).

Beta-adrenergic agonists (e.g., Alupent) work on beta-adrenergic receptors on the bladder resulting in bladder relaxation. **Smooth muscle relaxants** (e.g., Urispas) and **tricyclic antidepressants** (e.g., imipramine) also relax the detrusor muscle. These medications used alone or in concert are effective in 50% to 80% of patients.

There are no effective surgical procedures to treat detrusor instability.

KEY POINTS

1. Detrusor instability, or urge incontinence, results from involuntary and uninhibited bladder contractions.
2. Most cases of detrusor instability are idiopathic. Other cases are caused by UTI, bladder stones, cancer, diverticula, and neurologic disorders (stroke, multiple sclerosis, Alzheimer's).
3. Symptoms include urinary urge, frequency, and nocturia.
4. The goal of medical treatment is to relax the bladder and enhance urine storage.
5. Detrusor instability can be treated with medication (especially anticholinergics), bladder training, or a variety of other behavior modification strategies. When neurologic etiologies exist, treatment of the disorder may result in improved detrusor stability.
6. There are no effective surgical procedures for the treatment of detrusor instability.

◼ TOTAL INCONTINENCE

Pathogenesis

Total urinary incontinence (bypass incontinence) is typically the result of a **urinary fistula** formed between the bladder and the vagina (vesicovaginal fistula), as shown in Figure 19-7, or between the urethra and the vagina (urethrovaginal fistula) or the ureter and the vagina (ureterovaginal fistula).

In developing countries, the most common cause of urinary fistulas is **obstetric trauma** from a prolonged stage 2 or operative procedures (e.g., forceps). However, in the United States, genitourinary fistulas are most often caused by **pelvic radiation** or **pelvic surgery**. Ectopic ureters and urethral diverticula may also produce total incontinence.

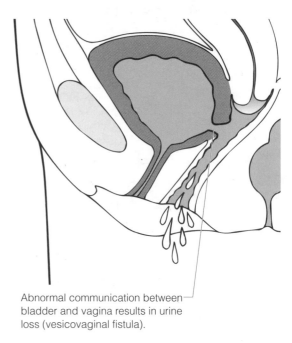

Abnormal communication between bladder and vagina results in urine loss (vesicovaginal fistula).

Figure 19-7 • Vesicovaginal fistula.

Epidemiology

Pelvic radiation and **pelvic surgery** account for over 95% of total urinary incontinence cases in the United States. In particular, simple abdominal hysterectomy and vaginal hysterectomy alone account for over 50% of vesicovaginal fistulas. Urethrovaginal fistulas may also occur as complications of surgery for urethral diverticula, anterior vaginal wall prolapse, or stress urinary incontinence. Ureterovaginal fistulas, as seen after 1% to 2% of radical hysterectomies, are usually due to devascularization rather than direct injury. Obstetric injuries associated with operative deliveries were once the leading cause of urinary fistulas but are now rare causes of total urinary incontinence in the United States, Canada, and Western Europe.

Risk Factors

The incidence of fistula formation after surgery is higher if the patient has a history of preoperative radiation, endometriosis, pelvic inflammatory disease (PID), or previous pelvic surgery.

History

Patients with a urinary fistula usually present with a history of **painless and continuous loss of urine**, usually after pelvic surgery or radiation. Fistulas caused by surgery become clinically apparent in 5 to 14 days.

Diagnostic Evaluation

Methylene blue dye instilled **into the bladder** will leak onto a sanitary pad if a vesicovaginal fistula is present. To diagnose a ureterovaginal fistula, **indigo carmine** is given intravenously. As the compound is filtered through the kidneys and passes through the ureters, it will stain the vaginal pad. If a ureterovaginal fistula is present, the methylene blue test will be negative and the indigo carmine test will be positive. **Cystourethroscopy** can then be used to identify the number and location of the fistulas. Intravenous pyelogram and retrograde pyelogram may also be used to localize ureterovaginal fistulas.

Treatment

Surgery is the main mode of treatment for urinary fistula. Most **obstetric fistulas** can be repaired immediately; however, it is typical to wait 3 to 6 months before attempting to repair **postsurgical fistulas**. This waiting period allows inflammation to decrease and vascularity and pliability of the area to increase. **Antibiotics** for urinary infection and **estrogen** for postmenopausal women are also used during this period. **Steroids** have been used to decrease inflammation, although their use is still controversial.

KEY POINTS

1. Total incontinence is usually due to vesicovaginal, urethrovaginal, or ureterovaginal fistulas.
2. Symptoms include painless, continuous urine leakage.
3. Total incontinence is caused by pelvic radiation and pelvic surgery in over 95% of cases in the United States.
4. In developing countries, total incontinence is attributable to obstetric trauma, often leading to urinary fistula.
5. Total incontinence is treated surgically with repair of the urinary fistula.

◼ OVERFLOW INCONTINENCE

Pathogenesis

Overflow incontinence in women is usually due to **detrusor insufficiency** (bladder hypotonia) or **detrusor areflexia** (bladder acontractility). As a result, bladder contractions are weak or nonexistent, causing incomplete voiding, urinary retention, and overdistension of the bladder (Figure 19-8). The causes of overflow incontinence due to detrusor insufficiency vary widely from fecal compaction, to use of certain medications, to neurological diseases including lower motor neuron disease, autonomic neuropathy (diabetes), spinal cord injuries, and multiple sclerosis (Table 19-6).

Outflow obstruction, typically due to surgical procedures that result in urethral kinking, stenosis, or obstruction, can also cause bladder overdistension and overflow incontinence, but it is rarely seen in women. **Postoperative overdistension** of the bladder due to unrecognized urinary retention and the use of epidural anesthesia are common causes of overflow incontinence.

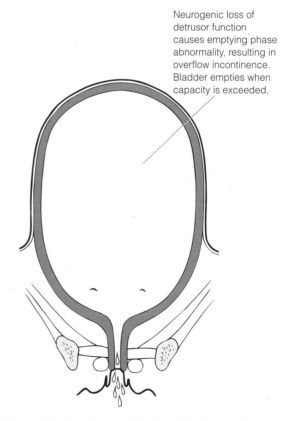

Neurogenic loss of detrusor function causes emptying phase abnormality, resulting in overflow incontinence. Bladder empties when capacity is exceeded.

Figure 19-8 • Overdistended bladder, inducing overflow incontinence.

▪ TABLE 19-6

Causes of Overflow Incontinence

Neurogenic causes
Lower motor neuron disease
Autonomic neuropathy (diabetes mellitus)
Spinal cord injuries
Multiple sclerosis

Obstructive causes
Postsurgical urethral obstruction
Postoperative overdistension (rare)
Pelvic masses

Pharmacologic causes
Anticholinergic drugs
α-adrenergic agonists
Epidural and spinal anesthesia

Other causes
Psychogenic (psychosis or severe depression)
Idiopathic
Fecal impaction

Clinical Manifestations

Patients with overflow incontinence may present with a wide variety of symptoms including frequent or constant urinary dribbling, along with the symptoms of stress incontinence and urge incontinence. Outflow obstruction (rare) involves a history of straining to void, poor stream, urinary retention, and incomplete emptying.

Treatment

Treatment strategy in overflow incontinence is geared toward relieving urinary retention, increasing bladder contractility, and decreasing urethral closing pressure.

Medical management of overflow incontinence includes the use of various agents to reduce urethral closing pressure (prazosin, terazosin, phenoxybenzamine) and **striated muscle relaxants** (diazepam, dantrolene) to reduce bladder outlet resistance. **Cholinergic agents** (bethanechol) are used to increase bladder contractility. Intermittent **self-catheterization** may also be used in overflow incontinence to avoid chronic urinary retention and infection.

Patients with overflow incontinence due to **urinary obstruction** may benefit from surgical correction of the obstruction. Postoperative overdistension of the bladder is typically temporary and may be managed by continuous bladder drainage for 24 to 48 hours.

KEY POINTS

1. Overflow incontinence is most commonly due to detrusor insufficiency caused by medications or neurologic disease; obstruction and postoperative overdistension occur less frequently in women.
2. Overflow incontinence is usually treated with self-catheterization and/or medications to increase bladder contractility (cholinergic agents) and lower urethral resistance (alpha-adrenergic agents).

Puberty, the Menstrual Cycle, and Menopause

■ PUBERTY

Puberty describes the series of events in which a child matures into a young adult. These changes include the development of secondary sex characteristics, the growth spurt, and achievement of fertility. Before any perceived phenotypic change, **adrenarche** occurs with regeneration of the zona reticularis in the adrenal cortex. **Gonadarche** follows with pulsatile gonadotropin-releasing hormone (GnRH) secretion stimulating the anterior pituitary to produce luteinizing hormone (LH) and follicle-stimulating hormone (FSH). Subsequently physical changes are triggered including breast development (**thelarche**), development of pubic and axillary hair (**pubarche**), the growth spurt (peak height velocity), and onset of menstruation (**menarche**) all occur, usually in that order (Figure 20-1). The length of time from breast bud development to menstruation is typically 2 years.

Adrenarche and Gonadarche

Adrenarche occurs between age 6 and 8. The adrenal gland begins regeneration of the zona reticularis, which had regressed shortly after birth, with concomitant enhancement of the P450 microsomal enzymes. This inner layer of the adrenal cortex is responsible for the secretion of sex steroid hormones. As a result, the adrenal androgenic steroid hormones—dehydroepiandrosterone sulfate (DHEAS), dehydroepiandrosterone (DHEA), and androstenedione—are increasingly produced from age 6 to 8 up until age 13 to 15.

Gonadarche begins around age 8, when pulsatile GnRH secretion from the hypothalamus is increased. This leads to stimulation of the gonadotrophs in the anterior pituitary, with subsequent secretion of LH and FSH. Initially, these increases occur mostly during sleep and fail to lead to any phenotypic changes. As a girl enters early puberty, the LH and FSH elevations eventually lead to stimulation of the ovary and subsequent estrogen release.

Thelarche

The first stage of thelarche, the development of breast buds, usually occurs around age 11. Thelarche is usually the first phenotypic sign of puberty and occurs in response to the increase in levels of circulating estrogen. Concomitantly, there is estrogenation of the vaginal mucosa and growth of the vagina and uterus. Further development of the breast will continue throughout puberty and adolescence, as described by Marshall and Tanner (Table 20-1 and Figure 20-2).

Pubarche

The onset of growth of pubic hair (Figure 20-3) usually occurs around age 12 and is often accompanied by growth of axillary hair. Pubarche usually follows thelarche, but a normal variant in order is seen with pubarche preceding thelarche, particularly in African American girls. The growth of pubic and axillary hair is likely secondary to the increase in circulating androgens.

Peak Height Velocity

The growth spurt is characterized by an acceleration in growth rate around age 9 to 10, leading to a peak height velocity around age 12 to 13. The increased rate of growth is likely secondary to the increased

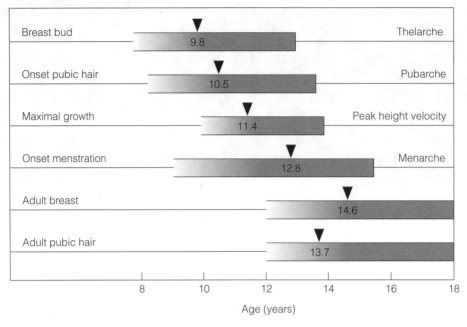

Figure 20-1 • Average age at onset and range given for the events of puberty.

TABLE 20-1		
The Tanner Stages of Breast Development		
Stage 1	Preadolescent: Elevation of papilla only	
Stage 2	Breast bud stage: Elevation of breast and papilla, areolar enlargement	
Stage 3	Further enlargement of breast and areola without separation of contours	
Stage 4	Projection of areola and papilla to form a secondary mound	
Stage 5	Mature stage: Projection of papilla only as areola recesses to breast contour	

Source: Adapted from Speroff L, Glass RH, Kase NG. Clinical Gynecologic Endocrinology and Infertility, 5th ed. Baltimore: Williams & Wilkins, 1994:377.

Menarche

The average age at onset of menstruation is between 12 and 13 or **2 years after the development of breast buds**. The adolescent menstrual cycle is usually irregular for the first 6 months to 1 year after menarche, reflecting anovulatory cycles. On average, it takes about 2 years after menarche before regular ovulatory cycles are achieved. Menarche is often delayed in gymnasts, distance runners, and ballet dancers. Some theories propose that this is due to an insufficient percentage of body fat that may be required for menstrual cycles. However, it is unclear whether it is the percentage of body fat or the exercise and stress on the body that interferes with menarche.

level of growth hormone and somatomedin-C, which increases in response to increasing levels of estrogen. However, this relationship is dose-related and excess levels of estrogen will lead to decreased growth hormone and somatomedin-C. Further, because estrogen causes fusion of the epiphyseal plate in long bones, a rapid growth spurt may be followed by growth cessation.

■ THE MENSTRUAL CYCLE

The hypothalamus, pituitary, ovaries, and uterus are all involved in maintaining the menstrual cycle (Figure 20-4). The menstrual cycle is divided into two 14-day phases: the **follicular** and **luteal phases** that describe changes in the ovary over the length of the cycle, and the **proliferative** and **secretory phases** that describe concurrent changes in the endometrium over the same period of time (Figure 20-4).

During the **follicular phase**, release of FSH from the pituitary results in development of a primary

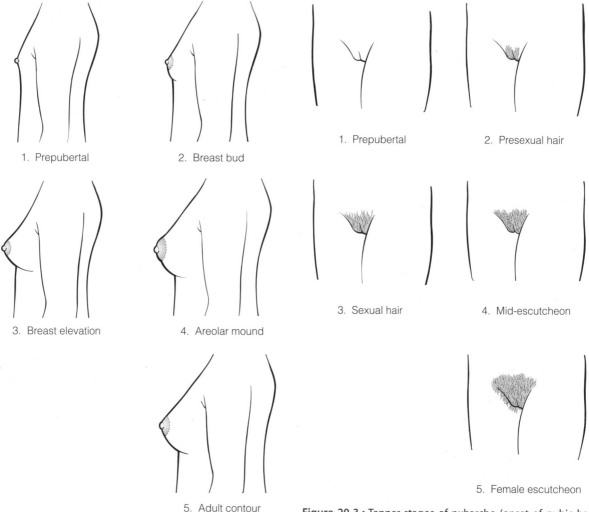

Figure 20-2 • Tanner stages of thelarche (breast development).

Figure 20-3 • Tanner stages of pubarche (onset of pubic hair growth).

ovarian follicle. The ovarian follicle produces estrogen, which causes the uterine lining to proliferate. At midcycle—approximately day 14—there is an LH spike in response to a preceding estrogen surge, which stimulates ovulation, the release of the ovum from the follicle (see Figure 20-4). After ovulation the **luteal phase** begins. The remnants of the follicle left behind in the ovary develop into the corpus luteum. This corpus luteum is responsible for the secretion of progesterone, which maintains the endometrial lining in preparation to receive a fertilized ovum. If fertilization does not occur, the corpus luteum degenerates and progesterone levels fall. Without progesterone, the endometrial lining is sloughed off, which is known as menstruation (see Figure 20-4).

Follicular Phase

The withdrawal of estrogen and progesterone during the luteal phase of the prior cycle causes a gradual increase in FSH. In turn, FSH stimulates growth of approximately 5 to 15 primordial ovarian follicles, initiating the follicular phase. Of these primordial follicles, one becomes the dominant follicle and develops and matures until ovulation. The developing follicle destined to ovulate produces estrogen that enhances follicular maturation and increases the production of FSH and LH receptors in an autocrine fashion. The estrogens are produced in a two-cell process with the theca interna cells producing androstenedione in response to LH stimulation and the granulosa cells converting this androstenedione to estradiol when stimulated by FSH. LH also rises

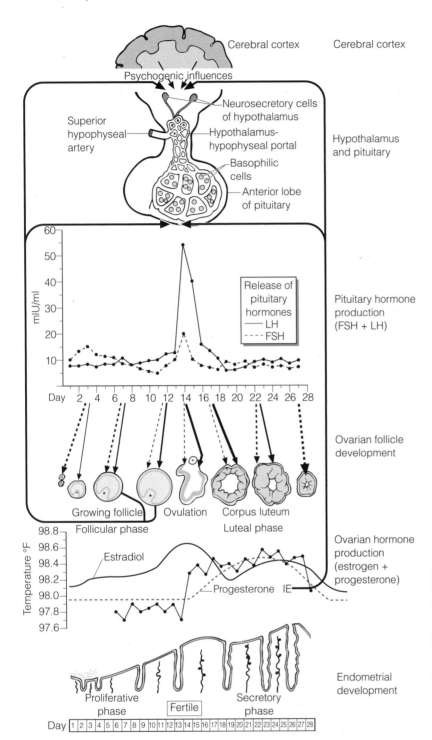

Figure 20-4 • Normal menstrual cycle, Day 1 to Day 28. The cyclic changes of FSH and LH and the resultant changes in the ovarian histology (follicular and luteal phases) in estrogen and progesterone levels, in basal body temperature and the endometrial histology (proliferative and secretory phases) are shown. Note how the LH surge near day 14 of a 28-day cycle triggers ovulation and a rise in basal body temperature dignifying the time of maximum fertility during the cycle.

and stimulates the synthesis of androgens, which are converted to estrogen. As rising estrogen levels negatively feedback on pituitary FSH secretion, the dominant follicle is protected from the decrease in FSH by its increased number of FSH receptors (Figure 20-5).

Ovulation

Toward the end of the follicular phase, estrogen levels eventually surge to reach a critical level that triggers the anterior pituitary to release an LH spike. Ovulation occurs as the increase in LH levels causes

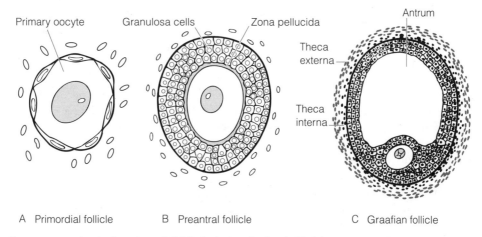

A Primordial follicle   B Preantral follicle   C Graafian follicle

Figure 20-5 • Changes occurring in the primordial follicle during the first half of the ovarian cycle. Under the influence of FSH, the primordial follicle (A) matures into the preantral follicle (B) and then into the graafian follicle (C). The oocyte remains a primary oocyte in the diplotene stage until shortly before ovulation. During the last few days of the growing period, the estrogen produced by the follicular and theca cells stimulate the formation of LH in the pituitary.

the follicle to rupture and release the mature ovum (Figure 20-6). The ovum usually passes into the adjoining fallopian tube and is swept down to the uterus by the cilia lining the tube. This process takes 3 to 4 days. **Fertilization of the ovum must occur within 24 hours of ovulation** or it degenerates.

Luteal Phase

After ovulation, the luteal phase ensues. The **granulosa** and **theca interna cells** lining the wall of the follicle form the corpus luteum under stimulation by

LH. The corpus luteum synthesizes estrogen and significant quantities of progesterone, which cause the endometrium to become more glandular and secretory in preparation for implantation of a fertilized ovum. If fertilization occurs, the developing trophoblast synthesizes **human chorionic gonadotropin (hCG)**—a glycoprotein very similar to LH—that maintains the corpus luteum so that it can continue production of estrogen and progesterone to support the endometrium until the placenta develops its synthetic function (at 8 to 10 weeks gestation). If fertilization, with its concomitant rise in hCG, does not

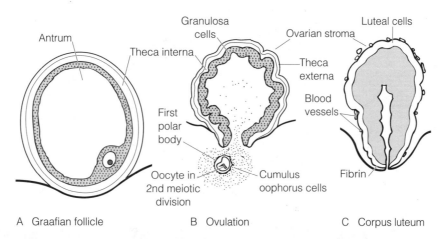

A Graafian follicle   B Ovulation   C Corpus luteum

Figure 20-6 • A: The graafian follicle just before rupture. B: Ovulation. The oocyte beginning its second meiotic division is discharged from the ovary together with a large number of cumulus oophorus cells. The follicular cells remaining inside the collapsed follicle differentiate into luteal cells. C: Corpus luteum. Note the large size of the corpus luteum caused by hypertrophy and accumulation of lipid in the granulose and theca interna cells. The remaining cavity of the follicle is filled with fibrin.

occur, the corpus luteum degenerates, progesterone levels fall, the endometrium is not maintained, and menstruation occurs.

Menstruation

The endometrium of the uterus undergoes cyclical changes during the menstrual cycle (Figure 20-4). During the follicular phase, the endometrium is in the **proliferative phase**, growing in response to estrogen. During the luteal phase, the endometrium enters the **secretory phase** as it matures and is prepared to support implantation. If the ovum is not fertilized, the corpus luteum degenerates after approximately 14 days, leading to a fall in estrogen and progesterone levels. The withdrawal of progesterone causes the endometrium to slough, initiating the **menstrual phase**. At the same time, FSH levels begin to slowly rise in the absence of negative feedback and the follicular phase starts again.

▨ MENOPAUSE AND POSTMENOPAUSE

The "**climacteric**" marks the termination of the reproductive phase in a woman's life. At this point, nearly all the oocytes have undergone atresia, although a few remain and can be found on histologic examination. The term "**menopause**" denotes the final menstruation and marks the cornerstone event during the climacteric. The average age at menopause in the United States is 50 to 51 years. Various physiologic and hormonal changes occur during this period, including a decrease in estrogen, increase in FSH, and classic symptoms such as "hot flashes." If menopause occurs before age 40, it is considered premature.

Etiology

Menopause is generally heralded by menstrual irregularity as the number of oocytes capable of responding to FSH and LH decrease and anovulation becomes more frequent. During this period, LH and FSH levels gradually rise because of decreased negative feedback from diminished estrogen production. The fall in estradiol levels leads to hot flashes, insomnia, depression, osteoporosis, atherosclerosis, and vaginal atrophy (Figure 20-7). Early menopause is associated with cigarette smoking. Premature menopause is often a result of premature ovarian failure and is usually idiopathic. If it occurs before age 35, chromosomal studies can be ordered to rule out a genetic basis (e.g., mosaicism).

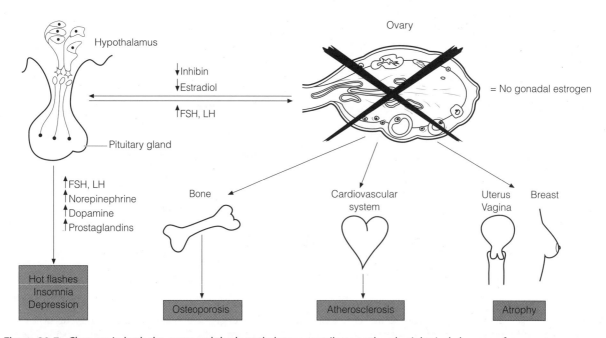

Figure 20-7 • Changes in both the ovary and the hypothalamus contribute to the physiological changes of menopause.

Diagnosis

The diagnosis of menopause can usually be made by history and physical examination and confirmed by testing FSH levels. Patients classically present between age 48 and 52 complaining of oligomenorrhea and vasomotor instability, sweats, mood changes, depression, dyspareunia, and dysuria. These symptoms generally disappear within 12 months, although a substantial proportion of women can remain symptomatic for years.

On physical examination there may be a decrease in breast size and change in texture. Vaginal, urethral, and cervical atrophy may all be seen, which are consistent with decreased estrogenation. If there is any question about the diagnosis, an elevated FSH is diagnostic of menopause.

Pathogenesis

Although menopause is a naturally occurring event, there are two important long-term consequences of the estrogen decrease. From a cardiovascular standpoint, the protective benefits of estrogen on the lipid profile (increased high-density lipoprotein [HDL], decreased low-density lipoprotein [LDL]) and the vascular endothelium (prevents atherogenesis, increases vasodilatation, inhibits platelet adherence) are lost and women are at **increased risk for coronary artery disease**. With menopause, **bone resorption accelerates** because estrogen plays an important role in regulating osteoclast activity. The increased bone resorption leads to osteopenia and finally osteoporosis (particularly in thin, fair, and Caucasian women) (Table 20-2).

Hormone Replacement Therapy (HRT)

The benefits of postmenopausal **hormone replacement therapy** (HRT) have been the center of multiple studies over time. Initial studies suggested that HRT may also be cardio-protective (reducing the risk of stokes and heart attacks) however, more recent studies do not support these findings. It is generally accepted that the **two major advantages to HRT** use are the **prevention of bone loss** and osteoporosis (and a subsequent reduction in the incidence of hip fractures and other complications of osteoporosis) and **the relief of symptoms** associated with menopause. Symptomatic relief involves reduction of vasomotor flushing, mood improvement, prevention of urogenital and vaginal atrophy, and improvement in skin and muscle tone.

Treatment must be considered carefully, however, and evidence of cholestatic hepatic dysfunction, known estrogen-dependent neoplasm (breast, ovary, uterus, cervix, vagina), history of thromboembolic disease, or undiagnosed vaginal bleeding are all **relative contraindications** to estrogen replacement therapy.

Estrogen replacement alone may cause endometrial hyperplasia and eventually cancer. Therefore progesterone is used in combination to offset the risks of unopposed estrogen in women who still have their uterus in situ. Either a combined continuous regimen of estrogen and progesterone or various combined sequential regimens can be used. The regimen of continuous progesterone is associated with more irregular breakthrough bleeding but may eventually lead to amenorrhea. Progesterone given periodically will result in regular withdrawal bleeding that is more predictable but will not always lead to amenorrhea.

Alternative Therapeutic Regimens

Alternative regimens for postmenopausal women who are unable or unwilling to take hormone replacement therapy should be targeted toward

---

■ **TABLE 20-2**

Treatment Options to Address the Various Symptoms of Menopause

Menopausal Symptoms	Treatment Options
Cardiovascular changes	Blood pressure and lipid control medications, smoking cessation, weight loss, exercise
Osteoporosis risk	HRT, calcium, calcitonin, bisphosphonates, raloxifene, weight-bearing exercise
Hot flashes	HRT, clonidine, SSRIs,* black cohosh, evening primrose, dong quai
Vaginal dryness/dyspareunia	HRT, vaginal estrogen, water-based lubricant, isoflavones, chasteberry, ginseng
Mood disturbances	HRT, SSRIs, St. John's wort, black cohosh

*Selective serotonin reuptake inhibitors.

treatment goals. **Vasomotor flushes** have been managed with behavioral therapy, herbal medications, clonidine, and selective seratonin reuptake inhibitors (SSRIs). **Vaginal atrophy** can be managed locally with lubricants and moisturizers. Topical estrogen can have excellent local effects on vaginal and urethral atrophy, with only minimal systemic absorption.

The treatment for **osteoporosis** has been refined over the past few years and includes calcium/vitamin D supplements, bisphosphonates, calcitonin, selective estrogen receptor modulators (SERMs), and exercise. A bone-density measurement may be determined to follow bone resorption. With respect to **cardiovascular risks**, improvement in lifestyle and diet are key factors, as well as optimal blood pressure control to decrease morbidity and mortality.

KEY POINTS

1. The mean age of menopause is 50.
2. Patients present with amenorrhea, "hot flashes," vaginal atrophy, mood and sleep changes; all consistent with decreased levels of estrogen.
3. Diagnosis is made with history and physical examination and can be confirmed by elevated levels of FSH.
4. Women who wish to use HRT and still have a uterus in place should use both estrogen and progesterone therapy to avoid endometrial cancer.
5. Two major advantages of HRT are the prevention of bone loss and osteoporosis and the relief of symptoms associated with menopause.

Amenorrhea

Amenorrhea—the absence of menses—is classified as either primary or secondary. **Primary** amenorrhea is the absence of menses in women who have not undergone menarche by age 16 or have not had menstruation by 4 years after thelarche (the onset of breast development). **Secondary** amenorrhea is the absence of menses for three menstrual cycles or a total of 6 months in women who have previously had normal menstruation. The pathophysiology underlying these two processes highly differs, as does the differential diagnoses.

■ PRIMARY AMENORRHEA

If menses have not occurred by age 16, the diagnosis of primary amenorrhea is made. In the United States, the prevalence of primary amenorrhea is 1% to 2%. The causes of primary amenorrhea include congenital abnormalities, hormonal aberrations, chromosomal abnormalities, hypothalamic-pituitary disorders, and the variety of causes of secondary amenorrhea that may present before menarche. These causes are divided into three categories: outflow tract obstruction, end-organ disorders, and central regulatory disorders (Table 21-1).

Outflow Tract Anomalies

Imperforate Hymen

The hymen sometimes fails to canalize during fetal development and remains as a solid membrane across the introitus. If the hymen is imperforate, it will not allow egress of menses. Thus, despite having begun to menstruate, patients appear to have primary amenorrhea. After a time, patients present with pelvic or abdominal pain from the accumulation and

subsequent dilation of the vaginal vault and uterus by menses. On physical examination these patients have a bulging membrane just inside the vagina, often with purple-red discoloration behind it consistent with hematocolpos. The treatment of imperforate hymen is surgical; usually a cruciate incision is made and the hymen is sewn open to allow the egress of menses.

Transverse Vaginal Septum

A transverse vaginal septum may result from failure of the müllerian-derived upper vagina to fuse with the urogenital sinus-derived lower vagina. Commonly found at the level of the midvagina, it is usually patent. However, in some cases it may be imperforate and cause primary amenorrhea. Diagnosis is made on careful examination of the female genital tract. The diagnosis is commonly mistaken as imperforate hymen, and can be differentiated by the presence of a hymeneal ring below the septum. Surgical correction involves resection of the septum.

Vaginal Agenesis

Patients with **Mayer-Rokitansky-Kuster-Hauser (MRKH)** syndrome have müllerian agenesis or dysgenesis. They may have complete vaginal agenesis and absence of a uterus or partial vaginal agenesis with a rudimentary uterus and distal vagina. This differs from **vaginal atresia** where the müllerian system is developed, but the distal vagina is composed of fibrosed tissue. Diagnosis is made with physical examination that reveals no patent vagina, chromosomes that are 46,XX, and ovaries visualized on ultrasound. With partial vaginal agenesis or vaginal atresia, a rectal examination may reveal a pelvic mass consistent with a uterus. The uterus can be visualized with ultrasound (US), computed

■ TABLE 21-1

Etiologies of Primary Amenorrhea

Outflow tract abnormalities
Imperforate hymen

Transverse vaginal septum

Vaginal agenesis
  Vaginal atresia
  Testicular feminization

Uterine agenesis with vaginal dysgenesis
  MRKH syndrome

End-organ disorders
Ovarian agenesis
  Gonadal agenesis 46,XX
  Swyer's syndrome/gonadal agenesis 46,XY

Ovarian failure
  Enzymatic defects leading to decreased steroid
    biosynthesis
  Savage's **syndrome—ovary** fails to respond to FSH
    and LH
  Turner's syndrome

Central disorders
Hypothalamic
  Local tumor compression
  Trauma
  Tuberculosis
  Sarcoidosis
  Irradiation

Kallmann's syndrome—congenital absence of GnRH

Pituitary
Damage from surgery or radiation therapy

Hemosiderosis deposition of iron in pituitary

---

tomography (CT), or magnetic resonance imaging (MRI). Creation of a vagina can be achieved either by serial dilation of the perineal body by the patient over an extended period of time or by reconstructive surgery. In true vaginal atresia, the neovagina created may be connected with the upper genital tract.

Testicular Feminization

Testicular feminization or androgen insensitivity results from a dysfunction or absence of the testosterone receptor that leads to a phenotypical female with 46,XY chromosomes. This syndrome occurs in 1:50,000 women. Because these patients have testes, **müllerian inhibiting factor** (MIF) was secreted early in development, and these patients therefore have an absence of all müllerian-derived structures. Of note, the testes may be undescended or have migrated

down to the labia majora. The diminished testosterone sensitivity commonly leads to an absence of pubic and axillary hair. Usually estrogen is produced, and these patients develop breasts but present with primary amenorrhea because they have no uterus. Patients commonly have a vagina that ends as a blind pouch. For those patients with the absence of or a foreshortened vagina, therapy involves creating a neovagina for sexual function; however, these patients are unable to reproduce.

End-Organ Disorders

Ovarian Failure

Primary ovarian failure results in low levels of estradiol but elevated levels of gonadotropins termed **hypergonadotropic hypogonadism**. There are a variety of causes of primary ovarian failure (Table 21-2). **Savage's syndrome** is characterized by failure of the ovaries to respond to follicle-stimulating hormone (FSH) and luteinizing hormone (LH) secondary to a

■ TABLE 21-2

Causes of Primary Gonadal Failure (Hypergonadotropic Hypogonadism)

Idiopathic premature ovarian failure

Steroidogenic enzyme defects (primary amenorrhea)
  Cholesterol side-chain cleavage
  3β-ol-dehydrogenase
  17-hydroxylase
  17-desmolase
  17-ketoreductase

Testicular regression syndrome

True hermaphroditism

Gonadal dysgenesis
  Pure gonadal dysgenesis (Swyer's syndrome)
    (46,XX and 46,XY)
  Turner's syndrome (45,XO)
  Turner variants

Ovarian resistance syndrome (Savage's syndrome)

Autoimmune oophoritis

Postinfection (e.g., mumps)

Postoophorectomy (also wedge resections)

Post irradiation

Post chemotherapy

Source: Adapted from DeCherney A, Pernoll M. Current Obstetric and Gynecologic Diagnosis and Treatment. Norwalk: Appleton & Lange, 1994:1009.

receptor defect. In **Turner's syndrome** (45,XO), the ovaries undergo such rapid atresia that by puberty there are usually no primordial oocytes. Defects in the enzymes involved in steroid biosynthesis, particularly 17-α-hydroxylase, can result in amenorrhea and absence of breast development because of lack of estradiol.

Gonadal Agenesis with 46,XY Chromosomes

If there is a defect in the enzymes that are involved in testicular steroid production—**17-α-hydroxylase** or **17,20 desmolase**—these patients will not produce testosterone. However, MIF will still be produced; hence, there will be no female internal reproductive organs. These patients will otherwise be phenotypically female, usually without breast development. Patients with an absence of or defect in the testosterone receptor develop testicular feminization syndrome.

While testicular feminization results from peripheral effects of diminished or absent sensitivity of testosterone receptors, another situation in which the patient is genetically male but phenotypically female is gonadal agenesis. The congenital absence of the testes in a genotypical male, **Swyer's syndrome**, results in a phenotypical picture similar to that of ovarian agenesis. Because the testes never develop, MIF is not released and these patients have both internal and external female genitalia. However, without estrogen they will not develop breasts.

Central Disorders

Hypothalamic Disorders

The pituitary will not release FSH and LH if the hypothalamus is unable to produce gonadotropin-releasing hormone (GnRH), transport it to the pituitary, or release it in a pulsatile fashion. Anovulation and amenorrhea result from this hypogonadotropic hypogonadism. **Kallmann's syndrome** involves a congenital absence of GnRH and is commonly associated with anosmia. GnRH transport may be disrupted with compression or destruction of the pituitary stalk or arcuate nucleus. This can result from tumor mass effect, trauma, sarcoidosis, tuberculosis, irradiation, or Hand-Schuller-Christian disease. There may be defects in GnRH pulsatility in cases of anorexia nervosa, extreme stress, athletics, hyperprolactinemia, and constitutionally delayed puberty.

Pituitary Disorders

Primary defects of the pituitary are a rare cause of primary amenorrhea. Pituitary dysfunction is usually secondary to hypothalamic dysfunction. It may be caused by tumors, infiltration of the pituitary gland, or infarcts of the pituitary. Surgery or irradiation of pituitary tumors may lead to decreases in or absence of LH and FSH. Hemosiderosis can result in iron deposition in the pituitary, leading to destruction of the gonadotrophs that produce FSH and LH.

Diagnosis

A patient who presents with primary amenorrhea can be worked up based on the phenotypic picture (Table 21-3, Figure 21-1). Lack of a uterus is seen in males because of the release of MIF by the testes and in females with müllerian agenesis. Breast development is dependent upon estradiol secretion by the ovaries. Patients who have neither uterus nor breasts are generally 46,XY males with steroid synthesis defects or varying degrees of gonadal dysgenesis, in which adequate MIF is produced by gonadal tissue but androgen synthesis is insufficient.

If breasts are present but no uterus, the etiologies can include congenital absence of the uterus (müllerian agenesis) in the female or testicular feminization in the male. In the latter case, estradiol from

■ TABLE 21-3

Diagnosis of Etiology of Primary Amenorrhea		
	Uterus Absent	**Uterus Present**
Breasts absent	Gonadal agenesis in 46,XY Enzyme deficiencies in testosterone synthesis	Gonadal failure/agenesis in 46,XX Disruption of hypothalamic-pituitary axis
Breasts present	Testicular feminization Müllerian agenesis or MRKH	Hypothalamic, pituitary, or ovarian Pathogenesis similar to that of secondary amenorrhea Congenital abnormalities of the genital tract

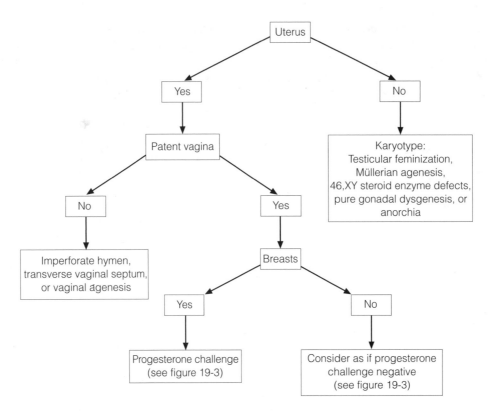

Figure 21-1 • Diagnostic flowchart for patients with primary amenorrhea.

direct testicular secretion as well as peripheral conversion of testosterone and androstenedione leads to breast development.

For patients who have a uterus but the absence of breast development, the differential includes (1) hypergonadotropic hypogonadism, as seen in gonadal dysgenesis in both sexes, and with defects in steroid pathways in 46,XX patients; and (2) hypogonadotropic hypogonadism, which is seen in central nervous system (CNS), hypothalamic, and pituitary dysfunction. A serum FSH level differentiates between these two, with elevation seen in hypergonadotropic hypogonadism.

The work-up for amenorrhea in phenotypic females with absence of either uterus or breasts must include karyotype analysis, followed by testosterone and FSH assays. Further biochemical and hormonal assays may be performed to elucidate specific enzyme defects. Patients with both uterus and breasts present should be evaluated to determine whether there is a patent outflow tract from the uterus. If the vagina, cervix, and uterus are continuous, these can be evaluated as if the patient were presenting with secondary amenorrhea.

Treatment

Patients with congenital abnormalities may be treated surgically with plastic procedures to allow egress of menses in those with a functional uterus or to create a functional vagina. Patients with absent uterus and breasts can be treated with estrogen replacement to effect breast development and prevent osteoporosis. Patients who have breast development but an absent uterus may not require medical intervention.

Patients with a uterus but without breast development and with hypergonadotropic hypogonadism often have irreversible ovarian failure and will require estrogen replacement therapy. Patients with hypogonadotropic hypogonadism require further work-up as patients with secondary amenorrhea.

KEY POINTS

1. Primary amenorrhea is the absence of menarche by age 16 or 4 years after the larche.
2. Primary amenorrhea can be caused by congenital abnormalities of the genital tract, chromosomal

abnormalities, enzyme or hormonal deficiencies, gonadal agenesis, ovarian failure, or disruption of the hypothalamic-pituitary axis.

3. The work-up of primary amenorrhea is usually organized into four categories based on the presence or absence of a uterus and the presence or absence of breast development.

4. In the absence of both uterus and breasts, karyotype usually reveals 46,XY.

5. In the absence of a uterus and presence of breasts, karyotype will differentiate between müllerian agenesis and testicular feminization.

6. In the absence of breasts and presence of a uterus, FSH will differentiate between hypergonadotropic and hypogonadotropic hypogonadism. Karyotype may be necessary to rule out gonadal agenesis in a 46,XY.

7. Patients with both a uterus and breasts should be evaluated as if presenting with secondary amenorrhea.

■ SECONDARY AMENORRHEA

Secondary amenorrhea is the absence of menses for more than 6 months or for the equivalent of three menstrual cycles in a woman who previously had menstrual cycles. **The most common cause of secondary amenorrhea is pregnancy.** Other causes can be categorized as anatomic abnormalities, ovarian dysfunction, prolactinoma and hyperprolactinemia, and CNS or hypothalamic disorders.

Anatomic Abnormalities

The common anatomic causes of secondary amenorrhea are Asherman's syndrome and cervical stenosis. **Asherman's syndrome** is the presence of intrauterine synechiae or adhesions, usually secondary to intrauterine surgery or infection. The etiology of Asherman's syndrome includes dilation and curettage (D&C), myomectomy, cesarean section, or endometritis. **Cervical stenosis** can manifest as secondary amenorrhea and dysmenorrhea. It is usually caused by scarring of the cervical os secondary to surgical or obstetric trauma.

Ovarian Failure

Ovarian failure may result from ovarian torsion, surgery, infection, radiation, or chemotherapy. Pre-

mature ovarian failure (POF) is often idiopathic. Anytime menopause occurs without another etiology before age 40, it is considered POF. Before age 35, chromosomal analysis is usually performed to diagnose a genetic basis for POF. Patients with either idiopathic POF or a known cause of early ovarian failure are generally treated with supplemental estrogen to decrease the risk of cardiovascular disease and osteoporosis.

Polycystic Ovarian Disease

Stein-Leventhal **syndrome** was described in 1935 and included the constellation of anovulation, oligomenorrhea or amenorrhea, hirsutism, obesity, and enlarged, polycystic ovaries. This syndrome is now understood to represent one end of the spectrum of patients with polycystic ovarian disease (PCOD), who have anovulation in common but can have any or all of the other findings. It is not entirely clear what precipitates the disease, but once it begins, a self-perpetuating cycle occurs.

Chronic anovulation leads to elevated levels of estrogen and androgen. The increased androgen released from the ovaries and the adrenal cortex are converted peripherally in the adipose tissue into estrone. Further, the elevated androgens lead to a decrease in the production of sex hormone binding globulin (SHBG), resulting in even higher levels of free estrogens and androgens. This hyperestrogenic state leads to an increased LH:FSH ratio, atypical follicular development, anovulation, and increased androgen production. Once again, the androgens are peripherally converted to estrogens, leading to a cyclical propagation of the disease. Many patients with PCOD who are hyperandrogenic and obese also develop insulin resistance and hyperinsulinemia. Not surprisingly, the incidence of type II diabetes mellitus is increased in these patients.

Treatment of these patients depends on the particular symptoms and the desires of the patient. For patients desiring fertility, ovulation induction (OI) using clomiphene citrate (Clomid) is begun. Patients with PCO are particularly resistant to OI and there is evidence that the probability of ovulation can be increased by weight loss or the concomitant use of corticosteroids. In patients with hyperinsulinemia, metformin has been shown to increase spontaneous ovulation. For patients who are not currently interested in fertility, either cyclic progestins or Depo-Provera should be used to decrease the risk of endometrial hyperplasia and cancer secondary to the unopposed estrogen. In addition, obese patients should be strongly urged to lose weight because this will decrease the risk of cardiovascular disease and diabetes and can actually break the cycle of anovulation.

Hyperprolactinemia-Associated Amenorrhea

Excess prolactin leads to amenorrhea and galactorrhea. Menstrual irregularities often result from abnormal gonadotropin (FSH and LH) secretion due to alterations in dopamine levels typically seen in hyperprolactinemia. The etiologies and consequences of excess prolactin are numerous. Prolactin release is inhibited by dopamine and stimulated by serotonin and thyrotropin-releasing hormone (TRH). Because of the constant suppression of prolactin release by hypothalamic release of dopamine, any disturbance in this process by a hypothalamic or pituitary lesion can lead to disinhibition of prolactin secretion.

Hyperprolactinemia has several possible etiologies (Table 21-4). Primary hypothyroidism that leads to elevated thyroid-stimulating hormone (TSH) and TRH can cause hyperprolactinemia. Medications that increase prolactin levels (by a hypothalamic pituitary effect) include dopamine antagonists (Haldol, Reglan, phenothiazines), tricyclic antidepressants, estrogen, monoamine oxidase (MAO) inhibitors, and opiates. A prolactin-secreting pituitary adenoma leads to elevated prolactin levels. The empty sella syndrome, in which the subarachnoid membrane herniates into the sella turcica, causing it to enlarge and flatten, which is another cause of hyperprolactinemia. Other conditions associated with high prolactin include pregnancy and breastfeeding. Any patient with an elevated prolactin level should have an imaging study to rule out prolactinoma.

Disruption of the Hypothalamic-Pituitary Axis

As in the hypothalamic and pituitary causes of primary amenorrhea, disruption in the secretion and transport of GnRH, absence of pulsatility of GnRH or acquired pituitary lesions will all cause hypogonadotropic hypogonadism (Table 21-5). Common causes of hypothalamic dysfunction include stress, exercise, anorexia nervosa, and weight loss.

■ TABLE 21-4

Differential Diagnosis of Galactorrhea-Hyperprolactinemia

Pituitary tumors secreting prolactin
Macroadenomas (>10 mm)
Microadenomas (<10 mm)

Hypothyroidism
Idiopathic hyperprolactinemia

Drug-induced hyperprolactinemia

Dopamine antagonists
  Phenothiazines
  Thioxanthenes
  Butyrophenone
  Diphenylbutylpiperidine
  Dibenzoxazepine
  Dihydroindolone
  Procainamide derivatives

Catecholamine-depleting agents

False transmitters (α-methyldopa)

Interruption of normal hypothalamic-pituitary relationship
Pituitary stalk section

Peripheral neural stimulation
Chest wall stimulation
  Surgery (e.g., mastectomy)
  Burns
  Herpes zoster
  Bronchogenic tumors
  Bronchiectasis/chronic bronchitis

Nipple stimulation
  Stimulation of nipples
  Chronic nipple irritation

Spinal cord lesion
  Tabes dorsalis
  Syringomyelia

CNS disease
  Encephalitis
  Craniopharyngioma
  Pineal and hypothalamic tumors
  Hypothalamic tumors
  Pseudotumor cerebri

Diagnosis

The approach to secondary amenorrhea always begins with a β-hCG (beta human chorionic gonadotropin) assay to **rule out pregnancy**. TSH and **prolactin** levels should then be checked to rule out hypothyroidism and hyperprolactinemia, both of

TABLE 21-5

Differential Diagnosis of Hypoestrogenic Amenorrhea (Hypogonadotropic Hypogonadism)

Hypothalamic dysfunction
Kallmann's syndrome
Tumors of hypothalamus (craniopharyngioma)
Constitutional delay of puberty
Severe hypothalamic dysfunction
Anorexia nervosa
Severe weight loss
Severe stress
Exercise

Pituitary disorder
Sheehan's syndrome
Panhypopituitarism
Isolated gonadotropin deficiency
Hemosiderosis (primarily from thalassemia major)

Source: Adapted from DeCherney A, Pernoll M. Current Obstetric and Gynecologic Diagnosis and Treatment. Norwalk: Appleton & Lange, 1994:1013.

which can cause amenorrhea. If both are elevated, the hypothyroidism should be treated and the prolactin level can be checked after thyroid studies have normalized to verify resolution.

If the prolactin level is elevated and TSH is normal, a work-up for the other causes of prolactinemia should ensue (Figure 21-2). In the diagnostic evaluation of the patient, a careful history should be taken, including a complete list of medications and clear documentation of the onset of symptoms. A thorough physical examination should include visual fields, cranial nerves, breast examination, and an attempt to express milk from the nipple. An MRI can rule out a hypothalamic or pituitary lesion.

If the prolactin level is normal, a **progesterone challenge test** (10 mg orally for 7 to 10 days to mimic progesterone withdrawal) should be performed to assess the adequacy of endogenous estrogen production and the outflow tract. Withdrawal bleeding occurring after the progesterone challenge indicates the presence of estrogen and an adequate outflow tract. In this case, amenorrhea is usually secondary to anovulation, which can be caused by a variety of endocrine disorders that alter pituitary/gonadal feedback such as polycystic ovaries, tumors of the ovary and adrenals, Cushing's syndrome, thyroid disorders, and adult-onset adrenal hyperplasia (Table 21-6).

Absence of withdrawal bleeding in response to progesterone alone must then be evaluated with estrogen and progesterone administration. If there is still no menstrual bleeding, an outflow tract disorder such as Asherman's syndrome or cervical stenosis is suspected. If menstrual bleeding does occur in response to estrogen and progesterone administration, this suggests an intact and functional uterus

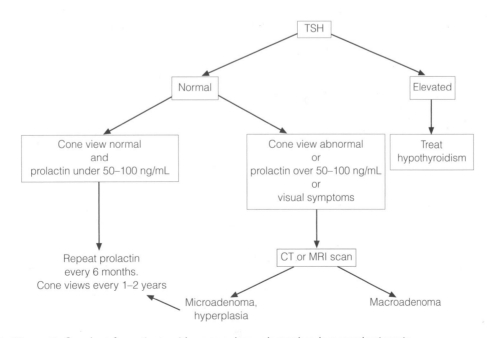

Figure 21-2 • Diagnostic flowchart for patients with amenorrhea-galactorrhea-hyperprolactinemia.

■ TABLE 21-6

Differential Diagnosis of Eugonadotropic Eugonadism (Progesterone Challenge Positive)

Mild hypothalamic dysfunction
Emotional stress
Psychologic disorder
Weight loss
Obesity
Exercise-induced
Idiopathic

Hirsutism-virilism
Polycystic ovary syndrome
Ovarian tumor
Adrenal tumor
Cushing's syndrome
Congenital and adult-onset adrenal hyperplasia

Systemic disease
Hypothyroidism
Hyperthyroidism
Addison's disease
Chronic renal failure
Many others seen in other chronic diseases

Source: Adapted from DeCherney A, Pernoll M. Current Obstetric and Gynecologic Diagnosis and Treatment. Norwalk: Appleton & Lange, 1994:1013.

without adequate endogenous estrogen stimulation. Measurement of FSH and LH will help differentiate between a hypothalamic/pituitary disorder (low/normal FSH and LH levels) and ovarian failure (high FSH and LH levels) (Figure 21-3).

Treatment

Patients with hypothyroidism are treated with thyroid hormone replacement. Those with pituitary macroadenomas are treated with surgical resection. Some patients with macroadenomas and most with microadenomas are treated with bromocriptine, a dopamine agonist that often causes tumor regression and the resumption of ovulation. Other hyperprolactinemic patients can also be treated with bromocriptine in order to resume ovulation. Further, this treatment should be followed with serial prolactin levels and cone view radiographs to diagnose development of a macroadenoma.

Patients who respond to progesterone challenge should be withdrawn with progesterone on a regular basis to prevent endometrial hyperplasia. Oral contraceptive pills (OCPs) are useful in this case and may be beneficial in the management of hirsutism. However, if the patient is a smoker over age 35, progesterone alone is indicated.

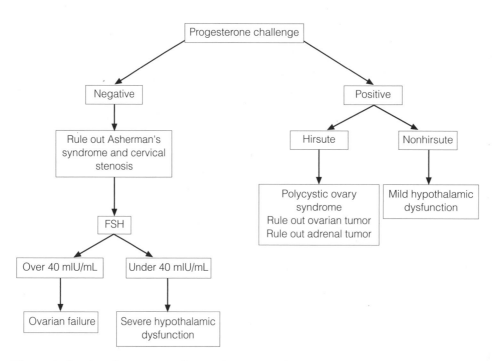

Figure 21-3 • Diagnostic flowchart for patients with secondary amenorrhea.

Patients who are hypoestrogenic should be treated with estrogen and progesterone for the effects these have on lipids, cardiovascular disease, bone density, and genital atrophy. OCPs are often used for women under age 35 or nonsmokers over age 35. For other patients, a regimen of 0.625 mg of conjugated estrogen cycled with 5–10 mg of medroxyprogesterone acetate is suitable. These patients should also receive 1.2 g of elemental calcium supplementation per day.

Ovulation Induction

Ovulation induction with bromocriptine can be used in patients with hyperprolactinemia. If the cause of hyperprolactinemia is medication related, discontinue or decrease the medication if possible. Patients who respond to the progesterone challenge have evidence of estrogenation. Any specific cause of this amenorrheic state should be corrected. If menses do not resume, ovulation induction may be performed with clomiphene citrate (Clomid), which acts as an antiestrogen to stimulate gonadotropin release. Patients with elevated androgens may need combined therapy with Clomid and corticosteroids.

Patients who do not respond to progesterone alone are presumed to have low estrogen levels; however, these patients will occasionally respond to Clomid as well. For patients who do not respond to Clomid, human menopausal gonadotropin (hMG) or recombinant GnRH can be used to stimulate ovulation. Careful monitoring with ultrasound and estradiol levels should be done in the case of gonadotropin ovulation induction because of the risk of ovarian hyperstimulation.

KEY POINTS

1. Anatomic abnormalities including Asherman's syndrome and cervical stenosis may lead to secondary amenorrhea. These patients fail to respond to estrogen and progesterone withdrawal.
2. Hyperprolactinemia is a common cause of secondary amenorrhea.
3. Patients with normal prolactin levels may be given a progesterone challenge to investigate whether or not the endometrium is estrogenized.
4. With progesterone challenge failure, the differential diagnosis becomes hypergonadotropic or hypogonadotropic hypogonadism that can be differentiated by an FSH measurement.
5. For patients not seeking current fertility, it is important to treat the specific cause of amenorrhea and to ensure that the hypoestrogenic patient receives hormone replacement therapy (HRT).
6. For patients who desire fertility, ovulation induction can usually be achieved. Patients with hyperprolactinemia require bromocriptine, whereas patients with other forms of hypogonadism may respond to clomiphene and gonadotropins.

Abnormalities of the Menstrual Cycle

■ DYSMENORRHEA

Dysmenorrhea is defined as pain and cramping during menstruation that interferes with the activities of daily living. Mild pain during menses is normal. Discomfort during menstruation ranges from mild discomfort to severe pain that causes some patients to be bedridden. Fifty percent of menstruating women suffer from dysmenorrhea, 10% of these are incapacitated for 1 to 3 days each month.

Dysmenorrhea is classified as primary or secondary. Primary or idiopathic dysmenorrhea is menstrual pain without identifiable pathology; secondary dysmenorrhea is painful menses without underlying pathology.

Primary Dysmenorrhea

Primary dysmenorrhea usually occurs before age 20. Although there is no obvious organic cause, primary dysmenorrhea is thought to result from **increased levels of endometrial prostaglandin production** derived from the arachidonic acid pathway. Additionally, there may be a psychological component involved for some patients that depends on attitudes toward menstruation learned from mothers, sisters, and friends.

Diagnosis

The diagnosis of primary dysmenorrhea is made on the basis of history and the absence of organic causes. Often, the pain of dysmenorrhea occurs with ovulatory cycles on the first or second day of menstruation. Associated symptoms include nausea, vomiting, and headache. On physical examination there are no obvious abnormalities but a generalized tenderness throughout the pelvis.

Treatment

The first-line treatment for primary dysmenorrhea is medical using **antiprostaglandin agents** and **nonsteroidal anti-inflammatory drugs** (NSAIDs). The most commonly used NSAIDs include aspirin, ibuprofen, and naproxen. These are all available without prescription; however, patients may need prescription-strength dosages to obtain adequate symptom relief. Patients should be advised to take the medications 24 hours prior to the onset of expected symptoms and continue throughout menses.

Oral contraceptive pills (OCPs) are the second-line of treatment for women who do not get relief from antiprostaglandin agents or who cannot tolerate them. More than 90% of women with primary dysmenorrhea find relief with oral contraceptives. The mechanism of relief is either secondary to the **cessation of ovulation** or the **decrease in endometrial proliferation** leading to decreased prostaglandin production. Most patients who have been cycled for 1 year on OCPs experience a reduction of symptoms even if the OCPs are discontinued.

Surgical therapies—including cervical dilation and neurectomies—have been used in the past but have little use in current management of true primary dysmenorrhea. Often, primary dysmenorrhea will decrease throughout a patient's 20s and early 30s. In addition, a pregnancy carried to viability will usually decrease the symptoms of primary dysmenorrhea. Most recently, the use of transcutaneous electrical nerve stimulation (TENS) has shown to relieve or decrease pain in women suffering from primary dysmenorrhea.

Secondary Dysmenorrhea

Secondary dysmenorrhea implies that any symptoms of dysmenorrhea are caused by endometriosis and adenomyosis (Chapter 15), fibroids (Chapter 14), cervical stenosis, or pelvic adhesions. Because the first three causes are discussed in other chapters, refer to those particular chapters for detailed management.

Cervical Stenosis

Cervical stenosis causes dysmenorrhea by obstructing blood flow during menstruation. The stenosis can be congenital or secondary to scarring from infection, trauma, or surgery. Patients often complain of scant menses associated with severe cramping pain that is relieved with increased menstrual flow. On physical examination there may be obvious scarring of the external os; often the physician is unable to pass a uterine sound through the cervical canal.

Treatment

Dilation of the cervix is the treatment for cervical stenosis. Either a surgical dilation can be performed or laminaria tents can be used. Surgical dilation is usually performed in the operating room, but can be attempted in the office with a paracervical block. Progressively larger dilators are placed through the cervical canal until a curette can be placed through and used to clean the endometrial cavity.

Laminaria may be placed in the cervix in the office setting. Made from seaweed, these dilate over a 24-hour period by absorbing water from the surrounding tissue. Slow dilation of the cervix results from expansion of the laminaria. Dilation will provide relief; however, symptoms often recur, requiring multiple dilations. Pregnancy with vaginal delivery often leads to a permanent cure.

Pelvic Adhesions

Patients with a history of pelvic infections including cervicitis, pelvic inflammatory disease, or tubo-ovarian abscess may have symptoms of dysmenorrhea secondary to adhesion formation. Patients with other local inflammatory diseases (appendicitis, endometriosis, or Crohn's disease) or prior pelvic surgery may also have adhesions leading to dysmenorrhea. Diagnosis is made via history of any of these problems in conjunction with laparoscopy revealing local adhesions. In some patients, pelvic adhesions can be so extensive as to cement the uterus into a fixed position, which may be noted on pelvic examination.

Treatment

These patients will occasionally respond to the **antiprostaglandins** prescribed for primary dysmenorrhea. For more severe cases that fail to respond to medical therapy, laparoscopy is indicated. At that time the diagnosis made and the adhesions, if accessible, can be surgically lysed. However, surgery can lead to further adhesions and further problems with dysmenorrhea.

KEY POINTS

1. Primary dysmenorrhea is severe pain with menses that cannot be attributed to any organic cause.
2. Most primary dysmenorrhea is managed with NSAIDs, OCPs, and/or TENS.
3. Secondary dysmenorrhea is usually caused by adenomyosis, endometriosis, fibroids, cervical stenosis, or pelvic adhesions, all of which can be diagnosed and treated.

■ PREMENSTRUAL SYNDROME (PMS)

Premenstrual syndrome (PMS) is a constellation of symptoms that occurs in the second half of the menstrual cycle including weight gain, edema, mood fluctuation, breast tenderness, and other depressive symptoms. Probably 90% of women suffer from some PMS symptoms and 5% of women are incapacitated at some point during the cycle.

Pathogenesis

The exact etiology of PMS has yet to be elucidated. However, it is likely due to both physiological and psychological causes. Hypotheses include abnormalities in the estrogen/progesterone balance, disturbance of the renin-angiotensin-aldosterone pathway, excess prostaglandin production, and reduction of endogenous endorphin production or receptor sensitivity.

Treatment

Treatments for premenstrual syndrome must often be tried as "hit or miss" therapies until an effective one is found. One-third of women experience sufficient improvement in symptoms with **dietary modification** alone. **NSAIDs** often bring symptomatic relief; this supports the excess prostaglandin hypothesis. **OCPs** sometimes provide relief, supporting the theory that symptoms are related to ovulation, low progesterone levels, or an imbalance in estrogen and progesterone levels. The idea that cyclic fluctuations in the steroid hormones affect PMS is supported by the fact that, in small trials, **GnRH agonists** such as leuprolide acetate (Depo Lupron) have been successful in treating symptoms. With severe edema, **diuretics** such as furosemide (Lasix) offer some relief. Patients with incapacitating depressive symptoms of sleep disturbance, depressed mood, withdrawal from society, and lack of appetite may be helped by **psychotropic medications** such as alprazolam (Xanax) and fluoxetine hydrochloride (Prozac).

KEY POINTS

1. PMS is most likely a multifactorial disease with physiological and psychological components.
2. Although the cause is unknown, a variety of palliative treatments including NSAIDs and OCPs offer some relief.

■ ABNORMAL UTERINE BLEEDING

Abnormal uterine bleeding refers to any departure from the norm in the menstrual cycle. It can involve too much bleeding as with heavy periods, frequent menses, or bleeding between periods. Abnormal bleeding may result in too little bleeding as with light periods, infrequent periods, or complete absence of periods.

Dysfunctional uterine bleeding (DUB) describes idiopathic heavy and/or irregular bleeding that cannot be attributed to another cause. Amenorrhea—complete absence of periods—is discussed in Chapter 21.

Menorrhagia

Menorrhagia, or hypermenorrhea, is defined as **heavy** or **prolonged menstrual bleeding**. The average blood loss during a menstrual cycle is approximately 35 mL; menorrhagia is when bleeding is greater than 80 mL in one menstrual cycle. Patients with menorrhagia occasionally describe the blood as "pouring" out or "gushing," and may have blood clots along with their excessive flow. The diagnosis can be made by weighing the menstrual pads used in a cycle and cal-

culating the volume of blood lost. Most gynecologists use a history of greater than 24 menstrual pads a day or soaking through a pad every hour as indicative of menorrhagia. Endometrial biopsy and pelvic ultrasound (US) can also be used to identify the source of menorrhagia. A hematocrit and iron studies should be checked and can contribute to the diagnosis. Bleeding from the cervix, vagina, or rectum should be ruled out with examination.

Menorrhagia can be caused by fibroids, adenomyosis, endometrial hyperplasia, endometrial polyps, endometrial or cervical cancer, dysfunctional uterine bleeding, primary bleeding disorders, or pregnancy complications.

Metrorrhagia and Menometrorrhagia

Metrorrhagia is characterized by **bleeding between periods**. This bleeding is usually less than or equal to menses. If the intermenstrual bleeding is heavy (greater than 80 mL) and associated with prolonged periods, it is described as **menometrorrhagia**. The usual causes include endometrial polyps, endometrial or cervical cancer, submucous fibroids, or complications of pregnancy.

Hypomenorrhea

Patients with hypomenorrhea have periods with unusually light flow. This is commonly caused by hypogonadotropic hypogonadism in anorexics and athletes. Atrophic endometrium can also occur in the case of Asherman's syndrome, intrauterine adhesions or synechiae secondary to congenital effects or intrauterine trauma. Patients on OCPs or Depo-Provera also have atrophic endometrium and often have light menses. Outlet obstruction secondary to cervical stenosis or congenital abnormalities also causes hypomenorrhea.

Polymenorrhea

Polymenorrhea, or frequent periods, can be confused with metrorrhagia. If all of the bleeding episodes are similar with fewer than 21 days between them, polymenorrhea should be considered. This is usually caused by anovulation.

Oligomenorrhea

Patients with periods greater than 35 days apart are described as having oligomenorrhea. The causes are similar to those for amenorrhea with disruption of the pituitary-gonadal axis by hypothalamic, pituitary, or gonadal abnormalities, or systemic disease (Chapter 21). The most common causes of oligomenorrhea are pregnancy, polycystic ovarian syndrome, and chronic anovulation.

Evaluation

The work-up for abnormal uterine bleeding includes a careful history and physical followed by diagnostic tests to determine the underlying etiology. The history should include timing of bleeding, quantity of bleeding, menstrual history with menarche and recent periods, and associated symptoms. It should also include a family history of bleeding disorders, particularly if menorrhagia appears at menarche.

On physical examination, vaginal and cervical causes of bleeding should be ruled out. The bimanual examination may reveal uterine or adnexal masses consistent with fibroids, adenomyosis, or cancer. A **Pap smear** is used to screen for cervical cancer. An **endometrial biopsy** is used to screen for endometrial hyperplasia and cancer. Sometimes a polyp or submucous fibroid will be diagnosed in this fashion.

All patients should have a **pregnancy test**. A **pelvic ultrasound** can be used to examine the intrauterine cavity in a noninvasive manner. Endometrial polyps, fibroids, and extensive cancers may be seen with this modality. A sonohystogram or **hysterosalpingogram** may show intrauterine defects. **Hysteroscopy** allows direct visualization of the intrauterine cavity. A **dilation and curettage** (D&C) provides tissue for diagnosis. The array of hormonal tests that can be performed are discussed with the work-up of amenorrhea included in Chapter 21.

Treatment

The treatment of abnormal uterine bleeding depends on the specific underlying etiology. A D&C may be therapeutic as well as diagnostic. Fibroids and polyps can be treated by removal. Cancer is diagnosed by biopsy and treated accordingly. Adenomyosis and the endocrinopathies sometimes respond to OCPs, as will dysfunctional uterine bleeding.

KEY POINTS

1. The most common cause of oligomenorrhea and secondary amenorrhea is pregnancy.
2. Structural abnormalities—polyps, fibroids, adenomyosis, and cancer—cause most of the menorrhagia, metrorrhagia, and menometrorrhagia except that which is related to pregnancy.

■ DYSFUNCTIONAL UTERINE BLEEDING (DUB)

If no pathologic cause of menorrhagia, metrorrhagia, or menometrorrhagia can be elucidated, the diagnosis of exclusion, DUB, is given. Most patients will be anovulatory, with disruption in the hypothalamic-pituitary-gonadal axis that leads to continuous estrogenic stimulation of the endometrium. The endometrium then sloughs off when it outgrows its blood supply rather than in any regular fashion. DUB usually occurs near menarche and menopause.

Diagnosis

Diagnosis is made by history and physical to rule out other causes of abnormal bleeding. A basal body temperature can be graphed daily to determine whether ovulation is occurring. This can also be accomplished with ovulation prediction kits, which are at-home tests for detecting the LH surge from urine samples. An appropriate day 23 to 25 serum progesterone level may also indicate if a patient is ovulating. Endometrial sampling is the gold standard to determine whether ovulation is occurring. If hemorrhage is a concern, a hematocrit and iron studies should be done.

Treatment

If patients are not hemorrhaging and are hemodynamically stable, OCPs are an effective means of regulating the menstrual cycle. Patients may also be cycled on progesterone alone. For patients with excessive blood loss, therapy to stop the bleeding should be initiated immediately. Conjugated estrogens given at 10 mg/day should control the bleeding within 24 to 48 hours. If this is not effective, the estrogens need to be increased. For hemodynamically unstable patients, intravenous estrogen can be used.

For patients with ovulatory DUB, NSAIDs have been shown to decrease menstrual blood loss by 20%

to 50% and may be used alone or in conjunction with estrogen and progesterone therapy.

Patients who do not respond to medical therapy require surgical intervention. D&C, the first treatment of choice, may be diagnostic and occasionally therapeutic. Endometrial ablation with laser, electrocautery, or heated roller may be performed to decrease uterine bleeding. Hysterectomy is the definitive surgery but should be reserved for those cases refractory to all other treatments.

DUB is most likely to occur with the anovulatory cycles more common in adolescence and near menopause. In adolescence, the risk of a structural cause is small. However, any congenital possibilities and bleeding disorders should be eliminated. In the reproductive years, there is an increased risk of other etiologies, ranging from structural to hormonal, that need to be eliminated. During perimenopause, the risk of DUB increases, as does the risk of other causes including cancer and fibroids. A careful work-up of abnormal uterine bleeding must therefore be performed before the diagnosis of DUB is given.

KEY POINTS

1. DUB is a diagnosis of exclusion when no other source for abnormal bleeding can be identified.
2. DUB is thought to be secondary to anovulation, and is therefore more prevalent near menarche and menopause.
3. Treatment includes initial medical therapy but may require surgical modalities for those patients whose symptoms are not controlled with medical management.

■ POSTMENOPAUSAL BLEEDING

Vaginal bleeding more than 12 months after menopause occurs is considered postmenopausal bleeding. Any bleeding after menopause is abnormal and should be investigated because patients in this age group are more likely to have cancer.

Bleeding in postmenopausal women can be due to nongynecologic etiologies, lower and upper genital tract sources, tumors, or exogenous hormonal stimulation. **Nongynecologic causes** include rectal bleeding from hemorrhoids, anal fissures, rectal prolapse, and lower gastrointestinal (GI) tumors. Urethral caruncles are another source of bleeding in the postmenopausal woman. These can be identified by history and physical with anoscopy and occult blood screening. Further work-up can include a barium enema or colonoscopy.

Vaginal atrophy is the most common source of lower genital tract bleeding. The thin vaginal mucosa is easily traumatized and therefore likely to bleed. Other causes of lower genital tract bleeding are lesions of the vulva, vagina, or exocervix.

Pathologic causes of postmenopausal bleeding from the upper genital tract include cervical cancer, endometrial hyperplasia, endometrial polyps, and endometrial cancer. Exogenous hormones are the most common cause of postmenopausal bleeding. However, bleeding that is abnormal with signs of menometrorrhagia should be worked up as abnormal postmenopausal bleeding.

Diagnosis

A careful history is important. Physical examination should include a careful inspection of the external anogenital region, the vagina, and cervix. A **Pap smear** should be performed as well as a digital rectal examination and occult blood screening.

Endometrial biopsy should be performed to rule out endometrial cancer if there is no obvious nongynecologic or lower genital tract etiology. With heavy bleeding, a hematocrit should be obtained.

Pelvic ultrasound can identify polyps and is used to examine the thickness of the endometrial stripe, which should be less than 5 mm in the postmenopausal woman. **Hysteroscopy**—either in the office or operating room—can further elucidate intrauterine abnormalities such as endometrial polyps. **D&C** is both diagnostic and therapeutic for some lesions of the uterus and cervix.

Treatment

If GI bleeding is suspected, referral to a gastroenterologist and colonoscopy are the routine management. Hemorrhoids and anal fissures should be referred to general surgeons for further management.

Lesions of the vulva and vagina should be biopsied. Lacerations of mucosa should be repaired. Atrophy should be treated with estrogen. Commonly, estrogen cream is used and may supplement hormone replacement therapy (HRT).

Endometrial hyperplasia can be simple, complex, or atypical (Chapter 14). Cases of simple endometrial hyperplasia will progress to carcinoma in 1%, complex in 3%, and atypical in 8% to 29%. Therapy therefore differs for each. Simple endometrial hyperplasia is often monitored with repeated endometrial biopsies. Complex and atypical hyperplasia is often treated with progestin therapy, which leads to reversal of lesions in greater than 85% of patients. Those without reversal or with recurrence are treated surgically with hysterectomy.

Endometrial polyps may be removed by hysteroscopic resection or D&C. Endometrial cancer is usually treated by hysterectomy that may or may not be performed in conjunction with chemotherapy and radiation therapy.

KEY POINTS

1. Postmenopausal bleeding should always be investigated to rule out cancer.
2. Causes of postmenopausal bleeding include cancer of the upper and lower genital tract, endometrial polyps, exogenous hormonal stimulation, vaginal atrophy, and nongynecologic sources.

Hirsutism and Virilism

Adults have two types of hair: vellus and terminal. Vellus hair is nonpigmented, soft, and covers the entire body. Terminal hair is, on the other hand, pigmented, thick, and covers the scalp, axilla, and pubic area. Androgens are responsible for the conversion of vellus to terminal hair at puberty, resulting in pubic and axillary hair. An abnormal increase in terminal hair is due to androgen excess or increased **5α-reductase** activity; this enzyme converts testosterone to the more potent dihydrotestosterone (DHT). DHT is believed to be the main stimulant of terminal hair development.

Hirsutism refers to the increase in terminal hair on the face, chest, back, lower abdomen, and inner thighs in a woman. Often, the pubic hair is characterized by the development of a male escutcheon, which is diamond shaped as opposed to the triangular female escutcheon. **Virilization** refers to the development of male features, such as deepening of the voice, frontal balding, increased muscle mass, clitoromegaly, breast atrophy, and male body habitus.

The evaluation of hirsutism and virilism in the female patient is complex and requires understanding pituitary, adrenal, and ovarian function with detailed attention to the pathways of glucocorticoid, mineralocorticoid, androgen, and estrogen synthesis.

■ NORMAL ANDROGEN SYNTHESIS

The adrenal gland is divided into two components: the adrenal cortex, which is responsible for glucocorticoid, mineralocorticoid, and androgen synthesis; and the adrenal medulla, which is involved in catecholamine synthesis. The adrenal cortex is composed of three layers. An outer **zona glomerulosa** layer produces aldosterone and is regulated primarily by the renin-angiotensin system. Because this zone lacks **17α-hydroxylase**, cortisol and androgens are not synthesized. In contrast, the inner layers, the **zona fasciculata** and the **zona reticularis**, produce both cortisol and androgens but not aldosterone because they lack the enzyme **aldosterone synthase.** These two inner zones are highly regulated by adrenocorticotropic hormone (ACTH).

ACTH regulates the conversion of cholesterol to pregnenolone by hydroxylation and side-chain cleavage. Pregnenolone is then converted to progesterone and eventually to aldosterone or cortisol or shunted over to the production of sex steroids (Figure 23-1).

In the adrenal glands, androgens are synthesized from the precursor **17α-hydroxypregnenolone**, which is converted to **dehydroepiandrosterone** (DHEA) and its sulfate (DHEAS), androstenedione, and finally to testosterone. DHEA and DHEAS are the most common adrenal androgens, whereas only small amounts of the others are secreted.

In the ovaries, the theca cells are stimulated by luteinizing hormone (LH) to produce androstenedione and testosterone. Both androstenedione and testosterone are then aromatized to estrone and estradiol, respectively, by the granulosa cells in response to follicle-stimulating hormone (FSH). Elevations in the ratio of LH to FSH may therefore lead to elevated levels of androgens.

Pathologic Production of Androgens

Elevation of androgens can be due primarily to adrenal or ovarian disorders. Because synthesis of steroid hormones in the adrenal cortex is stimulated by ACTH at a nondifferentiated step, elevated ACTH levels increase all the steroid hormones, including the androgens. If enzymatic defects are present, the pre-

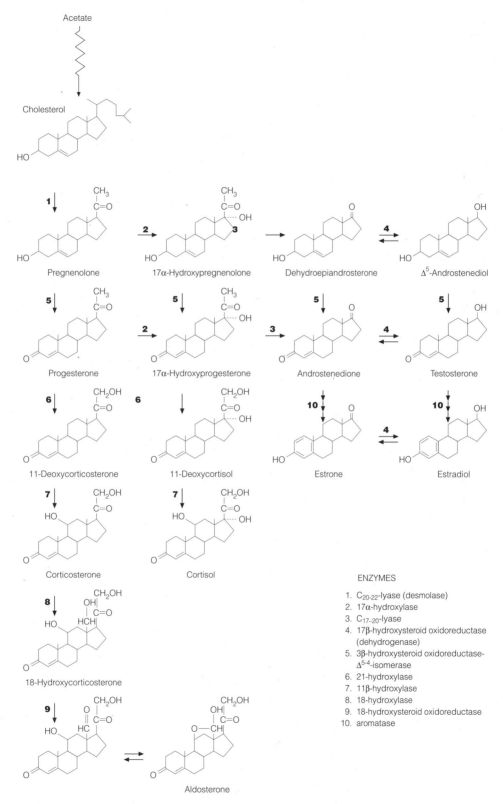

Figure 23-1 • Biosynthesis of androgens, estrogens, and corticosteroids.
(Reproduced with permission from Mishell DR, et al. Infertility, Contraception, and Reproductive Endocrinology. 3rd ed. Cambridge: Blackwell Science, 1991.)

cursor proximal to the defect accumulates and is shunted to another pathway. Thus, enzymatic blockade of either cortisol or aldosterone synthesis can lead to increased androgen production. Because DHEAS is derived almost entirely from the adrenal glands, its elevation is used as a marker for adrenal androgen production.

In the ovary, any increase in LH or in the LH:FSH ratio appears to lead to excess androgen production. Further, tumors of both the adrenal gland and the ovary can lead to excess androgens. Regardless of the source, elevated androgens lead to hirsutism and possibly virilism.

ADRENAL DISORDERS

The adrenal disorders leading to virilization in a woman are divided into two categories: nonneoplastic and neoplastic etiologies. Androgen-producing adrenal tumors may be either adenomas or carcinomas. Adrenal adenomas typically cause glucocorticoid excess and virilizing symptoms are rare. Carcinomas, on the other hand, can be more rapidly progressive and lead to marked elevations in glucocorticoid, mineralocorticoid, and androgen steroids.

Cushing's Syndrome

Cushing's syndrome is characterized by excess production of cortisol. Because the intermediates in production are androgens, there will be a concomitant hyperandrogenic state. Cushing's syndrome may be caused by pituitary adenomas, ectopic sources of ACTH, and tumors of the adrenal gland. **Cushing's syndrome** is caused by pituitary adenomas that hypersecrete ACTH. Paraneoplastic syndromes, such as nonpituitary ACTH-secreting tumors, also lead to increased ACTH levels. Adrenal gland tumors usually result in decreased levels of ACTH secondary to the negative feedback from the increased levels of adrenal steroid hormones. All three of these situations lead to the glucocorticoid excess characteristic of Cushing's syndrome, as well as hirsutism, acne, and menstrual irregularities related to adrenal androgen production.

When Cushing's syndrome is suspected, it can be diagnosed with the overnight dexamethasone suppression test. Essentially, if there is normal negative feedback from exogenous steroid hormone then the adrenal gland should decrease production in response to the dexamethasone. A plasma cortisol level is drawn the next morning and if it is <5 μg/dL the patient does not have Cushing's syndrome. A cortisol level >10 μg/dL is diagnostic, whereas a value between 5 and 10 is indeterminate. The diagnosis can be confirmed by collecting a 24-hour urine specimen and checking free cortisol.

Congenital Adrenal Hyperplasia

Congenital adrenal hyperplasia (CAH) refers to a constellation of enzyme deficiencies involved in steroidogenesis. The most common disorder is **21α-hydroxylase** deficiency. As seen in Figure 23-1, an enzymatic block at this step will lead to the accumulation of **17α-hydroxyprogesterone (17-OHP)**, which is then shunted to the androgen pathway. Patients with CAH do not synthesize cortisol or mineralocorticoids and thus present with salt-wasting and adrenal insufficiency at birth. Female infants will have ambiguous genitalia due to androgen excess. In milder or "adult-onset" forms, the degree of deficiency can vary, and often the only presenting sign is mild virilization and menstrual irregularities.

The other types of CAH that can be associated with virilization include **11β-hydroxylase** and **3β-hydroxysteroid dehydrogenase** (3β-HSD) deficiencies. Patients with 11β-hydroxylase deficiency present with similar symptoms of androgen excess as accumulated precursors are shunted to androstenedione and testosterone production pathways. Patients with 3β-HSD deficiency actually accumulate DHEA because they are unable to convert pregnenolone to progesterone or DHEA down the androgen synthesis pathway. DHEA and its sulfate, DHEAS, both have mild androgenic effects. Importantly, because this defect is also present in gonadal steroidogenesis, males have feminization and females have hirsutism and virilization. All patients have impaired cortisol synthesis and varying degrees of either mineralocorticoid excess or deficiency, depending on the location of the enzymatic block.

When CAH is suspected, a 17-OHP level should be checked because 21α-hydroxylase deficiency is the most common etiology. If 17-OHP is elevated (>200 ng/dL), the diagnosis can be confirmed with an ACTH stimulation test in which Cortrosyn (ACTH) is given IV and a 17-OHP level is checked after 1 hour. A marked increase in 17-OHP is consistent with CAH, with lower elevated values being seen in late-onset CAH and heterozygote carriers for the 21α-hydroxylase deficiency.

FUNCTIONAL OVARIAN DISORDERS

The ovarian disorders leading to virilization are divided into nonneoplastic and neoplastic etiologies. Polycystic ovaries, theca lutein cysts, stromal hyperplasia, and stromal hyperthecosis all involve nonneoplastic lesions. Neoplastic lesions vary and often cause rapid onset of virilization.

Non-neoplastic Ovarian Disorders

Polycystic Ovarian Syndrome

Polycystic ovarian syndrome (PCOS), previously known as the Stein-Leventhal syndrome, is a common disorder affecting up to 4% of reproductive age women. Patients present with a constellation of symptoms including hirsutism, virilization, anovulation, amenorrhea, and obesity. There is also an increased incidence of hyperinsulinemia, diminished insulin sensitivity, and type 2 diabetes mellitus in this population. The cause of androgen excess appears to be related to excess LH stimulation leading to cystic changes in the ovaries and increased ovarian androgen secretion. Typically, the LH:FSH ratio is greater than 2:1. What actually causes the elevation in LH levels is not clear, although it appears that any number of factors may be involved in this cycle including obesity, insulin resistance, and excessive adrenal androgen production.

Theca Lutein Cysts

The **theca cells** of the ovary are stimulated by LH to produce androstenedione and testosterone. These androgens are normally shunted to the **granulosa cells** for aromatization to estrone and estradiol. Theca lutein cysts produce an excess amount of androgens that are secreted into the circulation. These cysts may be present in either normal or molar pregnancy. The ovaries are enlarged, patients present with hirsutism and, occasionally, virilization. Diagnosis is made by ovarian biopsy.

Stromal Hyperplasia and Hyperthecosis

Stromal hyperplasia is common between age 50 and 70 and can cause hirsutism. The ovaries are uniformly enlarged. **Stromal hyperthecosis** is characterized by foci of utilization within the hyperplasic stroma. It is more likely than simple hyperplasia to result in virilization as the utilized cells continue to produce ovarian androgens. The ovaries typically appear enlarged and "fleshy," with the more florid cases seen in younger patients.

Neoplastic Ovarian Disorders

Functional Ovarian Tumors

Functional ovarian tumors that can produce varying amounts of androgen include the sex-cord mesenchymal tumors, Sertoli-Leydig cell tumors (arrhenoblastoma), granulosa-theca cell tumors, hilar (Leydig) cell tumors, and germ cell tumors (gonadoblastomas). Sertoli-Leydig cell tumors usually occur in young women and account for less than 1% of all ovarian neoplasms. Hilar cell tumors are even more rare than Sertoli-Leydig cell tumors and are usually seen in postmenopausal women. These tumors may secrete androgens, leading to hirsutism and virilism.

In pregnancy, there may be a luteoma—a benign tumor that grows in response to human chorionic gonadotropin. This tumor can result in high levels of testosterone and androstenedione and virilization in 25% of patients. There will also be virilization of 65% of female fetuses. These findings should resolve in the postpartum period.

Nonfunctional Ovarian Tumors

Androgen excess can also occur in the case of nonfunctional ovarian tumors (e.g., a cystadenoma or Krukenberg's tumor). Although these tumors do not secrete androgens themselves, they do stimulate proliferation in the adjacent ovarian stroma, which in turn may lead to increased androgen production.

DRUGS AND EXOGENOUS HORMONES

A variety of drugs can affect the circulating levels of sex hormone binding globulin (SHBG). SHBG is one of the major proteins that binds circulating testosterone, leaving a small proportion of "free" testosterone to interact at the cellular level. Androgens and corticosteroids decrease SHBG, leaving a greater percentage of free testosterone circulating. Patients who use anabolic steroids often present with hirsutism and virilization. In addition, drugs such as minoxidil, phenytoin, diazoxide, and cyclosporin will cause hirsutism without using androgenic pathways.

Idiopathic Hirsutism

Hirsutism is considered idiopathic in the absence of adrenal or ovarian pathology, an exogenous source of androgens, or use of the above-listed drugs. Patients may actually have occult androgen production, but many will have normal circulating androgen levels. There may be an increase in peripheral androgen production due to elevated 5α-reductase activity at the level of the skin and hair follicles.

Clinical Manifestations

A detailed history including time of onset, progression, and symptoms of virilization/hirsutism should be obtained, as well as a pubertal, menstrual, and reproductive history. Because various medications can affect androgen levels by affecting SHBG or intrinsic androgenic activity, a detailed drug history should be obtained. A family history is also important in order to look for genetic disorders such as CAH.

Physical Examination

On physical examination, the hair pattern should be noted, with attention to facial, chest, back, abdominal, and inner thigh hair, as well as the presence of frontal balding. The body habitus and presence or absence of female contours should be described. Breast examination may reveal atrophic changes, and a careful pelvic examination should include inspection of the escutcheon (pattern of pubic hair), clitoris (for clitoromegaly), and palpation for ovarian masses. Cushingoid features should be ruled out and inspection for acanthosis nigricans (velvety, thickened hyperpigmentation) in the axilla and nape of neck should be performed because this dermatologic finding is often associated with polycystic ovaries.

Diagnostic Evaluation

Laboratory evaluation should include free testosterone, 17-OHP, and DHEAS, the latter of which is normally exclusive to the adrenal gland. An elevation in free testosterone confirms androgen excess and a concomitant elevation in DHEAS suggests an adrenal source. An elevated 17-OHP is suggestive of CAH. If an adrenal source is suspected, an abdominal computed tomography (CT) should be performed to rule out an adrenal tumor, as well as further tests to diagnose Cushing's syndrome or CAH.

If the DHEAS is normal or minimally elevated, an ovarian source should be considered and a pelvic ultrasound or CT should be performed to rule out an ovarian neoplasm. An elevation in the LH:FSH ratio greater than 3 is suggestive of PCOS. Rapid onset of virilization and testosterone levels greater than 200 ng/dL may indicate an ovarian neoplasm.

At times the source of androgen excess is not readily evident and further diagnostic tests such as abdominal magnetic resonance imaging (MRI) and selective venous sampling need to be done for localization. In the hirsute woman with normal free testosterone, an assay for 5α-reductase activity is performed to determine whether increased peripheral enzymatic activity is responsible for the development of hirsutism.

Treatment

Adrenal non-neoplastic androgen suppression can be achieved with glucocorticoid administration, such as prednisone 5 mg qhs. Finasteride inhibits the 5α-reductase enzyme, thus diminishing peripheral conversion of testosterone to DHT. Antiandrogens such as spironolactone have been helpful as well, but are temporizing at best. In the case of ovarian or adrenal tumors, the underlying disorder should be treated. Often surgical intervention is required.

In general, ovarian non-neoplastic androgen production can be suppressed with oral contraceptives that will suppress LH and FSH as well as increase SHBG. Progesterone therapy alone may help patients with contraindications to estrogen use. Progesterone decreases levels of LH and thus androgen production; further, the catabolism of testosterone is increased, resulting in decreased levels. Gonadotropin-releasing hormone (GnRH) agonists can also be used to suppress LH and FSH. However, this leads to a hypoestrogenic state and requires concomitant estrogen replacement.

Patients using exogenous androgens or other drugs leading to increased androgens or hair growth should be advised to discontinue use. For patients with idiopathic hirsutism or contraindications to hormonal use, waxing, depilatories, and electrolysis will often provide cosmetic improvement.

KEY POINTS

1. Hirsutism is excess hair growth with a male pattern on the face, back, chest, abdomen, and inner thighs, usually in response to excess androgens.
2. Virilism is a constellation of symptoms including hirsutism, deepening of the voice, frontal balding, clitoromegaly, and increased musculature.
3. Primary causes of hirsutism and virilization include PCOS, ovarian tumors, adrenal tumors, CAH, and Cushing's syndrome.
4. Diagnosis is made by history and physical, serum assays for testosterone, DHEAS, and 17-OHP, and imaging studies.
5. Management involves primary treatment for the underlying cause; hormonal therapy with OCPs, GnRH, or progestins; and cosmetic treatment of hirsutism.

24 Contraception and Sterilization

Approximately 90% of women of childbearing age use some form of contraception. Despite this, nearly 55% of pregnancies in the United States are unintentional. Of these, 43% result in live births, 13% in miscarriages, and 44% end in elective abortion. In weighing the risks and benefits of contraception methods, couples must keep in mind that no contraceptive or sterilization method is 100% effective. Table 24-1 outlines relative failure rates or the number of women likely to become pregnant within the first year of using a particular method. **Theoretical efficacy rate** refers to the efficacy of contraception when used exactly as instructed. **Actual efficacy rate** refers to efficacy when used in "real life," assuming variations in the consistency of usage.

■ NATURAL METHODS

The methods of contraception described in this section—periodic abstinence, coitus interruptus, and lactational amenorrhea—are **physiology-based methods** that use neither chemical nor mechanical barriers to contraception. Many couples, for deeply held religious or philosophic reasons, prefer these methods to other forms of contraception. However, these are the **least effective methods** of contraception and should not be used if pregnancy prevention is a high priority.

Periodic Abstinence

Method of Action

Periodic abstinence (the rhythm method) is a physiologic form of contraception that emphasizes **fertility awareness** and **abstinence** shortly before and after the estimated ovulation period. This method requires instruction on the physiology of menstruation and conception and on methods of determining ovulation. **Ovulation assessment methods** may include the use of basal body temperature (Figure 24-1), menstrual cycle tracking, cervical mucus evaluation, and documentation of any premenstrual or ovulatory symptoms.

Effectiveness

The average effectiveness of periodic abstinence is relatively low (55% to 80%) compared to other forms of pregnancy prevention.

Advantages/Disadvantages

Periodic abstinence uses neither chemical nor mechanical barriers to conception and is therefore the method of choice for many couples for philosophic and/or religious reasons. However, this method requires a highly motivated couple willing to learn reproductive physiology, predict ovulation, and abstain from intercourse. Periodic abstinence is relatively unreliable compared to the more traditional methods of contraception. This low reliability may require prolonged periods of abstinence and regular menstrual cycles, making it less desirable for some couples.

Coitus Interruptus

Method of Action

Coitus interruptus, or withdrawal of the penis from the vagina before ejaculation, is one of the oldest methods of contraception. With this method, the majority of semen is deposited outside of the female reproductive tract with the intent of preventing fertilization.

TABLE 24-1

Failure Rates for Various Contraceptive Methods during the First Year of Use in the United States

	Percent of Women Who Become Pregnant	
Method	Theoretical Failure Rate	Actual Failure Rate
No method	85.0	85.0
Periodic abstinence	—	20.0
Calendar	9.0	
Ovulation method	3.0	
Symptothermal	2.0	
Postovulation	1.0	
Withdrawal	4.0	19.0
Lactational amenorrhea	2.0	15.0–55.0
Condom		
Male condom	3.0	12.0
Female condom	5.0	21.0
Diaphragm with spermicide	6.0	20.0
Cervical cap	6.0	18.0
Parous women	26.0	36.0
Nulliparous women	9.0	18.0
Spermicide alone	6.0	26.0
IUDs		
Copper-T IUD	0.6	0.8
Progesterone IUD	1.5	2.0
Levonorgestrel IUS	0.1	0.1
Combination pill	0.1	3.0
Progestin-only pill	0.5	3.0
Depo-Provera	0.3	0.3
Female sterilization	0.4	0.4
Male sterilization	0.1	0.15

Effectiveness

The failure rate for coitus interruptus is quite high (15% to 25%) compared to other forms of contraception. Failure can be attributed to the deposition of semen (pre-ejaculate) into the vagina before orgasm or the deposition of semen near the introitus after intracrural intercourse.

Advantages/Disadvantages

The primary disadvantage of coitus interruptus is its high failure rate and the need for sufficient self-control to withdraw the penis before ejaculation.

Lactational Amenorrhea

Method of Action

After delivery, the restoration of ovulation is delayed because of a nursing-induced hypothalamic **suppression of ovulation**. Continuation of nursing has long been a widespread method of contraception for many couples.

Effectiveness

The duration of ovulatory suppression during nursing is highly variable. In fact, 50% of lactating mothers will begin to ovulate between 6 and 12 months after delivery, even while nursing. As a result, 15% to 55% of lactating mothers become pregnant.

The effectiveness of lactational amenorrhea as a method of contraception can be enhanced by following certain principles. First, breast-feeding should be the only form of nutrition for the infant. Second, this method of contraception should be used only as long as the woman is experiencing amenorrhea and, even then, it should only be used for a **maximum of 6 months** after delivery. Following these guidelines, lactational amenorrhea as a method of contraception can have a failure rate as low as 2%.

Advantages/Disadvantages

Lactational amenorrhea has no effect on nursing. However, the efficacy rate is so low that it is an unacceptable and unreliable means of contraception.

KEY POINTS

1. Natural family planning methods are the least effective methods of contraception and should not be used if pregnancy prevention is a high priority.
2. These methods rely on physiology to prevent pregnancy and require highly motivated users.
3. Periodic abstinence relies on accurate prediction of ovulation and abstinence from intercourse during periods of maximal fertility.
4. Coitus interruptus has a high failure rate attributed to the need for sufficient self-control to withdraw the penis before ejaculation and the high likelihood of deposition of pre-ejaculate into the vagina.
5. The length of lactational amenorrhea varies widely during breast-feeding; therefore, breast-feeding should be used for contraception for a maximum of 6 months after delivery.

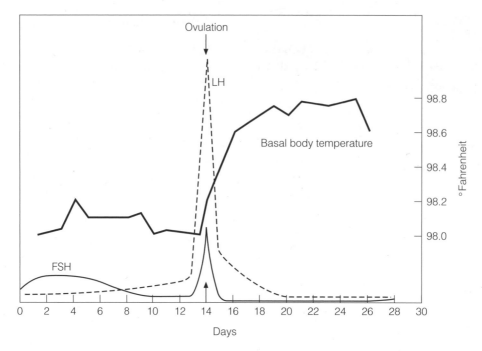

Figure 24-1 • The relationship between ovulation and basal body temperature.

■ BARRIER METHODS AND SPERMICIDES

These contraceptive methods work by preventing sperm from entering the endometrial cavity, fallopian tubes, and peritoneal cavity. Figure 24-2 shows the various barrier method contraceptives and spermicides.

Male Condoms

Method of Action

Condoms are latex sheaths placed over the erect penis before ejaculation. They prevent the ejaculate from being released into the reproductive tract of the woman.

Effectiveness

When properly used, the condom can be 98% effective in preventing conception. The actual efficacy rate in the population is 85% to 90%. To maximize effectiveness, it is important to leave a well at the tip of the condom to collect the ejaculate and to avoid leakage of semen as the penis is withdrawn. Efficacy is also increased by use of spermicide-containing condoms or by using a spermicide along with condoms.

Side Effects

Some individuals may experience an occasional hypersensitivity to the latex, lubricant, or spermicide in condoms.

Advantages/Disadvantages

Condoms are widely available for a moderate cost and carry the added benefit of preventing the transmission of many **sexually transmitted diseases** (STDs). Condoms are the only method of contraception that offers protection against human immunodeficiency virus (HIV). Drawbacks of the condom include coital interruption and possible decreased sensation or hypersensitivity.

Female Condoms

Method of Action

The female condom or **Reality Vaginal Pouch** is a pouch made of polyurethane that has a flexible ring at each end. One ring fits into the depth of the vagina, and the other stays outside the vagina near the introitus (Figure 24-3).

Effectiveness

Initial studies show that the failure rate of the female condom is 15% to 20%, somewhat higher than that of the male condom. However, these were short-term

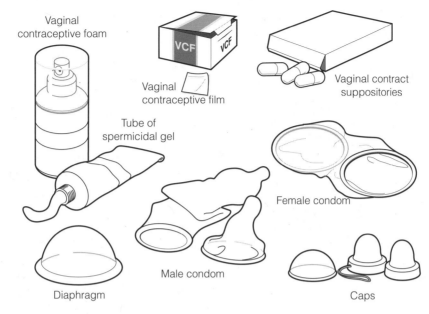

Figure 24-2 • Barrier methods and spermicides.

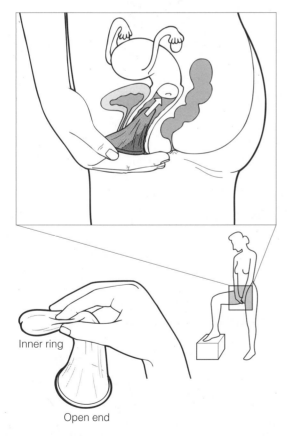

Figure 24-3 • Placement of the female condom.

studies and may not reflect the failure rate with long-term usage.

Advantages/Disadvantages

Female condoms protect against many STDs while also placing the control of contraception with the female partner. Major drawbacks include cost and overall bulkiness. The acceptability rating is somewhat higher for the male partner (75% to 80%) than for the female partner (65% to 70%).

Diaphragm

Method of Action

The vaginal diaphragm is a domed sheet of rubber or latex stretched over a thin coiled rim. Spermicidal jelly is placed on the rim and on either side of the diaphragm, and it is placed into the vagina so that it covers the cervix (Figure 24-4). The diaphragm and spermicide should be placed in the vagina before intercourse and left in place for **6 to 8 hours after intercourse**. If further intercourse is to take place within 6 to 8 hours after the first episode of intercourse, additional spermicide should be placed in the vagina without removing the diaphragm.

Effectiveness

The theoretical effectiveness of the diaphragm approaches 94%. The actual effectiveness rate of the diaphragm with spermicide is 80% to 85%.

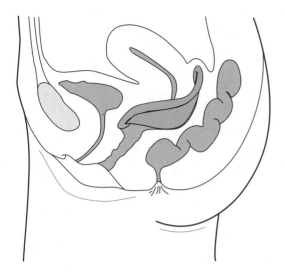

Figure 24-4 • Placement of the vaginal diaphragm.

Side Effects

Possible side effects include bladder irritation, which can lead to cystitis. If the diaphragm is left in place too long, colonization by *Staphylococcus aureus* may lead to the development of **toxic shock syndrome** (TSS). Some women also experience a hypersensitivity to the rubber, latex, or spermicide.

Advantages/Disadvantages

The diaphragm must be fitted and prescribed by a physician making its initial cost significantly higher than over-the-counter methods of contraception. The diaphragm should be replaced every 5 years and/or when the patient gains or loses more than 10 pounds. Women who are not comfortable with inserting the diaphragm or who cannot be properly fitted due to pelvic relaxation defects are poor candidates for the diaphragm.

Cervical Cap

Method of Action

The cervical cap is a small, soft, rubber cap that fits directly over the cervix (Figure 24-5). It is held in place by suction and acts as a barrier to sperm. The cap must be fitted by a physician and must be used with a spermicidal jelly. Because of the variability in cervix size, proper fit and usage of the cap is essential to its effectiveness. Although it is widely used in Britain and Europe, the cervical cap is not widely available in the United States.

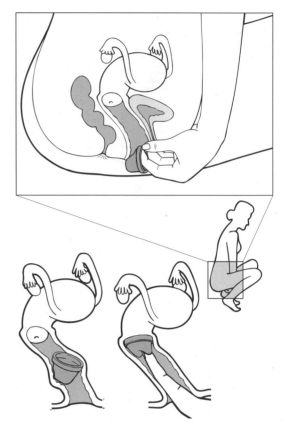

Figure 24-5 • Placement of the cervical cap.

Effectiveness

The actual efficacy rate of the cervical cap is 80% to 85%, similar to that of the vaginal diaphragm. **Dislodgment** is the most common cause of failure.

Advantages/Disadvantages

One advantage of the cervical cap is that it can be left in place for 1 to 2 days. However, a foul discharge often develops after the first day. Also, many women have a difficult time mastering the placement and removal techniques for the cervical cap; as a result, the continuation rate is low (30% to 50%).

Spermicides

Method of Action

Spermicidal agents come in varying forms—vaginal creams, jellies, suppositories, foams, and contraceptive film (Figure 24-2). The most widely used spermicides are **nonoxynol-9** and **octoxynol-9**. These agents both disrupt the cell membranes of spermatozoa and act as a mechanical barrier to the cervical canal. In general, spermicides should be placed in the vagina at least 30 minutes before intercourse to allow for dispersion throughout the vagina. Spermicides may be used alone but are far more effective when used in conjunction with condoms, cervical caps, diaphragms, or other contraceptive methods.

Effectiveness

When properly and consistently used with condoms, spermicides can have an effectiveness rate as high as 97%. However, in actual usage, the efficacy of spermicides when used alone is only 75% to 80%.

Side Effects

Occasionally, spermicides can irritate the vaginal mucosa and external genitalia.

Advantages/Disadvantages

Spermicidal agents are widely available in a variety of forms and are relatively inexpensive. Spermicides that contain nonoxynol-9 protect against STDs, including gonorrhea, syphilis, candida, trichomonas, and HIV.

KEY POINTS

1. Condoms, diaphragms, and cervical caps act as mechanical barriers between sperm and egg. Their efficacy is rate is 80% to 90% with practical use.
2. Condoms and spermicides containing nonoxynol-9 provide prophylaxis against STDs.
3. Diaphragms and cervical caps must be prescribed and fitted by a physician.
4. Spermicides come in a variety of over-the-counter forms at minimal cost. Spermicides have both a barrier and spermicidal effect.
5. Efficacy of spermicides is 75% to 80%, but variability in user technique can significantly lower efficacy.
6. Efficacy rates are greatly improved when using both barrier and spermicidal methods together.

■ INTRAUTERINE DEVICES (IUDS)

Intrauterine devices (IUDs) have been used to prevent pregnancy since the 1800s. In the 1960s and 1970s, IUDs became extremely popular in the United States. However, legal ramifications stemming from pelvic infections associated with one particular IUD—the Dalkon shield—resulted in consumer fear and limited availability of all IUDs. Currently, only three IUDs are available in the United States: the **Paragard** (Copper-T IUD), the **Progestasert** (progesterone T), and the **Mirena** (levonorgestrel intrauterine system). Despite previous fears, there are nearly 100 million IUD users globally making the IUD one of the most widely used methods of reversible contraception in the world (Figure 24-6).

The IUD is especially indicated for women in whom oral contraceptives are contraindicated, those who are low risk for STDs, and in monogamous multigravid women. Absolute and relative contraindications for IUD use are outlined in Table 24-2.

Method of Action

Intrauterine devices made of plastic and/or metal are introduced into the endometrial cavity using a cervical cannula (Figure 24-7). IUDs have one or two strings that extend through the cervix where they can be checked to detect expulsion or migration. The strings also facilitate removal of the device by the physician.

The mechanism of action for IUDs is not completely understood, but they are thought to elicit a sterile **spermicidal inflammatory response** resulting in sperm being engulfed, immobilized, and destroyed by inflammatory cells. This foreign-body reaction caused by IUDs is augmented by the addition of

■ TABLE 24-2

Contraindications for IUD Use

Absolute contraindications
Current pregnancy
Undiagnosed abnormal vaginal bleeding
Suspected gynecologic malignancy
Acute cervical, uterine, or salpingeal infection
History of PID

Relative contraindications
Nulliparity or desire for future childbearing
Prior ectopic pregnancy
History of STDs
Multiple sexual partners
Moderate or severe dysmenorrhea
Congenital malformation of the uterus

Source: Adapted from Speroff L, Darney P. A Clinical Guide for Contraception, 2nd ed. Baltimore: Williams and Wilkins, 1996:195.

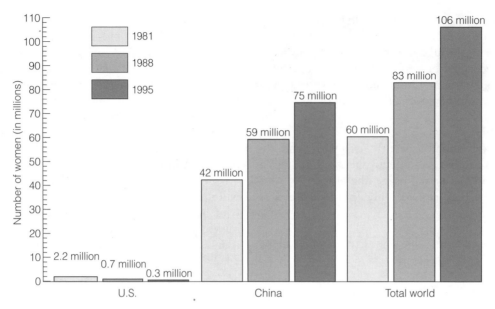

Figure 24-6 • Use of the IUD in the United States, China, and the rest of the world.

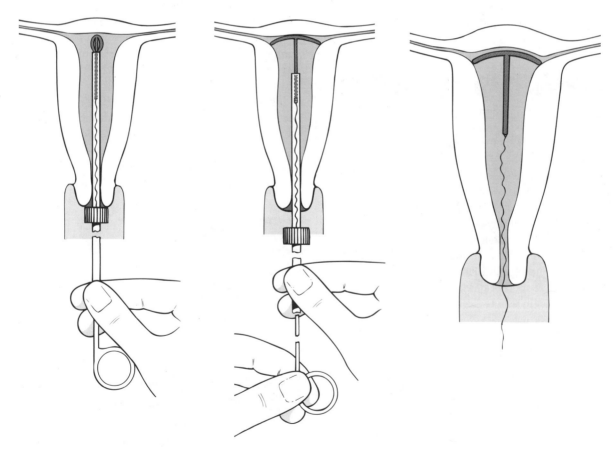

Figure 24-7 • Placement of an IUD.

progesterone in the Progestasert IUD, levonorgestrol in the Mirena IUD, or copper in the Paragard IUD. IUDs do not affect ovulation, neither do they act as abortifacients. Progesterone **thickens the cervical mucus** and **atrophies the endometrium** to prevent implantation. The IUD is also thought to **reduce tubal motility** that in turn inhibits sperm and blastocyst transport. Copper is thought to hamper sperm motility and capitation.

Effectiveness

The efficacy for IUDs rivals that of permanent sterilization with prolonged use. The failure rate is 2% for the Progestasert, 0.8% for the Paragard and 0.1% for the Mirena IUD. During the first year of use, however, the failure rate is near 3%. This is believed to be due to unrecognized expulsions.

Side Effects

Although extremely safe, uncommon side effects and complications of IUDs can be potentially severe and dangerous. These include pain and bleeding, pregnancy, expulsion, perforation, and infection.

Women who use IUDs appear to be at increased risk for **insertion-related PID**. This increased risk is now believed to be due to contamination of the endometrial cavity at the time of insertion. Otherwise, pelvic infection is rarely seen beyond the first 20 days after insertion. Prophylactic antibiotics (doxycycline or azithromycin) at the time of insertion provide protection against insertion-related infections. In addition, it is important to screen women for gonorrhea and *Chlamydia* prior to placement of the IUD.

The **spontaneous abortion rate** is increased to 40% to 50% for women who become pregnant with an IUD in place. Given this, if intrauterine pregnancy occurs while an IUD is in place, the device should be removed by **gentle traction on the string**. The risk of life-threatening, spontaneous septic abortion has only been seen with the Dalkon shield, which is no longer available. The IUD is not associated with any increased risk of congenital abnormalities.

Advantages/Disadvantages

The IUD must be prescribed, inserted, and removed by a physician. However, once in place, the user must do little other than periodically report for follow-up to check for expulsion and infection. The Mirena IUD must be replaced every 5 years; the Paragard every 10 years. The Progestasert IUD must be replaced annually. The IUD carries the added benefit of providing **protection against ectopic pregnancy** while in situ by preventing pregnancy. Although this decreased risk of ectopic pregnancy is not as low as that found with OCPs, use of an IUD lowers a woman's risk by 50% compared to that of noncontraceptive users. When a woman does become pregnant with an IUD in place, a higher percentage will be ectopic pregnancies compared to pregnancies conceived without an IUD in place.

KEY POINTS

1. IUDs are less well tolerated by nulliparous women but are ideal for the monogamous multiparous women for whom the pill is contraindicated.
2. The primary mechanism of action is a sterile spermicidal inflammatory response. Other mechanisms include inhibition of implantation and alteration in tubal motility.
3. The failure rates for IUD use are very low (<2%) with prolonged use but higher in the first year of use.
4. Potentially serious side effects include insertion-related salpingitis, spontaneous abortion, and uterine perforation.
5. The IUD provides protection against ectopic pregnancy while in situ.
6. The progesterone-containing IUD has the added benefit of decreasing bleeding and dysmennorhea.

■ HORMONAL CONTRACEPTIVE METHODS

Hormonal contraceptives are the most commonly used reversible means of preventing pregnancy in the United States and consist of combined (estrogen and progesterone) and progesterone-only methods. Currently, combined hormonal methods are available in oral, injectable, transdermal, and vaginal forms; whereas progesterone-only methods are available in oral, injectable, and intrauterine forms. Currently, there are several hormonal contraceptives in various stages of the FDA-approval process in the United States. These include the subdermal implant and a seasonal birth control pill.

Combined Hormonal Methods

Oral Contraceptive Pills (OCPs)

Method of Action

Oral contraceptive pills (OCPs) are composed of progesterone alone or a combination of progesterone and estrogen. (The progesterone-alone pill is described later in the progesterone-only section.) Over 150 million women worldwide—including one-third of sexually active women in the United States—use oral contraceptives. Oral contraceptives place the body in a **"pseudopregnancy"** state by interfering with the pulsatile release of follicle-stimulating hormone (FSH) and luteinizing hormone (LH) from the anterior pituitary. This pseudopregnancy state **suppresses ovulation** and prevents pregnancy from occurring. Figure 24-8 illustrates the serum levels of FSH and LH during the normal menstrual cycle, and Figure 24-9 shows FSH and LH levels during a cycle on the combination pill. Because the FSH and LH surges do not occur, follicle growth, recruitment, and ovulation do not occur.

Secondary mechanisms of action for OCPs include changing the **cervical mucus** to render it less penetrable by sperm and changing the **endometrium** to make it unsuitable for implantation.

Monophasic (Fixed Combination) Pills

Combination pills contain a fixed dose of estrogen and a fixed dose of progestin in each tablet. Nearly 30 combinations of estrogen and progestins are available in the United States. In general, the selection of a particular pill for each patient depends on

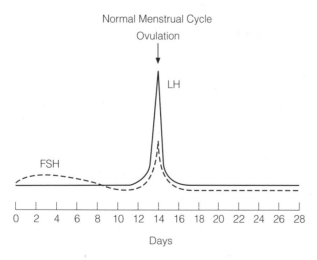

Figure 24-8 • Serum levels of FSH and LH during a normal menstrual cycle.

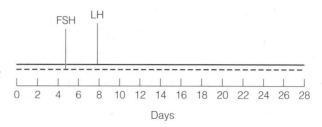

Figure 24-9 • Serum levels of FSH and LH while taking monophasic oral contraceptive pills.

the individual side effects and risk factors for each patient.

The combination pill containing both estrogen and progestin is taken for the first 21 days out of a 28-day monthly cycle. During the last 7 days of the cycle, a placebo pill or no pill is taken. Bleeding should begin within 3 to 5 days of completion of the 21 days of hormones. The hormone-containing pills may also be taken on a continuous basis, which is especially helpful for women with endometriosis who benefit from a continuous suppression of endogenous hormones. When taken continuously, women will not bleed since there is no placebo week and thus no withdrawal bleed.

Multiphasic (Dose Varying) Pills

Multiphasic oral contraceptives differ from monophasic pills only in that they **vary the dosage of progestin** each week during the 21 days of hormone pills. The advantage of the multiphasic dosing is that it may provide a lower level of estrogen and progestin overall but is still highly effective at preventing pregnancy.

Effectiveness

OCPs are remarkably effective in preventing pregnancy. In fact, the theoretical failure rate for the first year of use is less than 1%. However, the failure rate with actual "real life" usage is closer to 3%. Nausea, breakthrough bleeding, and the necessity of taking the pill every day are often cited as reasons for discontinuing the pill.

Several medications interact with oral contraceptives and reduce the effectiveness of the pill. Conversely, oral contraceptives can also reduce the efficacy of many medications (Table 24-3).

Side Effects

Table 24-4 lists some of the cardiovascular, neoplastic, and biliary complications associated with oral contraceptive use.

TABLE 24-3

Interactions of Oral Contraceptives with Other Medications

Medications that Reduce the Efficacy of Oral Contraceptives	Medications Whose Efficacies are Reduced by Oral Contraceptives
Penicillins	Folates
Tetracycline	Anticoagulants
Sulfonamides	Insulin
Rifampin	Methyldopa
Ibuprofen	Hypoglycemics
Phenytoin	Phenothiazides
Barbiturates	Tricyclic antidepressants

TABLE 24-4

Complications Associated with Oral Contraceptives

*Cardiovascular**
Thromboembolism
Pulmonary embolism
Cerebrovascular accident
Myocardial infarction
Hypertension

Other
Benign hepatic tumors
Increase in gallbladder disease

Note: *These complications occur mainly in smokers.
Source: Adapted with permission from Hacker N, Moore JG. Essentials of Obstetrics and Gynecology. Philadelphia: WB Saunders, 1998:519.

Oral contraceptives with estrogen doses greater than 50 μg can increase coagulability, leading to higher rates of myocardial infarction, stroke, thromboembolism, and pulmonary embolism, particularly in women who smoke. Even at lower doses of estrogen (35 μg or less), women over 35 who smoke more than one pack of cigarettes per day are still at increased risk of heart attack, stroke, DVT, and PE if they use OCPs. The progestins in oral contraceptives have been found to raise low-density lipoproteins while lowering high-density lipoproteins in pill users smoking more than 1 pack per day. For these reasons, oral contraceptives are **contraindicated in women over age 35 who smoke cigarettes**. The advent of new progestins and lower estrogen doses has led to pill formulations that are essentially neutral in terms of cardiovascular effect. However, oral contraceptive use is still contraindicated in women over age 35 who smoke.

Neoplastic complications of oral contraceptive use are rare. The effect of long-term oral contraceptive use on breast cancer has been studied extensively over the past decade with no conclusive findings. There is, however, an increased incidence of gallbladder disease and benign hepatic tumors associated with oral contraceptive use.

Table 24-5 outlines both the absolute and relative contraindications to oral contraceptive use.

Advantages and Disadvantages

The major advantages of oral contraceptive pills include their extremely high efficacy rates and the **noncontraceptive health benefits**, including a reduced incidence of ovarian cancer, endometrial cancer, ectopic pregnancy, pelvic inflammatory disease (PID), and benign breast disease (Table 24-6). By taking OCPs, nearly 50,000 women avoid hospi-

TABLE 24-5

Contraindications to Oral Contraceptives

Absolute Contraindications	Relative Contraindications	Other Relative Contraindications
Venous thrombosis	Uterine fibroids	An/oligo-ovulation
Pulmonary embolism	Lactation	Depression
Coronary vascular disease	Diabetes mellitus	Hyperlipidemia
Cerebrovascular accident	Sickle-cell disease	Acne
Breast/endometrial CA	Hypertension	Severe varicose veins
Melanoma	Age 35+ and smoking	Severe headaches (especially vascular)
Hepatic tumor	Age 40+ and high risk for vascular disease	
Abnormal liver function		

Source: Reproduced by permission from Hacker N, Moore JG. Essentials of Obstetrics and Gynecology. Philadelphia: WB Saunders, 1998:522.

TABLE 24-6

Noncontraceptive Health Benefits of Oral Contraceptives

Decreases life-threatening diseases
Ovarian cancer
Endometrial cancer
Ectopic pregnancy
Anemia
Pelvic inflammatory disease

Alleviates quality-of-life problems
Iron-deficiency anemia
Dysmenorrhea
Functional ovarian cysts
Benign breast disease
Osteoporosis

Source: Adapted from Hacker N, Moore JG. Essentials of Obstetrics and Gynecology. Philadelphia: WB Saunders, 1998:521.

talizations; of these, 10,000 avoid hospitalization for life-threatening illnesses. Disadvantages include cardiovascular complications, increased gallbladder disease, increased incidence of benign hepatic tumors, and the need to take a medication every day.

Monthly Injectable Combined Hormonal Contraception

Method of Action
The FDA approved the monthly injectable method of contraception with the brand name Lunelle in October 2000. However, due to problems with one of its delivery mechanisms, the manufacturer voluntarily removed Lunelle from the market temporarily at the time of this publication. Lunelle is administered intramuscularly by a doctor or nurse once a month and contains 5 mg of estradiol cypionate and 25 mg of medroxyprogesterone acetate. Its mechanism of action is the same as combined oral contraceptive pills in that it induces a pseudopregnancy state by decreasing the endogenous levels of FSH and LH and suppressing ovulation.

Effectiveness
Like oral contraception, combined injectable contraception is highly effective if received on time, every month. Since it is a new product, long-term studies have not been done, but it has been shown to have a 0.2% 1-year failure rate.

Advantages and Disadvantages
The noncontraceptive health benefits are the same as those with OCPs. Women do not have to remember to take a pill every day, but do need to visit their doctor every month to receive the injection. Depending on one's personality and lifestyle this may be viewed as an advantage or a disadvantage. Self-injectable forms of contraception are now being studied. As with OCPs the most frequent reasons for discontinuation are weight gain, bleeding, breast pain, menorrhagia, and dysmennorhea.

Transdermal Combine Hormonal Contraception

Mechanism of Action
The contraceptive patch with the brand name Evra releases progestin and ethinyl estradiol at a level similar to low-dose OCPs. The size of the patch determines the actual daily dose, but a common dose features 250 mcg per day of a progestin (norelgestromin) and 25 mcg per day of ethinyl estradiol. Women must change the patch weekly and then have a patch-free week every fourth week during which they will have bleeding like a period. Again, just like combined OCPs, the primary mechanism of action is suppression of ovulation by decreasing endogenous FSH and LH levels.

Effectiveness
The patch has been shown to have a 1% failure pregnancy rate if used correctly.

Advantages and Disadvantages
The same primary side effects and noncontraceptive health benefits of low-dose OCPs apply to the patch as well. The patch can cause skin irritation and should be discontinued if this arises. The patch has the added benefit of being self-administered only once a week.

Vaginal Ring

Method of Action
The hormone-releasing vaginal ring with the brand name of Nuvaring provides a daily dose of 120 mcg of etonogesterol and 15 mcg of ethinyl estradiol, stays in place for 3 weeks, and is removed for the fourth. During this time the woman will have a withdrawal bleed, like a period.

Effectiveness
Clinical studies are ongoing, but the vaginal ring has a high reported efficacy when used correctly, similar to other forms of combined hormonal contraception.

Advantages and Disadvantages
One size fits all women, therefore women do not have to be fitted for the vaginal ring. Women place the ring in the vagina themselves and remove it every

fourth week, so they do not have to visit a doctor for administration. Disadvantages include a woman's (or partners) concern with having a foreign body in the vagina and the potential for expulsion. Studies have shown that women do not feel the ring inside and can have intercourse without any difficulty or disturbance.

Progesterone-Only Contraception

Progesterone-only contraception consists of oral, injectable, and intrauterine options (the Progestasert IUD and Mirena IUS are discussed earlier in the IUD section). These all function primarily using the same mechanisms: thickening the cervical mucous, which inhibits sperm motility; and effecting the endometrial lining so that it is not suitable for implantation.

Progestin-Only Oral Contraception Pills (The Minipill)

Method of Action
Progestin-only pills are taken every day of the cycle to deliver a small daily dose of progestin. It is believed that the cervical mucus becomes less permeable to sperm and that the endometrium becomes less appropriate for implantation via progesterone-induced atrophy.

Effectiveness
Progestin-only pills are generally not as effective (failure rate is 3% to 6%) as combination or multiphasic regimens.

Side Effects
Side effects of the progesterone-only OCP include irregular ovulatory cycles, breakthrough bleeding, and ectopic pregnancy.

Advantages and Disadvantages
Because they contain no estrogen, progestin-only pills are ideal for nursing mothers and women for whom estrogens are contraindicated; particularly smokers over age 35.

Injectable Progesterone-Only Contraception—Depo-Provera

Method of Action
Although it was only approved for contraceptive use in the United States in 1992, Depo-Provera (**medroxyprogesterone acetate**) has been used in other countries since the mid-1960s. Depo-Provera is injected intramuscularly every 3 months in a vehicle that allows the slow release of progestin over a 3-month period. Depo-Provera acts by suppressing ovulation, thickening the cervical mucus, and making the endometrium unsuitable for implantation.

Effectiveness
With a first year failure rate of only 0.3%, Depo-Provera is one of the most effective contraceptive methods available.

Side Effects
The primary side effects experienced by Depo-Provera users include **irregular menstrual bleeding**, depression, weight gain, hair loss, and breast tenderness. Over 70% of patients experience spotting and irregular menses during the first year of use. This is the primary reason for discontinuing Depo-Provera.

Advantages and Disadvantages
The primary advantages of Depo-Provera are that it is highly effective, acts independent of intercourse, and only requires injections every 3 months. Irregular bleeding, weight gain, and mood changes are the major disadvantages. Its use is therefore discouraged in women with depression.

After 3 or 4 consecutive injections of Depo-Provera, most women no longer have any vaginal bleeding. After discontinuation of Depo-Provera injections, some women may experience a significant **delay in the return of regular ovulation** (6 to 18 months). This is independent of the number of injections but may be directly related to the weight of the patient. Within 18 months, however, fertility rates return to normal levels.

KEY POINTS

1. Hormonal contraceptives have extremely low failure rates and are available in oral, injectable, transdermal, vaginal, and intrauterine forms.
2. Combined hormonal contraception methods prevent pregnancy by suppressing ovulation, altering cervical mucus, and causing atrophic changes in the endometrium.
3. Serious complications from combined hormonal contraception use occur mainly in smokers over age 35, including pulmonary embolism, stroke, deep venous thrombosis (DVT), heart attack, and hypertension.
4. Benefits of combine hormonal contraception include protection from ovarian and endometrial cancer, and reduction in ectopic pregnancy, PID, osteoporosis, and benign breast disease.

5. Progesterone-only contraception (Depo-Provera, progestin-only OCPs, and the Mirena IUD) use progestins to suppress ovulation, thicken the cervical mucus, and make the endometrium unsuitable for implantation.
6. Primary side effects of Depo-Provera include irregular bleeding, weight gain, hair loss, and depression. Depo-Provera can be associated with significant delay in restoration of ovulation after discontinuation.
7. Other hormonal contraceptive devices and pills awaiting approval in the United States include the subdermal implant, and the seasonal oral contraceptive pill.

■ EMERGENCY CONTRACEPTION

Emergency contraception can **prevent pregnancy** after unprotected intercourse or in the case of contraceptive failure. It is used only if a woman is not already pregnant from a previous act of intercourse. Emergency contraception is used to prevent pregnancy by inhibiting ovulation, fertilization, or implantation (mechanism depends on timing of cycle and type of method utilized). Emergency contraception **does not cause an abortion**. It is available in two forms: (1) emergency contraceptive pills (also called the postcoital or the "morning after" pill), and (2) emergently inserted IUD.

Emergency Contraceptive Pills

Methods of Action

Emergency contraceptive pills use high doses of both estrogen and progestin or progesterone alone to prevent pregnancy *after* intercourse has taken place. Several differing regimens exist using high doses of regularly prescribed OCPs. Some prepackaged formulas are also available, such as "Plan B" (progestin only) and "Preven" (estrogen and progesterone). All regimens are taken in two doses, 12 hours apart. **The first dose must be taken within 72 hours of unprotected vaginal intercourse.** An anti-emetic is often prescribed at the same time to prevent nausea secondary to the high doses of estrogen. The mechanism of action for emergency contraceptive pills depends on the point during the cycle when the pills are taken. These act to either suppress ovulation or accelerate the ovum through the fallopian tube and endometrial cavity so that fertilization does not take place.

Effectiveness

When taken within 72 hours of intercourse, emergency contraceptive pills have a failure rate of 0% to 2.5%. These have been shown to reduce the risk of pregnancy between 75% to 90% for women who have had unprotected intercourse during the second or third week of their menstrual cycles, when they are most likely ovulating.

Side Effects

The primary side effects of emergency contraception includes bloating, nausea, and vomiting secondary to the high doses of estrogen in the combined regimens.

Advantages and Disadvantages

The emergency contraceptive pills are extremely effective in preventing pregnancy. The major disadvantages include the short window of time when they can be used (within 72 hours of intercourse) and possible teratogenic effects to the fetus in cases where a pregnancy ensues despite use of emergency contraception. Additionally, these cannot be used as long-term contraception.

Emergency IUD Insertion

Method of Action

The Copper T IUD can be inserted in the uterine cavity within 7 days of unprotected vaginal intercourse and functions primarily by eliciting a **sterile inflammatory response** within the uterus making the environment unsuitable for implantation.

Effectiveness

Emergency IUD insertion reduces the risk of pregnancy by 99.9%; therefore, only 1:1000 become pregnant after emergency IUD insertion.

Side Effects

The side effects are the same as those discussed in the IUD section.

Advantages and Disadvantages

Emergency IUD insertion is extremely effective. It differs from emergency contraceptive pills in that it can be used long term (10 years); whereas the pills have a one-time only use. Disadvantages are the IUD must be placed by a provider, and the potential (rare) complications such as infection and perforation that are described in the IUD section above.

■ SURGICAL STERILIZATION

The rate of surgical sterilization as a method of contraception has increased dramatically over the past three decades. Approximately 30% of reproductive-age couples in the United States and Great Britain choose female sterilization for contraceptive purposes. A similar number of men seek vasectomies each year. The rate of sterilization is higher in women who are married, divorced, over age 30, or African American.

Before performing any sterilization procedure, careful counseling should be provided and informed consent obtained based on the patient's understanding of the permanent nature of the procedure, operative risks, chance of failure, and possible side effects should be obtained. Sterilization is ideal in stable monogamous relationships where no additional children are desired.

Tubal Sterilization

Method of Action

Tubal sterilization prevents pregnancy by surgically occluding both fallopian tubes to prevent the ovum and sperm from uniting. There are a number of methods by which tubal occlusion can be accomplished, including banding (Figure 24-10) with Falope rings, clipping with Hulka clips (Figure 24-11) or Felchie clips, and ligation with electrocautery or sutures.

Tubal ligation can be performed immediately postpartum (**postpartum sterilization [PPS]**) through a small subumbilical incision using epidural or spinal anesthesia. The most commonly used method, the Pomeroy tubal ligation, is illustrated in Figure 24-12. When tubal ligation is performed outside the postpartum period, it is typically done via laparoscopy under general anesthesia (**laparoscopic tubal ligation [LTL]**).

Effectiveness

Tubal ligation has a failure rate of 0.2% to 0.4%. The highest success rates are achieved with PPS. When the LTL approach is undertaken, the Falope ring has found to be most effective in women under age 30.

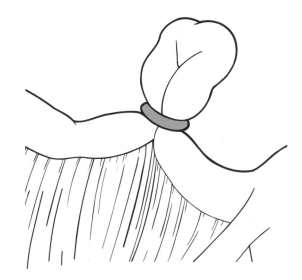

Figure 24-10 • Tubal occlusion with the Falope ring, which is typically performed via laparoscopy.

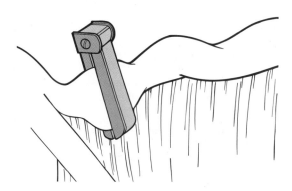

Figure 24-11 • Tubal occlusion with the Hulka clip, which is typically performed via laparoscopy.

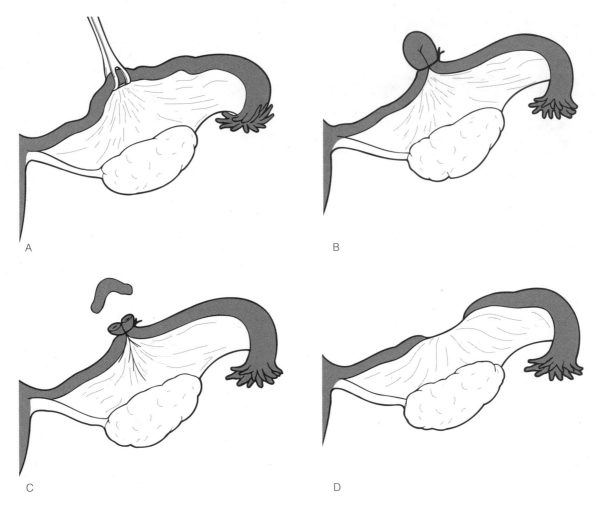

Figure 24-12 • A–D: The Pomeroy method of tubal sterilization. This technique is typically performed during the immediate post-partum period through a small subumbilical incision.

Electrocautery and Falope rings are equally effective in women over age 30. More recently, titanium Felchie clips have been used for tubal ligation but long-term efficacy rates are not yet available.

Side Effects

There are no side effects associated with tubal sterilization. Some women report pain and menstrual disturbances (post-tubal ligation syndrome) after the procedure. In most of these women, symptoms are due to discontinuation of oral contraceptives, which results in heavier baseline periods and dysmenorrhea.

Advantage and Disadvantages

Tubal ligation offers the advantage of permanent effective contraception without continual expense,

effort, or motivation. The mortality rate of bilateral tubal ligation is 4:100,000. Of those women who undergo tubal sterilization, 1:15,000 will have an ectopic pregnancy at some point after the procedure. However, nearly 1000 maternal lives are saved due to sterilization during the period from the time of sterilization to the end of the woman's reproductive life.

Of women who undergo permanent sterilization, regret is highest in women who were under age 30 when the procedure was performed. However, it is estimated that only 1% of women seek reversal of tubal sterilization. The success of reversal varies from 41% to 84% depending on the method (Table 24-7). When pregnancy is desired after tubal ligation, in vitro fertilization (IVF) offers a greater likelihood of

■ TABLE 24-7

Success Rates of Tubal Occlusion Reversal, by Method

Method of Tubal Sterilization	Success Rates for Reversal (in %)
Clips	84
Bands	72
Pomeroy	50
Electrocauterization	41

pregnancy than does tubal microplasty. However, when multiple future pregnancies are desired, tubuloplasty may be a more economical alternative than multiple IVF cycles.

Vasectomy

Method of Action

Vasectomy is a simple and safe option for permanent sterilization involving **ligation** of the **vas deferens**. This procedure may be performed in a physician's office under local anesthesia through a small incision in the upper outer aspect of each scrotum (Figure 24-13). In 1985, the **no-scalpel vasectomy** technique was introduced. With this procedure both vas are ligated through a single small midline incision that reduces the already low rate of complications associated with vasectomy. Unlike tubal ligation, **vasectomy is not immediately effective**. Because sperm can remain viable in the proximal collecting system after vasectomy, patients should use another form of contraception until azoospermia is confirmed by semen analysis, usually in 6 to 8 weeks.

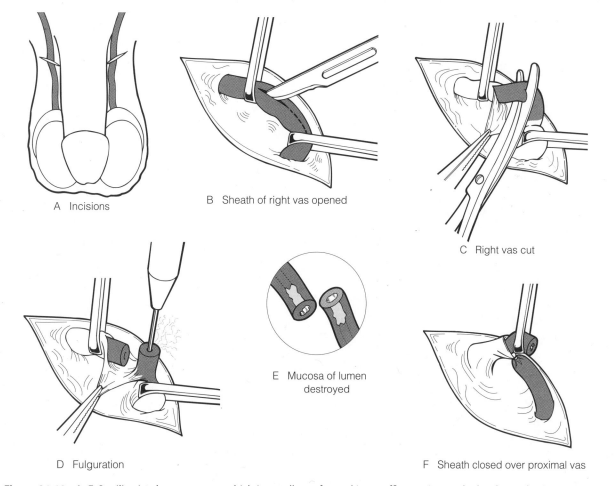

A Incisions

B Sheath of right vas opened

C Right vas cut

D Fulguration

E Mucosa of lumen destroyed

F Sheath closed over proximal vas

Figure 24-13 • A–F: Sterilization by vasectomy, which is usually performed in an office setting under local anesthesia.

Effectiveness

The failure rate for vasectomy is <1%. Many of these pregnancies are due to intercourse too soon after vasectomy rather than from recanalization.

Side Effects

Complications after vasectomy are rare and usually involve slight bleeding, skin infection, and reactions to the sutures or local anesthesia. Fifty percent of patients form **antisperm antibodies** after the procedure. However, there are no long-term side effects of vasectomy.

Advantages and Disadvantages

Vasectomy is a permanent, highly effective form of contraception with few, if any, side effects. Vasectomy is generally safer and less expensive than tubal ligation and can be performed as an outpatient under local anesthesia. Vasectomy offers permanent sterility; this may be considered a disadvantage for some couples. The success rate of vasal reanastomosis is 60% to 70%. Pregnancy rates after vasectomy reversal range from 18% to 60%.

KEY POINTS

1. Surgical sterilization has increased dramatically in the past 30 years.
2. Both vasectomy and tubal occlusion are highly effective forms of permanent sterilization.
3. Tubal ligations are performed under general anesthesia with few, if any, side effects.
4. Reversal rates for tubal occlusion vary from 41% to 84% depending on the method used for sterilization.
5. Complications after vasectomy are rare and minimal.
6. The success rate of vasal reanastomosis is 60% to 70% with pregnancy rates ranging from 18% to 60%.

Elective Termination of Pregnancy

It is estimated that 25% of all pregnancies worldwide end in elective abortion. Since its legalization in 1973, one legal abortion in the United States is performed for every four live births. Currently, over 1 million abortions are performed annually in the United States. One-third of all abortions are performed on women under age 20, one-third on women age 20–24, and the remaining one-third on women over age 25. Nearly 75% of all abortions are performed on unmarried women.

The abortion procedures used legally in the United States are both **safe and effective**. Risk of death from an abortion during the first 2 months of pregnancy is less than 1 : 100,000 procedures (Figure 25-1). In fact, first-trimester abortions have a lower mortality rate than using no birth control and giving birth. In general, however, maternal morbidity is lowest if legal abortion is performed before 8 weeks gestation (see Figure 25-1). The major cause of abortion mortality is from **general anesthesia**.

There are many surgical and medical procedures by which pregnancy termination can be achieved. First-trimester options include **surgical evacuation** of the uterus or a medical abortion using either **mifepristone** or **methotrexate**. Second-trimester options include **surgical evacuation** of the uterus and medical **induction of labor**. In general, the technique used for termination is determined by the duration of the pregnancy. Table 25-1 outlines the various options available during the first and second trimesters. Laws vary from state to state, but generally speaking, terminations are performed up until the fetus has reached what is considered to be the **stage of viability at about 24 weeks** gestation. After week 24, abortions are only allowed when necessary for the preservation of maternal life.

■ FIRST-TRIMESTER OPTIONS

Ninety percent of all abortions are performed **before 12 weeks gestation**. Suction curettage, manual vacuum extraction, and medical abortions are all methods of inducing abortion in the first trimester. Ninety percent of all abortions in the United States are achieved using suction curettage. However, this number may change since the recent FDA approval (September 2000) of the use of mifepristone for pregnancy termination in the United States. The mortality incidence from suction curettage is 1 : 100,000 patients. In general, the risk of complications after suction curettage is directly proportional to the gestational age.

Suction Curettage/Manual Vacuum Aspiration

Method of Action

Suction curettage (cervical dilation and vacuum aspiration) is both a safe and effective means of terminating a pregnancy at 12 weeks or less. This procedure involves **dilation of the cervix** and removal of the products of conception using a **suction cannula** (Figure 25-2). This is generally performed using a **paracervical block** with a local anesthetic possibly in combination with IV sedation. Less commonly, general anesthesia is used.

Manual vacuum aspiration can be performed only up until week 7 and involves the insertion of a cannula into the cervical os with manual extraction of the products of conception using a vacuum syringe instead of a suction machine; sharp curettage is not performed in this procedure.

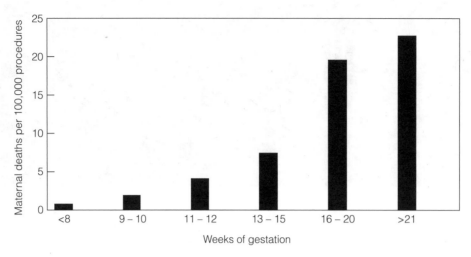

Figure 25-1 • The effects of gestational age on maternal mortality for legal abortions.

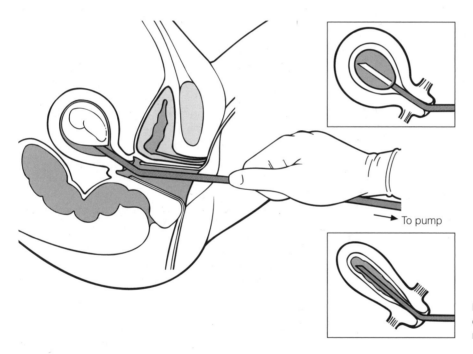

To pump

Figure 25-2 • Suction of uterine cavity for termination of pregnancy.

■ TABLE 25-1
Termination of Pregnancy Options, by Gestational Age
First-trimester terminations
Surgical evacuation of the uterus
Mifepristone (RU-486)
Methotrexate
Second-trimester terminations
Surgical evacuation of the uterus
Medical induction of labor

Effectiveness

When performed by a trained physician, the failure rate for suction curettage is extremely low. If the gestational age is less than 5 weeks, it is possible to fail to remove the small fetus with the suction curette.

Side Effects

Complications of suction curettage are rare and include infection (1%), excessive bleeding (2%), and uterine perforation (1%). Some data suggest that women who have three or more cervical dilation procedures (for terminations, hysteroscopies, D&Cs, etc.) are at higher risk for cervical incompetence and uterine scarring (Asherman's syndrome).

Medical Abortion

Method of Action

Mifepristone (RU 486) is a synthetic **antiprogestin** hormone that binds to progesterone receptors in the endometrium to block the effects of progesterone on its target tissue. By blocking the stimulatory effects of progesterone on endometrial growth, mifepristone essentially disrupts the pregnancy by making the endometrial lining unsuitable to sustain the pregnancy. Mifepristone is given orally up to 49 days from the last menstrual period (LMP). Mifepristone can be used alone or in conjunction with a **prostaglandin misoprostol** (Cytotec) that is taken orally or vaginally 2 days after the initial dose of mifepristone. Approximately 2 weeks after the procedure, the success of completion should be confirmed with **ultrasound** or a **serum β-hCG level**.

Effectiveness

When used alone, the efficacy rate of mifepristone is approximately 65% to 80%. However, when given with misoprostol, the success rate of expulsion using mifepristone within 49 days (7 weeks) since the LMP is approximately 95%. The efficacy rate for mifepristone declines significantly for pregnancies greater than 7 weeks gestation.

Methotrexate

Mechanism of Action

Methotrexate is a chemotherapeutic agent that **blocks folate** and thereby **prevents cell division** in the gestational trophoblastic tissue. Because methotrexate has been approved for use for a variety of medical conditions including ectopic pregnancy, it is often used by clinicians on an "off-label" basis as an abortofacient. Methotrexate is also used with a prostaglandin. Methotrexate is administered intramuscularly within 49 days of the LMP, then the misoprostol (Cytotec) is administered 3 to 7 days later.

Effectiveness

The efficacy rate increases with additional doses of misoprostol. Sixty-seven percent of patients will abort within 1 week with one dose of misoprostol and 80% to 85% of women will abort within 2 weeks with a second dose of misoprostol. Overall, this drug combination is believed to be 95% effective for

inducing abortion during the first seven weeks of pregnancy.

Side Effects

Side effects of medical abortion include nausea, cramps, vomiting, and prolonged uterine bleeding.

Advantages and Disadvantages

Medical abortion offers the advantages of being a highly effective noninvasive means of termination that can be achieved on an outpatient basis. In a medical abortion a miscarriage is induced and the woman must go through the experience of miscarrying a pregnancy, which generally involves substantial uterine cramping and bleeding. Medical abortion requires at least three total visits to a health provider: two for the treatment, then a 2-week follow-up visit.

KEY POINTS

1. First-trimester abortion options include suction curettage, manual vacuum extraction, and medical abortion up until week 7.
2. Ninety percent of all abortions in the United States are achieved using suction curettage.
3. Suction curettage can be performed anytime during the first trimester but is most effective after at least 6 weeks gestation.
4. Complications are rare but can include infection, bleeding, and perforation.
5. Mifepristone is an abortifacient that blocks progesterone.
6. Methotrexate is a chemotherapeutic agent that blocks folate thus preventing cell divison.
7. Both mifepristone and methotrexate may be used in combination with a prostaglandin and have high efficacy rates when used within 7 weeks of the LMP.

■ SECOND-TRIMESTER OPTIONS

Second-trimester abortions are elective terminations performed between weeks 12 and 24. **Congenital abnormalities** is the major reason for second-trimester abortions. Other indications include severe hyperemesis, previable preterm premature rupture of membranes (PPROM), life-threatening maternal condition, and undesired pregnancy.

Termination of pregnancy options for the second-trimester include **induction of labor** (with prostaglandins, oxytocin, or intra-amniotic instillation agents), and **dilation and evacuation** (D&E) (see Table 25-1). When a second-trimester termination is necessary, D&E has been found to be **safer** than induction of labor procedures completed through 16 weeks of gestation. At later gestational ages, D&E and induction of labor have similar morbidity and mortality.

Induction of Labor

Method of Action

Termination of a second-trimester pregnancy can be achieved with induction of labor. Although the greater majority of second-trimester terminations are achieved with D&E, the percentage of terminations with induction of labor **increases as gestational age increases**.

Termination through induction of labor is typically done using **cervical ripening agents, amniotomy** and **oxytocin**. Induction of labor can also be achieved with oral, vaginal, or intramuscular **prostaglandins** given every 3 to 4 hours until labor begins. Another method is the **instillation of agents** into the amnion to stimulate uterine contractions and the expulsion of the fetus and placenta hours later (Table 25-2). Instillation substances include hypertonic saline, prostaglandin F_{2alpha}, and hyperosmolar urea.

Effectiveness

The success rate for second-trimester abortions using induction of labor vary between 80% to 100% depending on the regimen used. The maternal mortality rate for second-trimester terminations using oxytocin, vaginal prostaglandins, or instillation agents is comparable to that of term delivery.

Side Effects

Induction of labor can often be a multi-day process and complications do exist (Table 25-3). Oral and vaginal prostaglandins have a higher incidence of

TABLE 25-2

Injection-Abortion Intervals for Amniotic Infusion

Amnioinfusion Agent	Injection-Abortion Interval (in hours)
Hypertonic (20%) saline	<48
Prostaglandin F_{2alpha}	19–22
Hyperosmolar (59.7%) urea	16–17

TABLE 25-3

Complications Associated with Second-Trimester Abortion by Induction of Labor

Complications	Side Effects
Retained placenta	Nausea
Incomplete abortion	Vomiting
Hemorrhage	Diarrhea
Emotional stress	Fever

live births and significant gastrointestinal side effects (**nausea, vomiting, diarrhea**), whereas instillation agents have a high rate of **retained placenta** (13% to 46%). Hypertonic saline may induce **hyperosmotic coma**, **hypernatremia**, and **diffuse intravascular coagulation** if inadvertent intravascular administration occurs. Because of this, urea and prostaglandin have largely replaced the use of hypertonic saline for amnioinfusion techniques.

Advantages and Disadvantages

Generally speaking, induction of labor is a longer process than a D&E; however, the potential for delivery of an intact fetus exists. For patients for whom the delivery of an intact fetus is emotionally important, this option is often preferred.

Dilation and Evacuation (D&E)

Method of Action

D&E is the general term to describe uterine curettage at 13 weeks gestational age or greater. This method of termination is very similar to suction curettage except that wider cervical dilation is required and forceps may be needed to assist in complete evacuation of the uterus.

Typically, D&E involves the gradual dilation of the cervix using **laminaria**, which are seaweed sticks placed into the cervix the day before the procedure (Figure 25-3). These osmotic dilators slowly expand over several hours to dilate the cervix prior to D&E. **Metal dilators** may also be used for cervical dilation. These techniques are followed by introduction of a large **suction cannula** into the uterus to extract the fetal tissue and placenta. At more advanced gestational ages, **forceps** are often needed in addition to suction curettage to remove fetal parts.

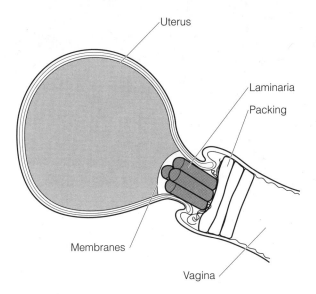

Figure 25-3 • Laminaria are placed inside the cervix through both the internal and external os. They slowly expand by absorbing moisture from the vagina thereby dilating.

Side Effects

Complications from D&E are uncommon but may include hemorrhage, perforation, infection, and retained tissues. These can be lessened by visual inspection of the fetal parts to ensure complete evacuation of the products of conception. For pregnancies through 16 weeks gestational age, D&E has been found to be safer than induction of labor for second-trimester terminations.

Advantages and Disadvantages

As a method of second-trimester abortion, D&E offers the advantage of being performed on an out-patient basis without the need to undergo labor and delivery. Also, complications from D&E occur at lower rates than those for intra-amniotic instillation or intravaginal prostaglandin abortions. Some patients may feel the **decreased amount of time** for this procedure is advantageous over an induction of labor; however, other patients may feel that the **delivery of a nonintact fetus** is unacceptable. Perceptions of advantages and disadvantages to these procedures greatly depends on patient preference and personal emotional situations.

KEY POINTS

1. During the second trimester, abortion may be achieved via induction of labor or D&E.
2. Induction of labor techniques include oxytocin, instillation agents such as hypertonic saline and urea, and intravaginal prostaglandins.
3. Complications from induction of labor include retained placenta, hemorrhage, coagulopathy, infection, and cervical laceration.
4. Intravaginal prostaglandins have an increased incidence of gastrointestinal side effects and, when used alone, live births.
5. D&E is similar to suction curettage and safer than induction of labor for second-trimester abortion.
6. Complications of D&E include hemorrhage, infection, perforation, and retained tissue.

Infertility and Assisted Reproduction

■ ETIOLOGY

Infertility is the inability to conceive after 1 year of unprotected intercourse. Although the overall incidence of infertility remained relatively unchanged over the past 30 years, the number of office visits to physicians by couples seeking infertility treatment nearly tripled, partially due to the availability of new treatment options for infertility. The first-line treatment options include ovulation induction (OI), intrauterine insemination (IUI), in vitro fertilization (IVF), gamete intrafallopian transfer (GIFT), intracytoplasmic sperm injection (ICSI), egg and sperm donation, and gestational surrogacy.

The normal fecundity rate (likelihood of achieving pregnancy in a given month) in a couple with normal fertility is approximately 20% to 25% per month; this means that 85% to 90% of couples are able to conceive within 18 months (Table 26-1). For the remaining 10% to 15% of couples who are incapable of conceiving on their own within that time frame, the factors contributing to infertility vary widely.

Of those couples who undergo evaluation for infertility, 30% are attributed purely to male factors and 30% to purely female factors. Both male and female factors are identified in 20% of the patient population (Figure 26-1). After evaluation, some 15% to 20% of couples will have no identifiable cause for their infertility. Fortunately, modern technologies make it possible to identify the one or more possible causes for infertility in 80% to 90% of cases. In these cases, appropriate therapy will result in pregnancy 50% of the time.

■ MALE FACTOR INFERTILITY

Pathogenesis

There are multiple causes of male factor infertility (Table 26-2): endocrine disorders, anatomic defects, problems with abnormal sperm production and motility, as well as sexual dysfunction.

Epidemiology

Thirty percent of infertility is due to purely male factors. An additional 20% of cases are caused by a combination of male and female factors (see Figure 26-1).

Risk Factors

Men with occupational or environmental exposure to chemicals, radiation, or excessive heat are at increased risk for infertility, as are those with a history of varicocele, mumps, hernia repair, pituitary tumor, anabolic steroid use, testicular injury, and impotence. Certain drugs have also been found to depress semen quantity and quality (Table 26-3).

Clinical Manifestations

History

The physician should ask about previous pregnancies fathered by the patient, environmental exposures, and any history of sexually transmitted diseases (STDs), mumps orchitis, hernia repair, or trauma to the genitals.

Physical Examination

The physical examination should include a search for signs of testosterone deficiency and varicocele, iden-

TABLE 26-1

Average Conception Rates for All Couples

Percent of Couples	Length of Time Before Conception (months)
20	conceive within 1
60	conceive within 6
75	conceive within 9
80	conceive within 12
90	conceive within 18

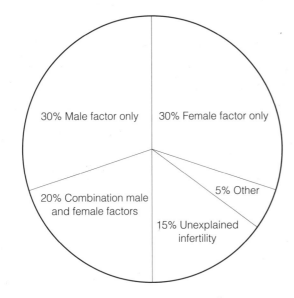

Figure 26-1 • Causes of infertility.

TABLE 26-2

Common Causes of Male Factor Infertility

Endocrine disorders
Hypothalamic dysfunction (Kallmann's)
Pituitary failure (tumor, radiation, surgery)
Hyperprolactinemia (drug, tumor)
Exogenous androgens
Thyroid disease
Adrenal hyperplasia

Abnormal spermatogenesis
Mumps orchitis
Chemical/radiation/heat exposure
Varicocele
Cryptorchidism

Abnormal motility
Varicocele
Antisperm antibodies
Kartagener's syndrome
Idiopathic

Sexual dysfunction
Retrograde ejaculation
Impotence
Decreased libido

Source: Adapted from DeCherney A, Pernoll M. Current Obstetric and Gynecologic Diagnosis and Treatment. Norwalk: Appleton & Lange, 1994: 998.

TABLE 26-3

Drugs that Decrease Semen Quality and Quantity

Cimetidine	Nitrofurans	Anabolic steroids
Sulfasalazine	Erythromycin	Chemotherapeutic agents
Spironolactone	Tetracyclines	Heavy marijuana/ alcohol use

tification of the urethral meatus, and measurement of testicular size.

Diagnostic Evaluation

A **semen analysis** is the primary investigative tool for male factor infertility. Sperm count, volume, motility, morphology, pH, and white blood cell count are analyzed.

In the case of an abnormal semen analysis, an **endocrine evaluation** should include thyroid function tests, serum testosterone, prolactin, and follicle-stimulating hormone (FSH) (may identify parenchymal damage to testes).

The **postcoital test** is less often performed but can be used to examine the interaction between sperm and the cervical mucus. A healthy **sperm-mucus interaction** occurs when a large number of forwardly moving sperm are seen in a thin acellular mucus.

Treatment

In general, the probability of conception can be enhanced by **improvements in coital practice**. This includes having intercourse every 2 days during ovulation with the female partner on the bottom placing more semen in contact with the cervix. The woman should lie on her back with her knees to her chest for at least 15 minutes after intercourse. Men should avoid the use of tight underwear, saunas and hot tubs, and unnecessary environmental exposures, such as radiation, excess heat, and certain medications (Table 26-3).

Low semen volume is most often treated by **washed sperm for intrauterine insemination**. Treatment of low sperm density or motility depends on the causal agent. Hypothalamic-pituitary failure can be treated with injections of human menopausal gonadotropins (hMGs) and varicoceles can be repaired by ligation. **ICSI** is another option for patients with low sperm density or impaired motility and has revolutionized the treatment of male factor infertility. This method involves retrieving sperm from the male, preparing it, individually injecting a single sperm directly into an egg (Figure 26-2), and then placing the fertilized egg into the uterus cavity (IVF) or fallopian tube (ZIFT). The sperm can be retrieved from the male by ejaculation, or by direct aspiration from the testis (**testicular sperm extraction [TSE]**) or epididymis (**microsurgical epididymal sperm aspiration [MESA]**).

In refractory cases of male factor infertility, artificial insemination with **donor sperm** is highly effective.

KEY POINTS

1. Male factor infertility is responsible for 30% of all infertility cases. An additional 20% are caused by a combination of male and female factors.
2. It may be idiopathic or due to improper coital practices; sexual dysfunction; endocrine disorders or abnormalities in spermatogenesis; or in sperm volume, density, or mobility.
3. Male factor infertility is diagnosed by semen analysis, a postcoital test, and endocrine evaluation.
4. The treatment depends on the causal agent and include improved coital practices, repair of anatomic defects, ICSI, and use of donor sperm.

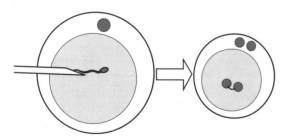

Figure 26-2 • Intracytoplasmic Sperm Injection (ICSI). A spermatid or spermatozoon is collected by ejaculation or aspiration from the epididymus or testis. One sperm is injected directly into each harvested egg. The embryos are then transferred back into the uterine cavity.

FEMALE FACTOR INFERTILITY

Thirty percent of infertility is attributed to purely female factors; another 20% is attributed to a combination of female and male factors (Table 26-4). Female factors can be divided into anatomic factors (Table 26-5) and ovulatory factors (Table 26-6).

Peritoneal and Tubal Factors

Pathogenesis

The primary peritoneal and tubal factors in infertility include endometriosis and pelvic adhesions.

TABLE 26-4

Common Causes of Infertility

Etiology		Incidence (in %)
Male factor	40	
Female factor	40	
Ovulatory factor		40
Peritoneal/tubal factor		40
Uterine factor		10
Cervical factor		10
Unexplained	15	
Other	5	

TABLE 26-5

Anatomic Causes of Female Factor Infertility

Anomalies of the cervix
DES exposure in utero
Müllerian duct abnormality
Cervical stenosis
Surgical treatment (cryotherapy, conization)
Cervicitis or chronic inflammation
Hostile cervical mucus

Abnormalities of the uterine cavity
Congenital malformations
Submucosal leiomyoma
Intrauterine synechiae (Asherman's syndrome)

Tubal occlusion
PID
Tubal ligation
Endometriosis

Peritoneal factors
Endometriosis
Pelvic adhesions

■ TABLE 26-6

Causes of Ovulatory Factor Infertility

Central defects
Pituitary insufficiency (trauma, tumor, congenital)
Hypothalamic insufficiency
Hyperprolactinemia (drug, tumor, empty sella)
PCOD (chronic hyperandrogenemic anovulation)
Luteal phase defects

Peripheral defects
Gonadal dysgenesis
Premature ovarian failure
Ovarian tumor
Ovarian resistance

Metabolic disease
Thyroid disease
Liver disease
Obesity
Androgen excess (adrenal, neoplastic)

Source: Adapted from DeCherney A, Pernoll M. Current Obstetric and Gynecologic Diagnosis and Treatment. Norwalk: Appleton & Lange, 1994:998.

Endometriosis is the presence of endometrial cells outside the uterine cavity (Chapter 15). It can invade local tissues and cause severe inflammation and adhesions. As a result, endometriosis can interfere with tubal mobility, cause tubal obstruction, or result in tubal or ovarian adhesions that contribute to infertility by holding the fallopian tube away from the ovary or by trapping the released oocyte. Infertility has also been diagnosed in women with minimal endometriosis.

Another major contributor to peritoneal and tubal factor infertility is **pelvic adhesions**. Pelvic adhesions, or scar tissue, can be formed as a result of prior pelvic surgery or acute inflammatory processes such as pelvic inflammatory disease (PID) or a ruptured viscus (appendicitis, diverticulitis, etc.). Similar to endometriosis, adhesions can interfere with tubal mobility and cause tubal occlusion resulting in the inability to conceive.

Epidemiology

Peritoneal factors account for 40% of female infertility cases (see Table 26-4). And, although the true prevalence is unknown, it is believed that in the United States, 7% to 10% of women of reproductive age have endometriosis.

Risk Factors

Endometriosis, prior PID, prior abdominal/pelvic infection, and prior pelvic surgery are the primary risk factors for peritoneal and tubal factor infertility.

Clinical Manifestations

History

Women with endometriosis give a history of **cyclic pelvic pain**, dysmenorrhea, dyspareunia, or abnormal bleeding. Pelvic adhesions may be asymptomatic or may be associated with varying degrees of pelvic pain, especially with movement or lifting.

Physical Examination

The findings associated with early endometriosis or pelvic adhesions may be subtle or nonexistent. When more extensive endometriosis is present, physical exam may reveal a fixed or retroverted uterus, uterosacral nodularity, or a tender, fixed adnexa.

Diagnostic Evaluation

Endometriosis or pelvic adhesions may be strongly suspected based on the patient's history, but **direct visualization** with laparoscopy or laparotomy is necessary to confirm the diagnosis. Ovarian endometriomas (cystic collections of endometrial cells on the ovaries) can be diagnosed on **pelvic ultrasound**. Tubal patency can be demonstrated with a **hysterosalpingogram** performed during the follicular phase or **tubal lavage** performed during laparoscopy.

Treatment

Symptomatic relief of endometriosis can be achieved medically or surgically. Medical treatments such as Danazol, gonadotropin-releasing hormone (GnRH) analogs, oral medroxyprogesterone (Provera), or continuous oral contraceptives can temporarily relieve symptoms but **do not increase fertility rates**. Fertility rates can be improved by surgical ligation of periadnexal adhesions during laparoscopy or laparotomy with excision, coagulation, fulguration, or **vaporization of endometrial implants**. Pregnancy rates after treatment depend on the extent of the disease, with conception rates as high as 75% for mild disease and as low as 30% to 40% for severe disease (Table 15-2).

Microsurgical tuboplasty with tubal reanastomosis or neosalpingostomy has proven to be effective for treating tubal occlusion due to prior infection or from prior tubal ligation. However, because it is more effective, most couples undergo IVF rather than attempt tuboplasty. The advantage of tuboplasty is that it allows for more than one future pregnancy without the cost and difficulty of multiple IVF cycles. Both IVF and tuboplasty are associated with an **increased risk of ectopic pregnancy**.

Uterine Cavity Factors

Pathogenesis

Varying uterine conditions can contribute to infertility including submucosal fibroids, intrauterine synechiae, and congenital malformations (especially uterine septums). Similarly, endometrial abnormalities such as hyperplasia, out-of-phase endometrium, and carcinoma can cause infertility. These factors may distort the uterine cavity, prevent implantation, or affect endometrial development.

Epidemiology

Uterine factors account for 10% of female factor infertility cases (see Table 26-4).

Risk Factors

Risk factors for uterine factor infertility include conditions that predispose to intrauterine adhesions such as history of pelvic inflammatory disease, infection after pregnancy loss, and multiple curettage of the uterus. Submucosal fibroids and diethylstilbestrol (DES) exposure in utero also predispose to uterine factor infertility.

Clinical Manifestations

History

The clinical presentation of uterine factor infertility varies with the etiology. For many of these factors, infertility may be the only symptom. Among the most common causes, endometritis may be seen with pelvic pain and fever; submucosal fibroids may be seen with recurrent pregnancy loss, heavy bleeding, and pain. A uterine septum may also present with recurrent pregnancy loss.

Physical Examination

The adnexa should be evaluated and the physician should look for leiomyoma and any signs of current or prior pelvic infection. Cervical cultures should also be collected.

Diagnostic Evaluation

The primary investigative tools for anatomic abnormalities of the female reproductive tract are **hysterosalpingogram** or **saline sonohystogram** (performed during the follicular phase), and **pelvic ultrasound**. **Hysteroscopy** and **laparoscopy** may also be used to directly visualize the uterus internally and externally.

Treatment

Uterine synechiae and septae can be treated with **surgical ligation** of adhesions via operative hysteroscopy, commonly followed by estrogen therapy to prevent recurrence of adhesions. Fertility is restored in 50% of cases. Most surgeons reserve **myomectomy** for treatment after recurrent pregnancy loss or when symptomatic fibroids have been identified.

Cervical Factors

Pathogenesis

Cervical problems can contribute to infertility through **structural abnormalities** of the cervix, **cervicitis**, and **abnormal cervical mucous production**. Cervical stenosis may be iatrogenic and may result from scarring after conization, multiple (four or more) mechanical dilations (abortions, dilation, and evacuations [D&Es]), or extensive laser or cauterization of the cervix. These procedures may result in stenosis as well as destruction of the endocervical epithelium, leading to inadequate mucous production.

Epidemiology

Cervical factors account for <10% of infertility cases (see Table 26-4).

Clinical Manifestations

History

A complete history should elicit information about prior cryotherapy, conization, cervical dilations, or in utero DES exposure.

Physical Examination

The patient should have a thorough pelvic examination with visualization of the cervix and evaluation of the amount, quantity, color, spinnbarkeit, fluidity, and ferning of the cervical mucous.

Diagnostic Evaluation

Cervical mucous studies and a postcoital test may be used to evaluate the quality of the cervical mucus.

This assesses both sperm quality and sperm-mucous interaction 2 to 8 hours after coitus.

Treatment

Treatment of cervical factor infertility varies with the cause. Cervical stenosis can often be treated with surgical or mechanical dilation of the endocervical canal. Both cervical stenosis and abnormal cervical mucous can be treated by bypassing the cervix with IUI. IUI appears to be the most effective treatment for cervical factor infertility. In cases that are refractory to other treatments, patients should be offered IVF, GIFT, or zygote intrafallopian transfer (ZIFT).

Ovulatory Factors

Pathogenesis

Disruption in the hypothalamic-pituitary-ovarian axis can result in amenorrhea, oligomenorrhea, menorrhagia, and infertility through impairment of folliculogenesis, ovulation, and endometrial development. Table 26-6 lists some of the many potential factors that may contribute to ovulatory abnormalities and infertility. The World Health Organization (WHO) has classified ovulatory factor infertility into three groups: (1) **Hypothalamic-pituitary failure** (hypothalamic amenorrhea), (2) **Hypothalamic-pituitary dysfunction** (polycystic ovarian syndrome [PCOS], anovulation, oligomenorrhea, luteal phase defects, hyperprolactinemia, thyroid dysfunction), and (3) **Ovarian failure** (premature ovarian failure, advanced maternal age).

Epidemiology

Ovulatory factors are responsible for female factor infertility in 40% of cases (see Table 26-4).

Clinical Manifestations

History

The medical history should include a thorough menstrual history and inquiries about spontaneous abortions, endometriosis, galactorrhea, weight changes, or hot flashes. Patients may report amenorrhea, oligomenorrhea, or menorrhagia.

Physical Examination

Physical examination should consider hirsutism, obesity, and signs of virilism, hypothyroidism, premature ovarian failure, and insulin resistance. The exam should also look for breast development as a sign of past estrogen secretion and a well-rugated, moist vagina with abundant clear stretchable cervical mucous as a sign of current estrogen secretion.

Diagnostic Evaluation

The primary tests for the evaluation of ovulatory factor infertility look for **evidence of ovulation** by tracking the menstrual cycle, measuring the basal body temperature (Figure 24-1), monitoring the cervical mucus, measuring the midluteal progesterone, and documenting any premenstrual or ovulatory symptoms. Over-the-counter **ovulation prediction kits** have made predicting the presence and timing of ovulation much easier.

An **endometrial biopsy** is sometimes used to evaluate the morphology of the glands and stroma of the endometrium to determine the adequacy of progesterone's effects on the endometrial lining. This is also the most accurate method for timing ovulation and looking for luteal phase defects.

A **progestin challenge test** may be used to demonstrate the endometrium's ability to respond with bleeding to appropriate stimulation. This involves administration of a progestin over 5 to 10 days to build up the endometrium. When the progestin is stopped, the patient should experience a withdrawal bleed within 1 week.

Finally, **endocrine evaluation** may include measurement of FSH, LH, prolactin, thyroid function tests, and thyroid antibodies. If Cushing's syndrome is suspected, serum testosterone, dehydroepiandrosterone sulfate (DHEAS), 17-hydroxyprogesterone, 24-hour urine cortisol levels, and an overnight dexamethasone suppression test are helpful. When intracranial lesions are suspected, **MRI** or **CT** imaging of the head should be done.

Treatment

The **underlying etiology** of ovulatory dysfunction should be identified and corrected. Regular ovulation can be restored in 90% of infertility cases that are due to endocrine factors by treating the underlying disorder.

For uncorrectable cases, ovulation induction with fertility drugs can be used. The most common etiology of ovulatory infertility is hypothalamic-pituitary dysfunction (WHO Group 2). For these patients, ovulation induction with **clomiphene citrate** is the first line of therapy. This nonsteroidal ligand binds to estrogen receptors in the hypothalamus, thus stimulating pulsatile release of GnRH (Table 26-7). This stimulates FSH and LH release from the pituitary and subsequently causes follicular development. If

TABLE 26-7

Drugs Used in the Treatment of Infertility and in Assisted Reproductive Technologies

Commercial Name	Generic Name	Mechanism
Clomid, Serophene	Clomiphene citrate	Antiestrogen, stimulates follicular development for ovulation induction
Pergonal, Humegon, Repronex	Human menopausal gonadotropins	Purified FSH/LH, stimulates follicular development during ovulation induction
Fertinex, Follistim, Gonal-F	Follistatins	Gonadotropins containing FSH that stimulates follicular development during ovulation induction
Danocrine	Danazol	Androgen derivative, decreases FSH and LH, used to treat endometriosis
Profasi, Pregnyl, Novarel	Human chorionic gonadotropin	Similar structure to LH, triggers ovulation after follicle stimulation
Lutrepulse	Pulsatile GnRH/gonadorelin	GnRH agonist, stimulates release of FSH/LH from pituitary
Lupron	Leuprolide acetate	GnRH agonist, decreases estrogen levels, shrinks fibroids, causes regression of endometriosis

this treatment is unsuccessful, ovulation induction and pregnancy can be attempted with a combination of **human gonadotropins** and some form of advanced reproductive technology such as IVF, GIFT, or ICSI.

For patients with hypothalamic-pituitary failure (WHO Group 1) ovulation can usually be achieved with **pulsatile GnRH therapy** or **human gonadotropins** (see Table 26-7). Of note, there is no treatment for WHO Group 3 patients with **ovarian failure** because these patients lack viable oocytes. Patients with this diagnosis should be offered the options of **egg donation**, **gestational surrogacy**, or **adoption**.

KEY POINTS

1. Female factor infertility is purely responsible for 30% of all infertility cases and partially responsible in 20% of cases. These can be divided into anatomic and ovulatory factors.
2. It may be due to peritoneal or tubal factors such as endometriosis and pelvic adhesions. These factors are diagnosed by history and laparoscopy or laparotomy and treated surgically to improve fertility rates. Tubal occlusion may be repaired with microsurgical tuboplasty, but most couples opt for IVF.
3. Female factor infertility may be due to uterine factors such as uterine synechiae, fibroids, endometritis, or polyps.
4. Uterine factors are diagnosed by pelvic ultrasound, hysterosalpingogram, saline sonogram, hysteroscopy, and laparoscopy.
5. Uterine factors are treated according to the cause of the infertility. Synechiae, fibroids, and polyps can be resected, endometritis is treated with antibiotics.
6. Female infertility may also be due to cervical factors such as cervical stenosis from surgical or mechanical dilation or poor cervical mucus. These factors are diagnosed by exam, mucous analysis, and the postcoital test, and treated with surgical or mechanical dilation of the endocervical canal or IUI to bypass the cervix.
7. Female factor infertility may be due to ovulatory factors that interrupt the hypothalamic-pituitary-ovarian axis such as intracranial tumors, polycystic ovarian syndrome, premature ovarian failure, and thyroid and adrenal diseases.
8. Ovulatory factors are diagnosed by confirming ovulation through menstrual history, basal body temperature measurements, mucous analysis, or midluteal progesterone followed by endocrine evaluation (TSH, prolactin, FSH, LH) and endometrial biopsy.

9. Ovulatory factors are best addressed by treating the cause of the ovulatory dysfunction, when refractory, by using ovulation induction agents along with IUI, IVF, or GIFT.

UNEXPLAINED INFERTILITY

Pathogenesis

For those couples who complete an initial assessment, 5% to 10% find no cause for their infertility. When the initial infertility evaluation reveals no cause for infertility, the problem often involves abnormalities in **sperm transport**, the presence of **antisperm antibodies**, or problems with penetration and fertilization of the egg. When problems in sperm transport, motility, or functional capacity are identified, **IVF, ICSI,** or **GIFT** may be used for treatment. If this fails, the use of donor sperm may result in pregnancy.

When no cause for infertility is identified after in-depth testing, studies show that most therapies have **no higher success rates** than no treatment at all. Although some patients with unexplained infertility may undergo three to six cycles of Pergonal stimulation with IUI before trying IVF or GIFT, many opt for no treatment. The eventual pregnancy rate for couples with unexplained infertility who receive no treatment approaches 60% over 3 to 5 years. Other options include use of donor sperm, surrogacy, adoption, or acceptance of childlessness.

KEY POINTS

1. Between 5% and 10% of couples find no explanation for infertility after their initial assessment.
2. Further assessment may be done to search for problems with sperm transport, ability to penetrate and fertilize the egg, and antisperm antibodies. IVF can be used to treat these patients.
3. Most therapies for unexplained infertility have not been shown to have higher success rates than no treatment.
4. Couples with unexplained infertility who choose no treatment will conceive up to 60% of the time over 3 to 5 years.

ASSISTED REPRODUCTIVE TECHNOLOGIES

Since their inception, the treatment of infertility with assisted reproductive technologies has progressed rapidly and now includes not only "fertility drugs" (Pergonal, Metrodin, and Clomid) that stimulate multiple follicular development, but also technologies that combine ovulation induction agents with IUI, IVF, GIFT, or ICSI. Ocytes may also be obtained via natural, nonstimulated cycles but the number of eggs per cycle is increased by ovulation induction.

Ovulation Induction

Method of Action

Clomiphene citrate (Clomid) is an **antiestrogen** that competitively binds to estrogen receptors in the hypothalamus. This results in increased GnRH. Subsequently, FSH and LH production is increased leading to follicular growth and ovulation (see Table 26-7). Clomid is generally administered orally during days 5 to 10 of the follicular phase of the menstrual cycle.

Absent or **infrequent ovulation** is the major indication for clomiphene citrate use such as women with PCOS or mild hypothalamic amenorrhea. Specific causes of anovulation should be ruled out first and patients should have normal TSH, FSH, and prolactin levels. Although Clomid is used as a first-line therapy in couples with unexplained infertility, it has no use in patients with premature ovarian failure.

The other major category of ovulation induction agents is **hMGs**. These are best used when the pituitary gland fails to secrete sufficient FSH and LH to stimulate follicular maturation and ovulation, and when clomiphene citrate is also incapable of stimulating ovulation. Patients with mild to severe hypothalamic dysfunction fall into this category and often require hMGs for ovulation induction.

One of the most frequently utilized hMGs is **Pergonal** (see Table 26-7), a purified preparation of FSH and LH from the urine of postmenopausal women. It is administered via intramuscular injection during the follicular phase of the menstrual cycle. The patient's response to ovulation induction should be monitored closely through serial estrogen levels and pelvic ultrasound to measure follicle size and number.

Both Clomid and Pergonal cause **multiple follicular development**. Once ovulation occurs, fertilization may be attempted by intercourse or IUI. Conversely, after ovulation induction, the oocytes may be aspirated transvaginally for fertilization via IVF, GIFT, ZIFT, or ICSI (Figure 26-3).

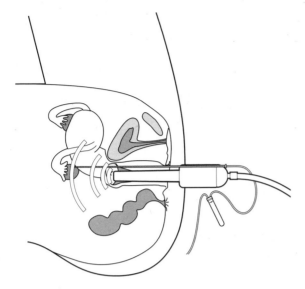

Figure 26-3 • Transvaginal Ultrasound-Guided Needle Aspiration of Oocytes. Following ovulation induction, multiple eggs are removed from the ovaries by placing a vaginal probe into the vagina. A fine needle is guided toward the ovary while the physician visualizes the follicles on ultrasound. Fluid around the follicles is them collected through a needle connected to a test tube.

Effectiveness

Clomiphene citrate is successful in inducing ovulation in 80% of correctly selected patients and 40% will become pregnant (Table 26-8). If pregnancy does not occur after 3 to 6 cycles of Clomid, more aggressive therapies are needed. Gonadotropins have an 80% to 90% ovulation success rate and a 10% to 40% pregnancy success rate per cycle depending on the diagnosis. The cumulative pregnancy rate over 6 cycles has reported at 90%. However, gonadotropins

■ TABLE 26-8

Percentage of Deliveries and Multiple Gestation Pregnancies per Cycle of ART

	Deliveries*	MGP
No procedure	25	1
Clomid	25	8
hMG	30	20
IVF	28	39
GIFT	30	34
ZIFT	30	36

Note: *Success varies by age of patient, type of infertility, and quality and quantity of sperm, egg, and embryo.

carry a much higher risk of **ovarian hyperstimulation** (1% to 3%) and **multiple gestation pregnancy** (20%).

Side Effects and Complications

The potential side effects of clomiphene citrate are related to its antiestrogen effect: hot flashes, abdominal distension and bloating, emotional lability, depression, and visual changes. These side effects are mostly mild and disappear after discontinuation of the medication.

Multiple gestation pregnancy is a major side effect of OI and assisted reproductive technologies. Multiple gestation pregnancies occur in 8% of Clomid-induced pregnancies and 20% of gonadotropin therapy.

The other major complications of OI with gonadotropins include **ovarian hyperstimulation** (1% to 3%), a potentially life-threatening condition caused by overstimulation of the ovaries. This completely iatrogenic disorder can range from ovarian enlargement and minimal symptoms to significant ovarian enlargement, torsion, or rupture. This may be complicated by ascites, pleural effusions, hemoconcentration, hypercoagulability, electrolyte disturbances, renal failure, and even death.

Advanced Reproductive Technologies (IVF, GIFT, ZIFT, ICSI)

Method of Action

Assisted reproductive technologies have advanced the treatment of infertility by allowing physicians to successfully bypass the normal mechanisms of gamete transportation and fertilization. In conjunction with OI, multiple oocytes may be harvested from the ovary using ultrasound or laparoscopic guidance (see Figure 26-3). **GIFT** involves laparoscopically placing mature eggs into the healthy fallopian tube along with washed sperm (Figure 26-4).

During **IVF** and **ZIFT**, however, the oocytes are allowed to mature briefly in vitro before washed sperm are added. Fertilization is verified 14 to 18 hours later by the presence of two pronuclei. In the case of IVF, the conceptuses are then placed into the uterus through the cervix using a catheter (Figure 26-5), making IVF a relatively noninvasive procedure when compared to ZIFT and GIFT. In the case of ZIFT, the zygotes are placed directly into the fallopian tubes via laparoscopy or transcervical fallopian tube catheterization.

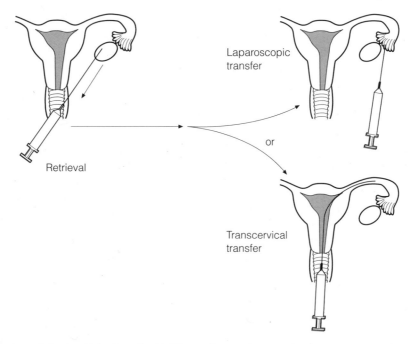

Figure 26-4 • Gamete Intra-Fallopian Tube Transfer (GIFT). A: After ovulation induction, oocytes are harvested transvaginally. B: The oocytes and washed sperm are then placed into the fallopian tube laparoscopically or transcervically where fertilization takes place.

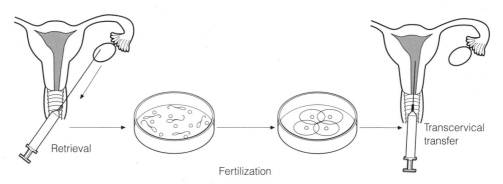

Figure 26-5 • In vitro fertilization (IVF). A: After ovulation induction, oocytes are harvested transvaginally. B: The egg and sperm are placed together in the laboratory and fertilization takes place. C: The fertilized embryos are transferred into the uterine cavity through the cervix.

ICSI has revolutionized the treatment of male factor infertility by allowing a single spermatid or spermatozoon to be directly injected into the cytoplasm of a harvested oocyte. The resulting embryos can then be placed back into the uterus for implantation (see Figure 26-2).

Effectiveness

The success rate of these advanced reproductive technologies varies from center to center. On average, with IVF, delivery is achieved in 28% of retrievals. GIFT and ZIFT have slightly higher delivery rates of 30% in properly selected couples (see Table 26-8). Success rates vary by maternal age; diagnosis; the number and quality of eggs, sperm, and embryos. The most favorable rates are seen in women under age 35 when there is no male factor infertility. Keep in mind that the normal fecundity rate in a couple with normal fertility is approximately 20% to 25% per month.

Again, **multiple gestation pregnancies** are a major complication of ART. The Society for Assisted Reproductive Technologies estimates the rates of multiple gestations at delivery to be 39% for IVF (33% twins,

5% triplets, 1% higher-order multiples), 34% for GIFT, and 36% for ZIFT (see Table 26-8). The rate of multiple gestations is important because these pregnancies carry much higher rates of **maternal complications** (preeclampsia, gestational diabetes, placenta previa, premature delivery, postpartum hemorrhage) and **fetal complications** (IUGR, respiratory distress syndrome [RDS], intraventricular hemorrhage, neonatal sepsis, low birth weight, stillbirth). The rate of multiple gestation pregnancies in ART can be reduced by close ultrasound surveillance and estradiol monitoring during ovulation induction and by limiting the number of oocytes, embryos, or zygotes transferred during ART.

KEY POINTS

1. Clomiphene citrate is an antiestrogen that binds to estrogen receptors in the hypothalamus to cause increased FSH and LH production, thereby promoting follicular maturation and ovulation.
2. Clomiphene citrate is best used for women with chronic anovulation or mild hypothalamic insufficiency after specific causes of hypothalamic dysfunction have been ruled out.
3. Human menopausal gonadotropins are forms of FSH or FSH and LH that directly stimulate follicular maturation in patients for whom Clomid has failed, or those with hypothalamic or pituitary failure or unexplained infertility.
4. The primary complications of fertility drugs include ovarian hyperstimulation and multiple gestation pregnancy.
5. IVF, GIFT, ZIFT, and ICSI may be used to bypass the normal mechanisms of gamete transport with fertilization with deliveries in about 30% of cases.

Neoplastic Disease of the Vulva and Vagina

PRE-INVASIVE NEOPLASTIC DISEASE OF THE VULVA

Benign lesions of the vulva and vagina are discussed in Chapter 13. This chapter discusses pre-invasive neoplasia of the vulva and vagina and cancer of the vulva and vagina (Table 27-1). It important to distinguish between benign disease and preinvasive disease so appropriate treatment and follow-up can be offered to patients.

Pre-invasive neoplastic disease of the vulva is divided into two categories: **Paget's disease** and **vulvar intraepithelial neoplasia** (VIN). Any time a pruritic area of the vulva does not respond to topical antifungal creams—particularly in the postmenopausal woman—further work-up with biopsy should be performed. If there are no obvious lesions, colposcopic-directed biopsy may be performed to reach a pathologic diagnosis. Histologically, Paget's disease, intraepithelial neoplasia, and melanoma of the vulva can all be quite similar (Table 27-2). Therefore, immunohistochemical staining can be used to assist in the diagnosis of vulvar lesions.

PAGET'S DISEASE OF THE VULVA

In the vulva, Paget's disease is an intraepithelial neoplasia of the skin overlying this region. In addition, about 20% of patients with Paget's disease will have **coexistent adenocarcinoma** underlying the outward changes. When this occurs, metastasis is common. Without the adenocarcinoma, Paget's disease can be treated locally without concern for metastases.

Diagnosis

The lesions of Paget's disease are consistent with chronic inflammatory changes. Commonly, there is a long-standing **pruritus** that accompanies **velvety-red lesions** of the skin that eventually become eczematous and scar into **white plaques**. These lesions may be focal on the labia, perineum, or perianal region; or may encompass the entire region. The disease is most common in patients over age 60, but the symptoms of vulvar pruritus and vulvodynia can precede the diagnosis by years. Absolute diagnosis is made with vulvar biopsy.

Therapy

Wide local excision of this intraepithelial lesion should be curative. Because microscopic Paget's disease often extends beyond the obvious gross lesions, wide margins should be taken and excised segments checked in pathology for clean margins. It is also important to rule out underlying adenocarcinoma with pathology. Finally, even with clean margins, Paget's disease has a **high recurrence rate** and may require multiple local excisions. Without nodal metastases, the disease is commonly cured with local excision; however, the disease is likely to be fatal if it spreads to nodes.

KEY POINTS

1. Paget's disease is an intraepithelial neoplasia; however, it is associated with adenocarcinoma 20% of the time.
2. These lesions are often velvety-red in appearance that eventually scar into white plaques.
3. Diagnosis is made by biopsy.
4. Treatment is with wide local excision; there is a high recurrence rate and close follow-up is important.

TABLE 27-1		
Classification of Neoplastic Disease of the Vulva and Vagina		
	Vulvar Disease	**Vaginal Disease**
Premalignant	VIN Paget's disease	VAIN
Malignant	SCC (80% to 90%) Melanoma (5% to 10%) Basal cell (2% to 3%) Sarcomas (<1%)	SCC (85% to 90%) Adenocarcinomas (5%)

VULVAR INTRAEPITHELIAL NEOPLASIA

Pathogenesis

As the incidence of cervical dysplasia has been rising in younger women, so has the incidence of premalignant disease of the vulva, or **VIN**. This concomitant rise is not surprising because both cervical and vulvar neoplastic disease is correlated with **human papillomavirus** (HPV) infection; 80% to 90% of VIN lesions will have DNA fragments from HPV. In fact, 60% of women with VIN have cervical neoplasia as well.

VIN lesions have also been associated with condylomata. Other risk factors for VIN include cigarette smoking and an immunocompromised state. This disease differs in younger and older patients. Younger women will have **multifocal lesions** that rapidly become invasive and more aggressive, whereas older women tend to have **single lesions** that are slow to become invasive.

Epidemiology

VIN has a peak incidence in postmenopausal women in their late 50s and early 60s, although lesions can be seen in many patients under age 35.

Diagnosis

As many as 50% of patients with VIN are **asymptomatic**, whereas other patients commonly present with complaints of **vulvar pruritus** or **vulvodynia**. Often, these women have been seen several times and diagnosed with candidiasis but will have no relief of symptoms with antifungal treatments or topical steroids. On physical examination there may be a variety of lesions that can be diffuse or focal; raised or flat; white, red, brown, or black. Extensive colposcopy of the entire vulvar region will often reveal multiple suspicious lesions that can be biopsied in order to make a pathologic diagnosis (Figure 27-1).

Treatment

It is assumed that VIN will progress to invasive vulvar cancer if not treated. If all of the biopsies taken reveal VIN without any evidence of invasion, then **wide local excision** is commonly used. The goal is to have a disease-free margin of at least 5 mm. When multifocal disease is diagnosed, split-thickness skin grafts are often used to replace the excised lesions. This process is known as "skinning." More recently, laser vaporization has been used to eradicate the lesions; this results in less scar tissue and decreased healing time, but it provides no pathologic specimen and should therefore only be used when nothing more extensive is suspected.

Follow-Up

These therapies are curative for VIN, but close follow-up is required. Patients should have follow-up colposcopies every 3 months until they have been disease-free for 2 years, at which time examinations are reduced to every 6 months.

TABLE 27-2			
Diagnostic Tests for Vulvar Disease			
Disease	**Carcino-Embryonic Antigen**	**S-100 Antigen**	**Melanoma Antigen**
Paget's	Positive	Negative	Negative
VIN	Negative	Positive	Negative
Melanoma	Negative	Negative	Positive

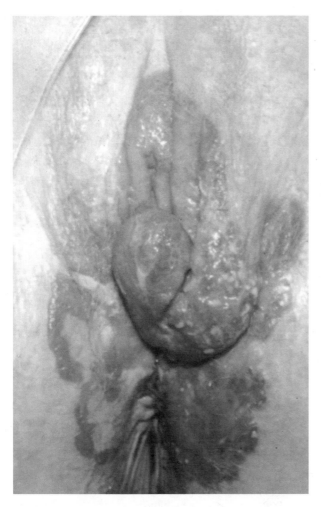

Figure 27-1 • Vulval intraepithelial neoplasia.
(Reproduced with permission from Singer A. Lower Genital Tract Precancer: Colposcopy, Pathology, and Treatment. Oxford: Blackwell Science, 1994:181.)

KEY POINTS

1. VIN is a premalignant disease of the vulva that will progress to cancer if not treated.
2. VIN is often asymptomatic but can present with vulvar pruritus and vulvodynia that are nonrefractory to treatment with antifungals or steroids.
3. The lesions are quite varied and are difficult to differentiate on the basis of physical examination; thus, diagnosis is made strictly by biopsy.
4. Treatments include wide local excision or laser vaporization of tissue with close colposcopic follow-up.

■ CANCER OF THE VULVA

Pathogenesis

The most common type of vulvar cancer is **squamous cell carcinoma** (SCC), which occurs in 85% to 90% of cases. This lesion ranges in appearance from a cauliflower-like mass to a hard indurated ulcer. Spread of disease is primarily via the **lymphatics** to the superficial lymph nodes with a smaller degree of spread via direct extension to vagina, urethra, and anus.

The other types of vulvar cancers include malignant melanoma (5% to 10%), basal cell carcinoma (2% to 3%), and sarcomas (>1%) including leiomyosarcomas and fibrous histiocytomas.

Epidemiology

Vulvar cancer accounts for only **5% of gynecologic malignancies**. It is more common in older patients and those of lower socioeconomic status. It has a peak incidence in patients in their 60s. Associated conditions include diabetes, hypertension, obesity, non-neoplastic disorders of the vulva, and any granulomatous pelvic infection. Poor personal hygiene has also been found to contribute to the occurrence of vulvar cancer.

Diagnosis

Annual screening of the vulva by a physician is an important component in the diagnosis of vulvar cancer. Patients with vulvar cancer often present with long histories of **vulvar pruritus, pain,** and **bleeding.** They may also present with a vulvar mass. Focal lesions tend to be merely inflamed and erythematous in early cancers and heaped up or ulcerated as the lesions progress. Final diagnosis is made by pathologic examination of a **biopsy** specimen.

Staging

Vulvar carcinoma is surgically staged using the International Federation of Gynecology and Obstetrics (FIGO) staging criteria based on tumor size and invasiveness, nodal involvement, and distant metastases (Table 27-3). That is why, without doing a **lymph node dissection** of the groin, it is impossible to definitely stage vulvar cancer. Staging may be approximated by a thorough examination for palpable lymph nodes, although 27% of those with positive

■ **TABLE 27-3**

Staging of Vulvar Cancer

Ia	Lesions 2 cm or less in size confined to the vulva or perineum and with stromal invasion no greater than 1.0 mm (no nodal metastasis)	III	Tumor any size with (a) adjacent spread to the lower urethra and/or distal vagina and/or anus; (b) unilateral regional lymph node metastasis
Ib	Lesions 2 cm or less in size confined to the vulva or perineum and with stromal invasion greater than 1.0 mm (no nodal metastasis)	IVa	Tumor invades any of the following: upper urethra, bladder, mucosa, bone, bilateral regional node metastasis
II	Tumor confined to the vulva and/or perineum— more than 2 cm in greatest dimension (no nodal metastasis)	IVb	Any distant metastasis including pelvic lymph nodes

nodes will have no palpable nodes on physical examination. Metastasis to the intraabdominal lymph nodes is very unlikely if the groin nodes are disease-free.

Treatment

For a primary occurrence of squamous cell carcinoma of the vulva carcinoma, **wide local excision** with regional **lymph node dissection** is the treatment of choice. Stage I disease rarely has positive contralateral lymph nodes, thus ipsilateral lymphadenectomy is sufficient. Most stage II and III disease can be treated with separate inguinal incisions for resection of lymph nodes. Stage IV disease and advanced stage III disease may require radical vulvectomy with en bloc lymphadenectomy, chemotherapy, and radiation therapy.

If lymphadenectomy reveals metastatic disease, **pelvic radiation** is used as adjunct therapy. In patients for whom extensive surgery is contraindicated, the procedure may be confined to vulvectomy. In these patients, preoperative radiation therapy with and without chemotherapy has been used to reduce tumor burden. For recurrence, secondary excision or radiation therapy can be used.

Prognosis

The 5-year survival rate for all patients after surgical treatment of invasive SCC is approximately 75%. The most important prognostic factor is the number of positive lymph nodes. In patients with metastases to local lymph nodes, 5-year survival rates are 90% to 95% for one positive lymph node, 75% to 80% for two positive lymph nodes, and less than 15% for three or more positive lymph nodes.

Melanoma of the vulva can be treated similarly to SCC, except that lymphadenectomy is rarely performed. Depth of invasion is the key prognostic factor. Once the melanoma has metastasized, the mortality rate is near 100%; these patients will not therefore benefit from further surgery to document the spread of the disease. **Basal cell carcinoma** can be treated with wide local excision. These lesions rarely metastasize to the lymph nodes; thus, lymphadenectomy is not required.

KEY POINTS

1. Patients with vulvar cancer often present with symptoms and lesions similar to those of VIN.
2. Diagnosis is made by biopsy.
3. Most treatment includes wide excision and regional lymphadenectomy; radiation therapy is used to reduce tumor burden and for recurrence.
4. Five-year survival rates are excellent for two or fewer positive nodes, but drops to 15% for three or more positive nodes.

■ PRE-INVASIVE DISEASE OF THE VAGINA

Pathogenesis

Vaginal intraepithelial neoplasia (VAIN) is a premalignant lesion similar to that of the vulva and cervix. It is designated VAIN I or II depending on its thickness; carcinoma in situ of the vagina is designated VAIN III. VAIN occurs most commonly as multifocal lesions in the vaginal apex. VAIN is associated with cervical intraepithelial neoplasia (CIN), cervical cancer, condylomas, and history of **infection with HPV**.

Epidemiology

The peak incidence occurs in patients in their mid to late 40s, younger than patients with VIN and older than patients with CIN. At least 50% of patients with VAIN will have **coexistent neoplasia** of the lower genital tract; usually cervical intraepithelial neoplasia.

Diagnosis

Patients with VAIN are usually asymptomatic and typically diagnosed as an abnormality on **Pap smear**. In particular, suspicion of vaginal neoplasia should be raised in patients with persistently abnormal Pap smears but no cervical neoplasia on cervical biopsy. Patients who have undergone hysterectomy should continue to have annual Pap smears to screen for VAIN. In the case of an abnormal Pap, **colposcopy** should follow. Suspicious lesions are often diagnosed with acetic acid application. These lesions should then be **biopsied** to give a final pathologic diagnosis.

Treatment

For focal lesions, **local resection** is curative. If lesions are found on the cervix and extend into the upper third of the vagina, they can be removed with hysterectomy. If invasive disease has been ruled out with extensive biopsies, the lesions can be vaporized with CO_2 **laser** or treated with application of topical **5-fluorouracil (5-FU)**. Many of these patients tend to have multifocal lesions of both the vulva and cervix as well and need close follow-up with colposcopy every 3 months until they have been disease-free for 2 years.

KEY POINTS

1. VAIN lesions are often asymptomatic and are usually found only with careful Pap smear screening.
2. Diagnosis is made by biopsy.
3. Local excision, laser vaporization, and topical 5-FU are common therapies.
4. Patients need close follow-up with colposcopy to rule out recurrence.

■ CANCER OF THE VAGINA

Pathogenesis

Vaginal cancer is extremely rare and most likely represents metastasis or direct extension from cervical cancer rather than a primary vaginal cancer. The most common type of vaginal cancer is **SCC** (85% to 90%); **adenocarcinoma** is found in a much smaller percent of patients (5%). In the 1970s, **clear cell adenocarcinoma** was found to be associated with in utero exposure of diethylstilbestrol (DES).

Epidemiology

Invasive cancer of the vagina has a peak incidence in women in their 50s (mean age of 55). This pertains primarily to the most common cancer of the vagina: SCC. However, women who were exposed in utero to DES have a propensity to develop clear cell adenocarcinoma of the vagina, which can be found in these women under age 30.

Diagnosis

Many patients with vaginal cancer are asymptomatic. The most common presenting symptoms are increasing **vaginal discharge**, **bleeding**, and **pruritus**. As in VAIN, diagnosis is screened for with Pap smear and follow-up colposcopy, and pathologic diagnosis is made with biopsy of suspicious lesions.

Staging and Treatment

Invasive **SCC** of the vagina is often complicated by involvement with local structures such as the rectum or bladder. Stage I and II lesions of the upper third of the vagina are amenable to **surgical resection**, but those of the lower two-thirds of the vagina and stage III and IV lesions are treated with **radiation therapy** alone (Table 27-4). Lesions that are invading into local structures often require palliative surgical therapy, but this does not in any way affect survival rates.

Adenocarcinoma of the vagina is treated similarly to SCC. However, a clear-cut therapy for clear cell carcinoma has not been established. These lesions are often treated similarly with resection of earlier staged lesions and radiation for stage III and IV lesions or those involving the lower vagina.

■ **TABLE 27-4**

FIGO Staging for Carcinoma of the Vagina

Stage	Clinical/Pathologic Findings
Stage 0	Carcinoma in situ, intraepithelial carcinoma
Stage I	The carcinoma is limited to the vaginal wall
Stage II	The carcinoma has involved the subvaginal tissue but has not extended to the pelvic wall
Stage III	The carcinoma has extended to the pelvic wall
Stage IV	The carcinoma has extended beyond the true pelvis or has clinically involved the mucosa of the bladder or rectum; bullous edema as such does not permit a case to be allotted to stage IV
Stage IVa	Spread of the growth to adjacent organs and/or direct extension beyond the true pelvis
Stage IVb	Spread to distant organs

Prognosis

The 5-year survival rate for SCC of the vagina is highly dependent upon the clinical stage. Stage I and II lesions have a 5-year survival rate of 70% to 75%. Stage III has a 5-year survival rate of approximately 30%. Stage IV has few survivors.

KEY POINTS

1. Vaginal cancer is often asymptomatic, with the most common presenting symptoms being vaginal pruritus, discharge, or bleeding.
2. Diagnosis is made by biopsy.
3. Stage I and II lesions of the upper vagina can be treated with excision; all other lesions are treated with radiation therapy.

28 Cervical Cancer

■ NEOPLASTIC DISEASE OF THE CERVIX

In the United States, cervical cancer was the leading cause of death from malignancy in women in the early 1900s. Since the advent of the **Papanicolaou (Pap) smear**, which gained widespread acceptance in the 1950s and 1960s, it has been easier to detect cervical cancer in earlier premalignant or nonlethal stages. It is estimated that annual Pap smear screening reduces a woman's risk of dying of cervical cancer by 90%.

Although cervical cancer has decreased to the sixth leading cause of death from cancer in women in the United States, it still accounts for nearly 5000 deaths per year and is the number one cancer killer of women in the developing world. Cervical cancer and premalignant cervical dysplasia are correlated with onset of sexual activity at an early age and increasing number of sexual partners, whereas it is notably decreased by celibacy. Therefore, for years, it was suspected that cervical cancer was caused by a sexually transmitted agent.

Human Papillomavirus (HPV)

Human papillomavirus (HPV) is now accepted as the **primary causative agent** in cervical cancer. DNA fragments of HPV have been found incorporated into the DNA of cells from invasive cervical cancer in over 90% of cases studied. Further, male partners of patients with cervical cancer are often found to have subclinical infections of HPV. Although **serotypes 6 and 11** seem to **predispose to condylomas**, serotypes such as **16, 18, 31, and 45** are considered "**high-risk types**" and are **correlated with cervical cancer**. We are now able to test for high-risk HPV types in Pap smear specimens. This testing allows physicians to more accurately predict which precancerous lesions have the potential to progress to cancer if left untreated.

Epidemiology

There are approximately 15,000 cases of cervical cancer diagnosed annually in the United States, leading to an estimated 4600 deaths. Risk factors for cervical cancer and dysplasia include **HPV infection**, **cigarette smoking**, high number of sexual partners, early age at onset of sexual activity, and a history of sexually transmitted diseases (STDs). Additionally, patients with human immunodeficiency virus are considered at risk for cervical neoplasia and invasive cervical cancer is considered an AIDS-defining illness.

Pap Smear

The Pap smear involves scraping cells from the external os of the cervix with a blunt spatula to gain cells from the **transformation zone**. Because the squamocolumnar junction may be in the endocervical canal, it is important to also sample the **endocervical canal** with a cytobrush. The sample is then placed directly on a slide or into a liquid-based medium that is then used to make a slide ("thin-prep" Pap smear). The latter has proved to be a more sensitive Pap smear method because the cells do not clump on top of each other and there is **less debris** on the resulting slide. Additionally, **fewer cells are required** to make an adequate liquid-based specimen than with a conventional Pap smear. As a result, with thin-prep Pap smears, more intraepithelial lesions are identified and fewer Pap smears are considered nondiagnostic secondary to "insufficient material." The prepared slides are examined by a cytopathologist.

Current recommendations call for annual Pap smears in **anyone who has begun sexual activity or has reached the age of 18**. Pap smears may show findings consistent with normal cellular material, infection, inflammatory changes, dysplasia, carcinoma in situ, or invasive carcinoma.

In 1988, the Bethesda system of reporting Pap smears was created. This system has since been revised twice; the most recent revision was in 2001. The Bethesda system is utilized by over 95% of U.S. pathology laboratories. The Pap smear is a screening test for cervical cancer and cancer precursors; a "negative" test is titled "Negative for Intraepithelial Lesion or Malignancy." In addition to other categories such as "organisms," "glandular cells," and "other," this system gives four interpretations of epithelial squamous cell abnormalities:

1. Atypical squamous cells (ASC); atypical squamous cells of undetermined significance (ASC-US) and atypical squamous cells cannot exclude high-grade squamous intraepithelial lesion (ASC-H)
2. Low-grade squamous intraepithelial lesion (LSIL)
3. High-grade squamous intraepithelial lesion (HSIL)
4. Squamous cell carcinoma (SCC)

The cellular changes in ASC may represent benign inflammatory response to infection or trauma but may also herald a pre-invasive neoplastic lesion. In fact, it is estimated that **10% to 15% of ASC and LSIL Pap smears harbor high-grade histology** that should be treated. Women with these Pap smear results must therefore be followed closely. Fortunately, with close observation, **80% to 85% of ASC** and **LSIL lesions resolve** spontaneously over 1 to 2 years. While ASC and LSIL usually represent a transient infection with HPV, **HSIL is more likely** to be **associated with persistent infection** and **progression to cancer**.

With the advent of **HPV DNA testing**, it is now recommended that women with an ASC-US result should be tested immediately for HPV: **reflex HPV testing**; that is, when the initial Pap smear sample (it must be liquid-based) gets automatically tested for HPV after having been read as ASC-US. This aids the clinician to predict a patient's risk for a high-risk lesion with more accuracy and to better direct the plan of care. If the woman tests positive for a high-grade HPV type she should then proceed to colposcopy where directed biopsies can be performed. However, if the patient tests negative for a high-grade

HPV type, she can be followed by another Pap smear in 1 year.

Since HPV testing and these guidelines are new, not everyone is utilizing HPV testing in their management of ASCUS Pap smears; some physicians repeat the cytology in 4 to 6 months and then refer to colposcopy if the repeat Pap smear results are ASC or higher. Patients who receive an **ASC-H, LSIL**, or **HSIL result** should **proceed directly to colposcopy**.

Prior to the advent of the Bethesda system, many different ways of describing cervical cytologic changes existed. Since the Bethesda system is most frequently used today, the other methods of describing Pap smears have been correlated with Bethesda terminology as follows. Cytologic changes consistent with HPV infection, mild cervical dysplasia, and cervical intraepithelial neoplasia (CIN-I) all correspond to LSIL. Moderate dysplasia (CIN-II), and severe dysplasia (CIN-III)—known as carcinoma in situ—correspond to HSIL. Patients with any description of dysplasia, ASC-H, HSIL, LSIL, or CIN, as well as those with two consecutive ASC-US results, should proceed to colposcopy for further work-up of their abnormal Pap smears.

Colposcopy

To determine the severity of dysplasia or to identify any invasive carcinoma, colposcopy can be performed and directed biopsies taken. The colposcope gives a magnified view of the cervix and, when stained with acetic acid, cervical lesions can be noted. Changes may include acetowhite epithelium, mosaicism, punctuations, and atypical vessels. These lesions should be biopsied and the specimens sent to pathology where more definitive diagnoses can be made.

The **cytologic classification** of Pap smears uses two-tiered LSIL/HSIL terminology, but the three-tiered CIN system is still sometimes used as an additional descriptor for **histopathologic findings** in cervical biopsies. Cervical dysplasia in these biopsies is categorized as mild (CIN-I), moderate (CIN-II), or severe (CIN-III) depending on the depth and involvement of the epithelium. In general, **CIN-I** can be followed with repeat Pap smears and colposcopies, whereas **CIN-II** and **CIN-III biopsies** should be **treated** with **conization of the cervix**.

■ CERVICAL INTRAEPITHELIAL NEOPLASIA (CIN)

Cervical dysplasia is believed to be the **precursor to cervical cancer**. On average, it takes about 7 years for LSIL to become cervical cancer, and about 4 years to become HSIL. Because of the severity of this disease and the rapidity of progression of an occasional lesion, HSIL is often treated by surgical excision.

Treatment of Cervical Dysplasia

When the diagnosis is made by biopsy of a CIN lesion, several treatments may ensue. ASC-H or LSIL are commonly followed with colposcopy every 4 to 6 months. With resolution of this CIN lesion, patients can return to annual exams after 2 years of normal Pap smears and biopsies.

In patients with biopsies showing HSIL, destruction or excision of the lesion(s) is usually performed. The same is true for patients with LSIL that persists for more than 1 to 2 years. Historically, a **cold knife cone** (CKC) biopsy (Figure 28-1) was performed, which removed a wedge-shaped portion of the cervical stroma and endocervical canal. The **loop electrosurgical excision procedure** (LEEP) or **large loop excision of the transformation zone** (Lletz) is now more commonly performed to remove HSIL lesions. LEEP, loop, or Lletz all refer to the same procedure that involves removing a cone-shaped piece of cervix (conization), typically with a cauterized fine-wire loop or with a laser. The LEEP can be performed as an office procedure under local anesthesia and is quicker and has less blood loss than the CKC.

For small lesions confined to the **exocervix** with invasive disease ruled out, **LEEP, cryotherapy**, or **laser therapy** may be used to destroy the epithelial tissue without causing extensive damage to the cervix. If the lesion involves the **endocervix**, surgical excision of the transformation zone and distal endocervical canal must ensue. This can be accomplished with a two-level LEEP procedure where the first LEEP is performed to remove the exocervix and a second smaller LEEP is then done to remove a portion of the endocervical canal. This is also known as a "top hat" because the resulting defect in the cervix resembles the shape of a top hat. Lesions that involve the endocervix can also be treated using a laser or CKC.

In general, cervical conization procedures remove cervical tissue without causing extensive damage to the stroma of the cervix, although scarring of the endocervical canal may still ensue. Other complications include cervical stenosis, cervical incompetence, infection, or bleeding.

■ CERVICAL CANCER

Pathophysiology

SCC accounts for about 90% of all cervical cancers. It can be subdivided into large-cell keratinizing,

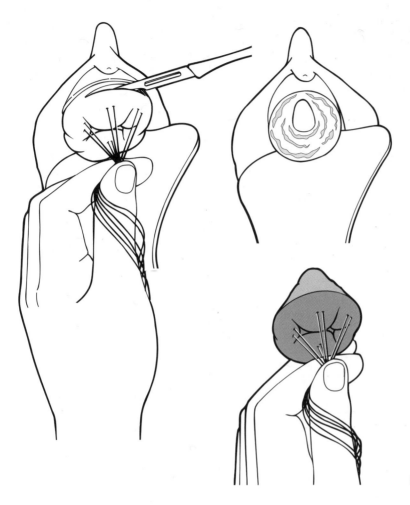

Figure 28-1 • Cold knife cone of the cervix.

large-cell nonkeratinizing, and small cell. **Adeno-carcinoma** accounts for most of the remaining 10% of cervical cancers. One type of adenocarcinoma is clear-cell carcinoma, which is correlated with **in utero diethylstilbestrol (DES) exposure**. A malignancy of the cervix is rarely a sarcoma or lymphoma.

Clinical Manifestations

Even though the Pap smear has proved to be an excellent screening method for cervical cancer, patients still occasionally present with advanced stages of this disease. The classic presentation is with **postcoital bleeding**. Other signs and symptoms that accompany cervical cancer include any **abnormal vaginal bleeding**, watery discharge, **pelvic pain** or pressure, and rectal or urinary tract symptoms. On speculum examination, an **exophytic lesion** on the cervix or invading into the upper vagina may be visible. On bimanual examination, a mass within the cervix may be palpated as well as invasive lesions into the upper vagina, cul-de-sac, or adnexa.

Diagnostic Evaluation

If a lesion is found, it should be **biopsied**. If the Pap smear is abnormal, the cervix should be biopsied colposcopically. If the physical examination is abnormal, **ultrasound** (US) or **computed tomography** (CT) may be performed to confirm the findings and define the extent of disease. However, for a pathologic diagnosis, tissue still needs to be obtained if there are lesions to biopsy.

Clinical Staging

Cervical cancer is one of the few gynecologic cancers that are still **clinically staged** (Table 28-1). This is due in large part to the fact that it is the leading cause of cancer death in women in developing nations where many diagnostic tools are not readily available. Clin-

■ TABLE 28-1

FIGO Staging for Carcinoma of the Cervix Uteri

Stage	Clinical/Pathologic Findings
0	Carcinoma in situ, intraepithelial carcinoma.
I	The carcinoma is strictly confined to the cervix (extension to the corpus should be disregarded).
Ia	Invasive cancer identified only microscopically. All gross lesions—even with superficial invasion—are stage Ib cancers. Invasion is limited to measured stromal invasion with maximum depth of 5.0 mm and no wider than 7.0 mm.*
Ia-1	Measured invasion of stroma no greater than 3.0 mm in depth and no wider than 7.0 mm.
Ia-2	Measured invasion of stroma greater than 3.0 mm and no greater than 5.0 mm and no wider than 7.0 mm.
Ib	Clinical lesions confined to the cervix or preclinical lesions greater than stage Ia.
Ib-1	Clinical lesions no greater than 4.0 cm in size.
Ib-2	Clinical lesions greater than 4.0 cm in size.
II	The carcinoma extends beyond the cervix but has not extended to the pelvic wall. The carcinoma involves the vagina but not as far as the lower third.
IIa	No obvious parametrial involvement.
IIb	Obvious parametrial involvement.
III	The carcinoma has extended to the pelvic wall. On rectal examination, there is no cancer-free space between the tumor and the pelvic wall. The tumor involves the lower third of the vagina. All cases with hydronephrosis or nonfunctioning kidney are included unless they are known to be due to other causes.
IIIa	No extension to the pelvic wall.
IIIb	Extension to the pelvic wall and/or hydronephrosis or nonfunctioning kidney.
IV	The carcinoma has extended beyond the true pelvis or has clinically involved the mucosa of the bladder or rectum. A bullous edema as such does not permit a case to be allotted to stage IV.
IVa	Spread of the growth to adjacent organs.
IVb	Spread to distant organs.

Note: *The depth of invasion should be no more than 5 mm taken from the base of the epithelium, either surface or glandular, from which it originates. Vascular space involvement, either venous or lymphatic, should not alter the staging.

ical staging involves predicting the amount of **invasion into adjacent structures** and **metastatic involvement** (Figure 28-2). Acceptable diagnostic tools for staging of cervical cancer include exam under anesthesia, chest x-ray, cystoscopy, proctoscopy, intravenous pyelography (IVP), and barium enema. **Magnetic resonance (MR) imaging** and **CT** may be used to define the extent of the disease but **cannot** be used to **determine the stage** of the disease.

Stage I is confined to the cervix (see Table 28-1 and Figure 28-2). Stage II extends beyond the cervix but not to the pelvic sidewalls or the lower third of the vagina. Stage III extends to the pelvic sidewalls or lower third of the vagina. Extension beyond the pelvis, invasion into local structures including the

bladder or rectum, or distant metastases all lead to the diagnosis of stage IV disease.

Treatment

Pre-invasive and Microinvasive Disease

In the case of **pre-invasive carcinoma** (stage 0) and **microinvasive carcinoma** (stage Ia-1), the **standard of care** is **simple hysterectomy**. A **cone biopsy** may be adequate therapy if the patient wants to maintain fertility (Table 28-2).

Early Disease

Early disease (stages Ia-2–IIa) may be treated with either **radical hysterectomy** (with bilateral pelvic

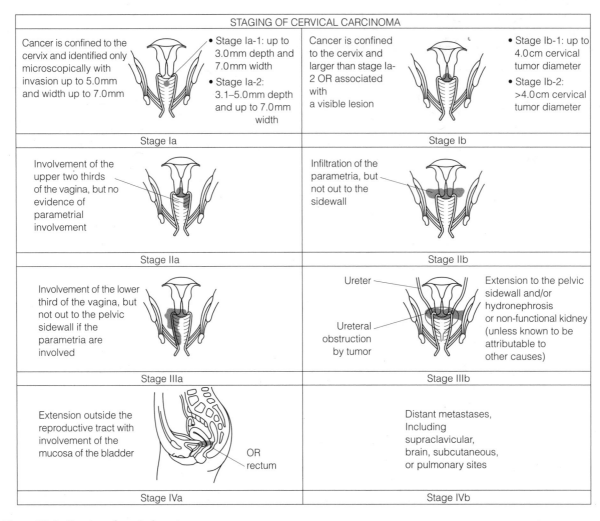

Figure 28-2 • Staging of cervical carcinoma.

TABLE 28-2	
Treatment of Cervical Cancer by Stage	
Stage	**Treatment**
0–Ia-1	CKC biopsy or simple hysterectomy
Ia-2–IIa	Radical hysterectomy or radiation
IIb–IV	Chemoradiation*

Note: *External beam radiation, cisplatin-based chemotherapy, and intracavitary radiation.

lymph node dissection) or **radiation therapy** (see Table 28-2) with similar recurrence and survival rates. The choice of treatment depends on the patient's age, ability to tolerate surgery, and proximity to radiation facilities. Young patients who are otherwise healthy are often treated with surgery to maintain ovarian function that would be diminished or terminated by radiation therapy.

Advanced Disease

For **more advanced lesions** (stages IIb–IV) that have spread to the parametria or beyond, the treatment is **chemoradiation therapy** (see Table 28-2). Both external beam radiation and intracavitary radiation are used in combination with **cisplatin-based chemotherapy**. The goals of chemoradiation are to eradicate local disease and prevent metastatic disease. This combined treatment regimen has led to significantly prolonged disease-free survival when compared to radiation therapy alone.

Recurrent Disease

When cervical cancer recurs in a patient initially treated with surgery alone, **radiation** can be used to treat the recurrence. When the cancer recurs in a patient already treated with radiation, surgical treatment with **pelvic exenteration** can be used if the recurrence is centrally located. Exenteration involves removal of the pelvic organs including the bladder, rectum, uterus, vagina, and supporting ligaments.

Palliative Care

Palliative **radiation** with external beam or intracavitary therapy may be used to control bleeding or for pain management. Cisplatin **chemotherapy** may also be used for palliative care.

Survival

Overall survival rates for cervical cancer are shown in Table 28-3.

■ TABLE 28-3

Overall 5-Year Survival for Cervical Cancer

Stage	5-Year Survival (in %)
I	85–90
II	60–75
III	35–45
IV	15–20

KEY POINTS

1. Pre-invasive (stage 0) and microinvasive disease (stage Ia-1) can be treated with cone biopsy or simple hysterectomy. Stage Ia-2 should be treated with radical hysterectomy.
2. Early disease—stages Ia-2 to IIa—is equally responsive to radical hysterectomy or radiation therapy.
3. More advanced lesions—stage IIb or greater—are treated with radiation therapy, usually in combination with cisplatin chemotherapy.
4. Radiation and/or chemotherapy may be used for palliative care.
5. Five-year survival rates for cervical cancer vary from 85% to 90% for stage I disease, and 15% to 20% for stage IV disease.

Endometrial Cancer

Endometrial carcinoma is the **most common gynecologic cancer** in the United States and the fourth most common cancer in American women today, exceeded only by cancer of the breast, bowel, and lung. Over 35,000 women are diagnosed with this disease each year in the United States alone. Fortunately, early symptoms and easy and accurate diagnosis modalities make endometrial cancer only the third most common cause of gynecologic cancer deaths (behind ovarian and cervical cancer) accounting for 6000 deaths each year in the United States.

Endometrial carcinoma is known as an "estrogen-dependent neoplasm" because of the strong association between **estrogen exposure** in the absence of progesterone and the development of endometrial carcinoma. Factors such as obesity, chronic anovulation, low parity, and late menopause lead to an increased exposure to unopposed estrogen and subsequently to an increased risk of endometrial carcinoma. These same factors place women at an increased risk of **endometrial hyperplasia** as well (see Table 14-5). The degree of risk of malignant transformation of endometrial hyperplasia to endometrial cancer depends on the type of hyperplasia. The most severe form—atypical complex hyperplasia—poses a 29% risk of developing endometrial cancer if left untreated (see Table 14-4).

PATHOGENESIS

There are **two distinct pathogenic types** of endometrial cancer. The most common type occurs in younger perimenopausal women with a history of chronic estrogen exposure. These are referred to as **estrogen-dependent** neoplasias. These tumors are initially endometrial hyperplasia and progress to carcinomas. The tumors tend to be well differentiated and usually have a favorable prognosis.

The second pathogenic type of endometrial cancer is believed to be **estrogen-independent.** These tumors are not generally associated with endometrial hyperplasia and tend to occur in older, postmenopausal, thin women. These cancers are less differentiated and occur more frequently in African American and Asian women.

The most common type of endometrial cancer (80%) is **endometrioid adenocarcinoma**. Other types are mucinous carcinomas (5%), clear-cell carcinoma (5%), squamous carcinoma (1%), and papillary serous carcinoma (4%). Invasive adenocarcinoma usually results from **proliferation of the glandular cells** of the endometrium rather than stromal proliferation. The degree of abnormality in these glandular cells is used to determine the grade of the tumor (Table 29-1).

Endometrial carcinoma has four primary routes of spread. The most common route is **direct extension** of the tumor downward to the cervix or outward through the myometrium and serosa. When there is significant myometrial penetration, cells may spread through the lymphatic system to the pelvic and periaortic lymph nodes. Exfoliated cells may also be shed transtubally through the fallopian tubes to the ovaries, parietal peritoneum, and omentum. Hematogenous spread occurs less frequently but can result in metastasis to the liver, lungs, and/or bone.

Histologic grade is the most important prognostic factor for endometrial carcinoma (see Table 29-1). Poorly differentiated tumors have a higher grade and a much poorer prognosis due to the likelihood of spread outside of the uterus. Depth of **myometrial invasion** is the second most important prognostic factor. The prognosis is dramatically wors-

■ TABLE 29-1

Histologic Grading System for Endometrial Cancer

Grade 1 (G1)	5% or less of the tumor shows a solid growth pattern
Grade 2 (G2)	6% to 50% of the tumor shows a solid growth pattern
Grade 3 (G3)	More than 50% of the tumor shows a solid growth pattern

■ TABLE 29-2

Risk Factors for Endometrial Cancer

Risk Factor	Relative Risk
Nulliparity	2–3
Late menopause	2–4
Diabetes mellitus	2–8
Tamoxifen use	2–3
Obesity	
21–50 lbs overweight	3
>50 lbs overweight	10
Unopposed estrogen therapy	4–8

ened when the cancer has invaded greater than one-third of the thickness of the myometrium. The **histologic type** of carcinoma also affects prognosis. In general, adenosquamous (found in older women), clear-cell squamous, and papillary serous carcinomas have worse prognoses than the far more common adenocarcinoma. Other important prognostic factors are pelvic node metastases, original tumor volume, extension to the cervix, adnexal metastases, and positive peritoneal washings.

■ EPIDEMIOLOGY

Endometrial cancer occurs in both premenopausal (25%) and postmenopausal (75%) women. The median age of diagnosis is 61; the largest affected group is between age 50 and 59. Most tumors are caught early when they are of low grade and low stage; therefore, the overall prognosis for the disease is good and overall mortality rates are declining.

■ RISK FACTORS

Most women with endometrial cancer have a history of unopposed estrogen exposure, including obesity (>30 lbs overweight), nulliparity or low parity, chronic anovulation, menopause after age 50, or a history of unopposed exogenous estrogen use (Table 29-2). Other risk factors include diabetes mellitus, hypertension, cancer of the breast or ovary, and a family history of endometrial cancer. Conversely, oral contraceptive pills (OCPs) may help prevent endometrial cancer in women who have taken them for at least 12 months.

Despite these known risk factors, there are no effective screening mechanisms for endometrial carcinoma. Neither annual Pap smears nor endometrial biopsies have been shown to offer cost-effective screening in asymptomatic patients.

■ CLINICAL MANIFESTATIONS

History

The most common symptom of endometrial cancer is **irregular bleeding** (postmenopausal bleeding, menorrhagia, postcoital spotting, or intermenstrual bleeding). Some form of abnormal vaginal bleeding occurs in 90% of patients with endometrial cancer.

Physical Examination

The physical examination may reveal hypertension, obesity, or stigmata of diabetes. The clinician should look for signs of metastatic disease including pleural effusion, ascites, hepatosplenomegaly, general lymphadenopathy, and abdominal masses.

Women with endometrial carcinoma typically have a **normal pelvic examination**. In more advanced stages of the disease, the cervical os may be patulous and the cervix may be firm and expanded. The uterus may be of normal size or enlarged and the adnexae should be carefully examined for evidence of extrauterine metastasis and/or coexistent ovarian carcinoma.

Differential Diagnosis

The differential diagnosis for postmenopausal bleeding includes uterine and cervical polyps, uterine fibroids, endometrial hyperplasia, exogenous estrogen use, and atrophic vaginitis (Table 29-3). The

TABLE 29-3

Differential Diagnosis of Postmenopausal Bleeding

Cause of Bleeding	Frequency (in %)
Endometrial atrophy	60–80
Exogenous estrogens/HRT	15–25
Endometrial cancer	**10**
Endometrial or cervical polyps	2–12
Endometrial hyperplasia	5–10
Miscellaneous*	10

Note: *For example, cervical cancer, uterine sarcoma, trauma.
Source: Adapted from Hacker N, Moore JG. Essentials of Obstetrics and Gynecology. Philadelphia: WB Saunders, 1998:635.

older the patient, the more likely it is that malignancy is the cause of bleeding.

DIAGNOSTIC EVALUATION

Although dilation and curettage (D&C) was once the gold standard for evaluating irregular bleeding, modern office endometrial biopsy has an accuracy of 90% to 98% without the need for anesthesia and operative time. The **endometrial biopsy** has therefore become the standard of care. If an adequate endometrial biopsy cannot be performed due to patient discomfort, cervical stenosis, or insufficient tissue sample, a **hysteroscopy** and **D&C** should be done to visualize and sample the endometrium.

In addition to endometrial sampling, the initial work-up for a postmenopausal woman with vaginal bleeding should also include a **Pap smear**, although only 30% to 40% of patients with endometrial cancer will have an abnormal Pap smear. A **pelvic ultrasound** should also be performed to rule out fibroids, polyps, and endometrial hyperplasia. If bone pain is present, a chest radiograph and bone scan should also be performed.

TREATMENT

Although endometrial cancer was once clinically staged, in 1988 the International Federation of Gynecology and Obstetrics (FIGO) changed to a **surgical staging system** that more accurately identifies the true degree of disease progression. This system relies on pathologic confirmation of the extent of spread of the disease (Table 29-4).

In general, treatment for endometrial carcinoma includes **surgical staging**, **total abdominal hysterectomy and bilateral salpingo-oophorectomy** (TAHBSO), and postoperative **radiation** treatment. **High-dose progestins** are the first line of treatment for advanced and recurrent disease. Single-agent non-hormonal chemotherapy may be used in advanced or recurrent disease but has a low efficacy.

TABLE 29-4

FIGO Surgical Staging of Endometrial Carcinoma (1988)

Stages		Extent of Disease
Ia	G123	Tumor limited to endometrium
Ib	G123	Invasion to less than half of the myometrium
Ic	G123	Invasion to greater than half of the myometrium
IIa	G123	Endocervical glandular involvement only
IIb	G123	Cervical stromal invasion
IIIa	G123	Tumor invades serosa and/or positive peritoneal cytology
IIIb	G123	Vaginal metastases
IIIc	G123	Metastases to pelvic and/or para-aortic lymph nodes
IVa	G123	Tumor invasion of bladder and/or bowel mucosa
IVb	G123	Distant metastases including intraabdominal and/or inguinal lymph nodes

Because most endometrial cancers are stage I at diagnosis, the overall 5-year survival is 65%. Survival rates for the various stages of endometrial cancer are 73% for stage I, 56% for stage II, 32% for stage III, and 10% for stage IV.

■ FOLLOW-UP

Seventy-five percent of recurrences of endometrial carcinoma will occur within the first 2 years after treatment and 85% by the end of the third year. Follow-up should occur every 3 months for 2 years, then twice a year for 3 years, and then annually. The first line of treatment for recurrent disease is high-dose progestin therapy. These therapies, typically megestrol (Megace) or medroxyprogesterone (Provera), have been used with a 30% response rate.

The use of **estrogen replacement therapy** in patients treated for endometrial carcinoma is controversial and usually reserved for those patients whose cancer was well-differentiated and minimally invasive. Even then, estrogen replacement therapy is usually only used after the patient has been cancer-free for 5 years.

KEY POINTS

1. Endometrial cancer is the most common gynecologic cancer and the fourth most common cancer in women.
2. Endometrial cancer can be caused by prolonged exposure to exogenous or endogenous estrogen in the absence of progesterone.
3. The most common type of endometrial cancer (80%) is endometrioid adenocarcinoma.
4. Endometrioid cancer is diagnosed at a median age of 61 with 25% of patients being diagnosed premenopausally and 75% postmenopausally.
5. The major risk factors for endometrial cancer include unopposed estrogen exposure such as obesity, chronic anovulation, nulliparity, late menopause, and unopposed exogenous estrogen use. Hypertension and diabetes are also important risk factors.
6. The most common presenting symptom is abnormal vaginal bleeding.
7. Endometrial biopsy is the standard of care for diagnosing endometrial cancer.
8. Currently, there are no cost-effective screening tools for endometrial cancer; however, because of abnormal bleeding most women are diagnosed early with 75% of lesions being at stage I at the time of diagnosis.
9. Treatment may involve TAHBSO followed by radiation depending on the stage; recurrent disease is treated with high-dose progestin therapy.
10. Overall 5-year survival rate is 65% with 85% of recurrences occurring in the first 3 years after treatment.

Ovarian and Fallopian Tube Tumors

There are many types of benign and malignant tumors of the ovaries (Table 30-1), each possessing its own characteristics (Table 30-2). Fortunately, 80% of ovarian tumors are benign. While fallopian tube carcinoma is extremely rare, ovarian cancer is the fifth most common cancer in women in the United States and the third most common cancer of the female genital tract, second only to endometrial and cervical cancer (Figure 30-1).

Although ovarian carcinoma accounts for 25% of all gynecologic malignancies (28,000 new cases per year), it is responsible for nearly 50% of deaths from cancer of the female genital tract (15,000 deaths per year). This high mortality is due in part to the lack of effective screening tools for early diagnosis and in part to the spread by direct extension into the peritoneal cavity. Because the overall 5-year survival rate for women with ovarian carcinoma is only 25% to 30%, a high degree of suspicion and prompt diagnosis and intervention are critical.

PATHOGENESIS

Tumors of the ovaries are derived from one of the three distinct components of the ovary: the surface coelomic epithelium, the ovarian stroma, or the germ cells (Figure 30-2). Over 65% of all ovarian tumors and 90% of all ovarian cancers originate from **coelomic epithelium** in the ovary capsule. About 5% to 10% of ovarian cancer is metastatic from other primary tumors in the body, usually from the gastrointestinal tract, breast, or endometrium, and are known as **Krukenberg tumors**.

Ovarian carcinoma is primarily spread by **direct exfoliation** of malignant cells from the ovaries. As a result, the sites of metastasis often follow the circulatory path of the peritoneal fluid, and the regional lymph nodes are often involved. **Hematogenous spread** is responsible for more rare and distant metastases to the lung and brain. In advanced disease, intraperitoneal tumor spread leads to accumulation of ascites in the abdomen and encasement of the bowel with tumor. This results in intermittent bowel obstruction known as a carcinomatous ileus. In many cases, this progression results in malnutrition, slow "starvation," cachexia, and death.

Although the cause of ovarian carcinoma is unclear, it is believed to result from malignant transformation of ovarian tissue after prolonged periods of **chronic uninterrupted ovulation**. Ovulation disrupts the epithelium of the ovary and activates the cellular repair mechanism. When ovulation occurs for long periods of time without interruption, this mechanism is believed to provide the opportunity for somatic **gene deletions** and **mutations**. Ten percent of women with ovarian cancer have a familial cancer syndrome (e.g., familial breast-ovarian syndrome, Lynch II syndrome). Mutations in the **BRCA1 or BRCA2** generally account for most of these cases. High dietary fat, mumps virus, and agents such as talc and asbestos have also been proposed as possible etiologic agents in the pathogenesis of ovarian carcinoma.

EPIDEMIOLOGY

The average woman has a 1:60 chance of developing ovarian carcinoma over her lifetime. The median age of diagnosis is 61 years of age.

■ **TABLE 30-1**

Benign and Malignant Ovarian Tumors

Epithelial tumors	Serous tumors
	Serous cystadenoma
	Borderline serous tumor
	Serous cystadenocarcinoma
	Adenofibroma and cystadenofibroma
	Mucinous tumors
	Mucinous cystadenoma
	Borderline mucinous tumor
	Mucinous cystadenocarcinoma
	Endometrioid carcinoma
	Clear cell adenocarcinoma
	Brenner tumor
	Undifferentiated carcinoma
Germ cell tumors	Teratoma
	Benign (mature, adult)
	Cystic teratoma (dermoid cyst)
	Solid teratoma
	Malignant (immature)
	Monodermal or specialized (e.g., carcinoid, struma ovarii)
	Dysgerminoma
	Endodermal sinus tumor
	Choriocarcinoma
	Others (embryonal carcinoma, polyembryoma, mixed germ cell tumors)
Sex cord-stromal tumors	Granulosa-theca cell tumors
	Granulosa cell tumor
	Thecoma
	Fibroma
	Sertoli-Leydig cell tumor (androblastoma)
	Gonadoblastoma
Unclassified	Ex. Lipoid-cell tumors and tumors sarcomas
Metastatic tumors	Ex. From GI tract, female genital tract, or breast

Source: *Reproduced with permission from Robbins S, Cotran R, Kumar V. Robbins Pathologic Basis of Disease. Philadelphia: WB Saunders, 1991:1158.*

■ RISK FACTORS

Women at the highest risk for ovarian cancer are those with a **family history** of the disease and those with a history of **uninterrupted ovulation**, including nulliparous women, and women with decreased fertility, delayed childbearing, or late onset menopause. Other risk factors include the use of talc on the perineum, a high fat diet, lactose intolerance, and a history of colon cancer. Women with breast cancer also have a twofold increase in the incidence of ovarian cancer. It has been suggested that women who undergo ovulation induction may be at increased risk of developing ovarian carcinoma. These findings have not been proved.

Oral contraceptives (OCPs) have been found to have a protective effect against ovarian cancer that is attributed to suppression of ovulation. Breast-feeding, multiparity, and chronic anovulation have also been found to be protective agents that act by interrupting or suppressing ovulation.

■ CLINICAL MANIFESTATIONS

History

Patients with ovarian cancer are often **asymptomatic** until the disease has progressed to the advanced stages. Some patients may present with vague lower abdominal pain, abdominal enlargement, and early

TABLE 30-2

Frequency of the Major Ovarian Tumors

Type	Percentage of Malignant Ovarian Tumors	Percentage of Bilateral Ovarian Tumors
Serous	60	
Benign (60%)		25
Borderline (15%)		30
Malignant (25%)		65
Mucinous	10	
Benign (80%)		5
Borderline (10%)		10
Malignant (10%)		20
Endometrioid carcinoma	5	40
Undifferentiated carcinoma	5	—
Clear cell carcinoma	6	40
Granuloma cell tumor	5	5
Teratoma		
Benign (96%)		15
Malignant (4%)	1	Rare
Metastatic	6	<50
Other	3	—

Source: Reproduced with permission from Robbins S, Cotran R, Kumar V. Robbins Pathologic Basis of Disease. Philadelphia: WB Saunders, 1991:1159.

satiety. As the tumors progress, other symptoms may develop, including gastrointestinal complaints, urinary frequency, dysuria, and pelvic pressure. Ascites may develop in later stages. Ventral hernia may also be seen due to increased intra-abdominal pressure.

Physical Examination

There is no evidence to suggest that routine pelvic examination improves the early diagnosis of ovarian cancer. As the disease progresses, the primary findings on examination are a **solid, fixed pelvic mass** that may extend into the upper abdomen and **ascites** (Table 30-3).

Diagnostic Evaluation

Pelvic ultrasound is the primary diagnostic tool for investigating an adnexal mass (Table 30-4). These physical and radiographic findings help to distinguish between benign and malignant tumors. Other studies, including computed tomography (CT) and magnetic resonance imaging (MRI) of the pelvis and abdomen, can assist in diagnosis and in delineation of the spread of disease. Because malignant cells can spread via direct exfoliation, paracentesis and cyst aspiration should be avoided. Once the diagnosis is made, studies are undertaken to look for **metastatic disease** and to distinguish between primary and sec-

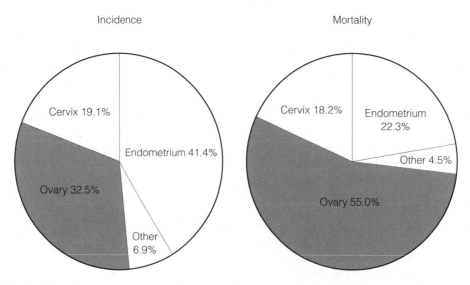

Figure 30-1 • Relationships of ovarian cancer to other gynecologic cancer for incidence and mortality; United States, 1996. (Modified from Parker SL, Tong T, Bolden S, Wingo PA. Cancer Statistics, CA Cancer J Clin 1996;46:5–27.)

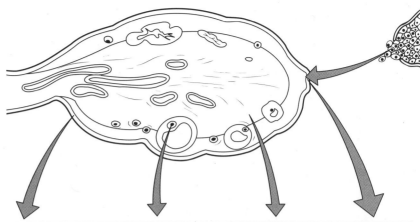

Origin	Surface epithelial cells (common epithelial tumors)	Germ cell	Sex cord–stroma	Metastasis to ovaries
Percent of all ovarian tumors	65–70%	15–20%	5–10%	5%
Age group affected	20+ years	0–25+ years	All ages	Variable
Types	• Serous tumor • Mucinous tumor • Endometrioid tumor • Clear cell tumor • Brenner tumor • Undifferentiated	• Teratoma • Dysgerminoma • Endodermal sinus tumor • Choriocarcinoma • Embryonal carcinoma	• Granulosa–theca cell tumor • Sertoli-Leydig cell tumor • Fibroma	

Figure 30-2 • Classification of various ovarian neoplasms (benign, borderline, and malignant).

■ TABLE 30-3

Characteristics of Pelvic Mass on Physical Examination

	Benign	Malignant
Mobility	Mobile	Fixed
Consistency	Cystic	Solid or firm
Bilateral or unilateral	Unilateral	Bilateral
Cul de sac	Smooth	Nodular

Source: Adapted from De Cherney A, Pernoll M. Current Obstetric and Gynecologic Diagnosis and Treatment. Norwalk: Appleton & Lange, 1994:960, Table 49-3.

■ TABLE 30-4

Radiographic Characteristics of Adnexal Masses

	Benign	Malignant
Size	<8 cm	>8 cm
Consistency	Cystic	Solid or cystic and solid
Septation	Unilocular	Multilocular
Bilateral or unilateral	Unilateral	Bilateral
Other	Calcification, esp. teeth	Ascites

Source: Adapted from De Cherney A, Pernoll M. Current Obstetric and Gynecologic Diagnosis and Treatment. Norwalk: Appleton & Lange, 1994:961, Table 49-4.

ondary ovarian cancer. Ovarian cancer metastasis to the umbilicus is known as **Sister Mary Joseph's nodule**.

Depending on the type of tumor, ovarian malignancies can be monitored using the **serum tumor markers** CA-125, α-fetoprotein (AFP), lactate dehydrogenase (LDH), and human chorionic gonadotropins (hCG).

■ SURGICAL STAGING

Ovarian carcinoma is **surgically staged** (Table 30-5). Primary staging includes total abdominal hysterectomy bilateral oophorectomy (TAHBSO), omentectomy, collection ascites and peritoneal washings, Pap smear of the diaphragm, and sampling the regional lymph nodes. Because there are no reliable screening tools for ovarian cancer and few early symptoms, nearly 75% of patients present with stage III or more advanced disease. The different forms of ovarian cancer are discussed below.

■ EPITHELIAL TUMORS

Pathogenesis

Epithelial cell tumors of the ovaries are derived from the surface mesothelial cells of the ovary (Figure 30-2). The six primary types of epithelial tumors are serous, mucinous, endometrioid, clear cell, Brenner's, and undifferentiated. The neoplasms in this group range in malignant potential from benign to borderline to frankly malignant.

Malignant epithelial tumors extend through the capsule of the ovary to seed the peritoneal cavity and rarely invade the underlying ovary. These are **slow-growing tumors** that often remain undiagnosed until they are very large and at an advanced stage. In over 75% of patients, tumors have spread beyond the ovary at the time of diagnosis; thus, the prognosis is very poor.

■ TABLE 30-5

Staging of Ovarian Carcinoma

Stage I: Growth limited to the ovaries
　Ia—one ovary involved
　Ib—both ovaries involved
　Ic—Ia or Ib and ovarian surface tumor, ruptured capsule, malignant ascites, or peritoneal cytology positive for
　　malignant cells

Stage II: Disease extension from the ovary to the pelvis
　IIa—extension to the uterus or fallopian tube
　IIb—extension to other pelvic tissues
　IIc—IIa or IIb and ovarian surface tumor, ruptured capsule, malignant ascites, or peritoneal cytology positive for
　　malignant cells

Stage III: Disease extension to the abdominal cavity
　IIIa—abdominal peritoneal surfaces with microscopic metastases
　IIIb—tumor metastases <2 cm in size
　IIIc—tumor metastases >2 cm in size or metastatic disease in the pelvic, para-aortic, or inguinal lymph nodes

Stage IV: Distant metastatic disease
　Malignant pleural effusion
　Pulmonary parenchymal metastases
　Liver or splenic parenchymal metastases (not surface implants)
　Metastases to the supraclavicular lymph nodes or skin

Source: Reproduced with permission from American College of Obstetricians and Gynecologists. Prolog: Gynecologic Oncology and Surgery, 3rd ed. Washington, DC, 1996:181.

Epidemiology

Epithelial tumors tend to occur in patients who are in their 50s. **Epithelial cell cancers account for 65% to 70% of all ovarian tumors** and more than 90% of ovarian cancers. **Serous tumors** are the most common type of epithelial ovarian cancer. These tumors are bilateral 65% of the time.

Clinical Manifestations

The serum tumor marker **CA-125** is elevated in 80% of epithelial cell cancers. Because CA-125 levels correlate with the progression and regression of these tumors, it has been useful in tracking the effect of treatment for epithelial ovarian carcinoma. Its value as a screening tool for the detection of ovarian cancer has not yet been established. One reason for this is the high number of benign and malignant gynecologic and nongynecologic conditions associated with an elevated CA-125 level (Table 30-6).

Treatment

Surgery is the mainstay of treatment for epithelial cell tumors, including TAHBSO, omentectomy, and cytoreductive surgery.

After surgery, epithelial cell carcinoma is treated with a cisplatin-based combination chemotherapeutic regimen of **carboplatin** and **paclitaxel** (Taxol). After chemotherapy, a "second look" laparotomy may be performed to evaluate the patient's response to treatment. In the past, the **second look laparotomy** was used to evaluate patient response to treatment, but it is no longer accepted as the standard of care. The tumor marker **CA-125** is used to evaluate the success of treatment and to diagnosis recurrent disease. Unfortunately, the tumors frequently recur despite aggressive treatment.

The overall 5-year survival for patients with epithelial cell carcinoma is less than 20% (80% to 95% for stage I, 40% to 70% for stage II, 30% for stage III, and less than 10% for stage IV disease).

KEY POINTS

1. Epithelial tumors of the ovary account for 90% of ovarian cancers.
2. These tumors are derived from the coelomic epithelium on the surface of the ovary.
3. Epithelial tumors of the ovary are slow-growing but aggressive tumors that may cause few symptoms until they are significantly advanced.
4. Over 75% of patients are diagnosed at stage III or higher.
5. Tumors are staged surgically and treated with surgery followed by taxol and carboplatin chemotherapy.
6. The tumor marker CA-125 can be used to evaluate the success of treatment and look for recurrence of disease.
7. The 5-year survival rate for epithelial ovarian cancer is less than 20%.
8. Ovarian cancer metastasis to the umbilicus is known as Sister Mary Joseph's nodule.
9. Krukenberg tumors are ovarian tumors that are metastatic to the ovary from another primary cancer usually from the colon, breast, or uterus.

■ TABLE 30-6

Gynecologic and Nongynecologic Conditions Associated with Elevated CA-125 Levels

Gynecologic cancers
Epithelial ovarian cancer
Fallopian tube cancer
Endometrial cancer
Endocervical cancer

Nongynecologic cancers
Pancreatic cancer
Lung cancer
Breast cancer
Colon cancer

Benign gynecologic conditions
Normal and ectopic pregnancy
Endometriosis
Fibroids
Pelvic inflammatory disease

Benign nongynecologic conditions
Pancreatitis
Cirrhosis
Peritonitis
Recent laparotomy

■ GERM CELL TUMORS

Pathogenesis

Germ cell ovarian tumors are thought to arise from totipotential germ cells capable of differentiating into the three germ cell layers: yolk sac, placenta, and fetus (Figure 30-3). Ovarian germ cell tumors are

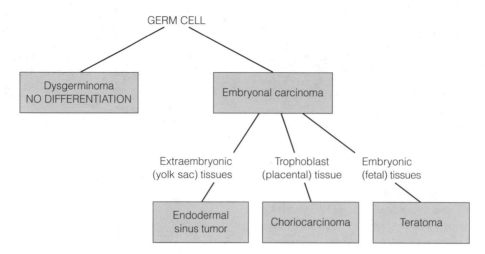

Figure 30-3 • Histogenesis of tumors of germ cell origin.

very similar to germ cell tumors in the testis. The most common types of germ cell cancers are **dysgerminomas** and **immature teratomas**. Embryonal cell carcinoma, endodermal sinus (yolk sac) tumors, nongestational choriocarcinoma, and mixed-germ cell tumors are less common. Many of these tumors produce **serum tumor markers** that can be used to assess response to therapy (Table 30-7). Although there is wide variation in the type of serum tumor markers produced by ovarian tumors, in general, dysgerminomas produce LDH, embryonal sinus tumors produce AFP, and choriocarcinomas produce β-hCG.

In contrast to epithelial tumors, most germ cell tumors are in the **early stage** at the time of diagnosis. The prognosis for germ cell tumors is therefore far better than that for epithelial tumors. In most cases, these tumors are considered curable.

Epidemiology

Germ cell tumors account for 15% to 20% of all ovarian tumors. Although **95% are benign**, the remaining 5% of germ cell tumors are malignant and found primarily in children and young women. Germ cell tumors tend to occur in women in their teens and twenties.

Clinical Manifestations

Unlike epithelial ovarian cancer, the signs and symptoms of germ cell tumors are from the primary tumor rather than from metastatic disease. Patients with germ cell carcinoma present with **rapidly enlarging adnexal mass** and **abdominal pain**. Functional germ cell tumors may produce hCG, AFP, LDH, and/or CA-125 depending on the cell type (Table 30-5).

Treatment

Because most germ cell tumors are diagnosed in the early stage and are rarely bilateral, surgery is typically limited to **removal of the involved ovary**. However, complete surgical staging should still be performed. Most cases of germ cell cancer are considered curable with **multidrug chemotherapy** (e.g., cisplatin, vinblastine, and bleomycin or bleomycin, etoposide, and platin).

Radiation therapy is not a major component of treatment for germ cell tumors except in the case of dysgerminomas, which are exquisitely sensitive to whole abdominal radiation.

The 5-year survival rate is 85% for dysgerminomas, 70% to 80% for immature teratomas, and 60% to 70% for endodermal sinus tumors.

TABLE 30-7

Serum Tumor Markers for Germ Cell Neoplasia

Tumor	hCG	AFP	LDH	CA-125
Mixed germ cell tumor	+	+	+	+
Embryonal carcinoma	+	+		+
Endodermal sinus tumor		+		
Dysgerminoma			+	+
Immature teratoma				+
Choriocarcinoma	+			

Source: Adapted from Frederickson H, Wilkins-Haug L. OB/GYN Secrets, 2nd ed. Philadelphia: Hanley & Belfus, 1997:132.

KEY POINTS

1. Germ cell tumors arise from totipotential germ cells.
2. The most common types of germ cell tumors are dysgerminomas and immature teratomas.
3. Germ cell tumors produce serum tumor markers (AFP, LDH, CA-125, and/or hCG) that can be used to assess response to therapy.
4. These occur primarily in women under the age 20, who present with a unilateral, rapidly enlarging adnexal mass.
5. Germ cell tumors are usually diagnosed at an early stage.
6. Most germ cell tumors are chemosensitive and thus treated by combination chemotherapy and removal of the affected ovary. Dysgerminomas are extremely sensitive to radiation therapy.
7. The 5-year survival rate is 60% to 85% depending on the type of tumor.

■ SEX CORD-STROMAL TUMORS

Pathogenesis

These tumors originate from either the **sex cords** of the embryonic gonad (before the differentiation into male or female) or from the **ovarian stroma** (Figure 30-2). Granulosa-theca cells are the most common (70%) type of tumor in this group and are low-grade malignancies. Both granulosa-theca cell tumors and Sertoli-Leydig cell tumors are characterized by **hormone production**. Ovarian stroma can develop into an ovary or a testis. As a result, ovarian **granulosa-theca cell tumors** resemble fetal ovaries and produce large amounts of estrogens, whereas ovarian **Sertoli-Leydig cell tumors** resemble fetal testes and produce testosterone and other androgens.

The **ovarian fibroma** is derived from mature fibroblasts and, unlike the other stromal cell neoplasms, is not a functioning tumor. Occasionally, fibromas are associated with ascites. The presence of ovarian tumor, ascites, and right hydrothorax is known as **Meigs' syndrome**.

Epidemiology

Stromal cell ovarian carcinoma typically affects postmenopausal women between age 40 and 70.

Clinical Manifestations

Granulosa-theca cell tumors often produce **estrogen and inhibin** that can cause feminization, precocious puberty, or postmenopausal bleeding. Sertoli-Leydig cell tumors produce **androgens** that can cause virilizing effects including hirsutism, deepened voice, acne, and clitoromegaly.

Treatment

Because most stromal cell tumors occur in postmenopausal women, treatment typically includes **TAHBSO**. Chemotherapy is ineffective in treating stromal cell carcinoma. Even with aggressive treatment, the tumor **typically recurs**. Postoperative pelvic radiation is occasionally used in early stage disease.

The 5-year survival rate for patients with stromal cell carcinomas is 90% for stage I disease. However, these tumors are slow growing and recurrences can be detected 15 to 20 years after removal of the primary lesion.

KEY POINTS

1. Sex cord-stromal tumors are derived from the sex cords of the embryonic gonad or from the ovarian stroma. Granulosa cell tumors are the most common type (70%).
2. These tumors are characterized by hormone production.
3. Granulosa-theca cell tumors secrete inhibin and estrogen as tumor markers, whereas Sertoli-Leydig cell tumors secrete testosterone as a tumor marker.
4. Sex cord-stromal tumors are slow-growing tumors with low malignant potential and are often found only incidentally, usually in postmenopausal women in their 50s to 70s.
5. The tumors are treated surgically, including TAHBSO, but recurrences can be detected 15 to 20 years later.

■ CANCER OF THE FALLOPIAN TUBES

Pathogenesis

The cause of fallopian tube carcinoma is unknown. Most fallopian tube cancers are **adenocarcinomas** arising from the mucosa. Sarcomas and mixed tumors are less common. The disease progression of these tumors is similar to that of ovarian cancer, including wide **peritoneal spread** and ascites accumulation. The cancer is bilateral in 10% to 20% of cases and is often the result of metastasis from other primary tumors.

Epidemiology

Primary fallopian tube carcinoma is extremely rare, accounting for less than 0.5% of gynecologic malignancies. These tumors can occur at any age (18–80), but the mean age is 52.

Clinical Manifestations

The diagnosis of fallopian tube cancer is almost never made preoperatively. The disease is typically **asymptomatic** and is usually diagnosed during laparotomy for other indications. The classic triad of **pain, profuse watery discharge,** and **menorrhagia** is known as **hydrops tubae profens** and, although rare, is considered pathognomonic for fallopian tube carcinoma. Some patients may also report a history of vague lower abdominal pain.

Treatment

Treatment of fallopian tube cancer is the same as that of epithelial ovarian cancer including TAHBSO, omentectomy, and cytoreduction. Adjunctive chemotherapy includes cisplatin and cyclophosphamide. Whole-abdominal radiation is given for patients with completely resected disease. The prognosis for fallopian tube cancer is similar to that of ovarian cancer.

KEY POINTS

1. Fallopian tube cancers are rare malignancies that can occur at any age.
2. These are usually adenocarcinomas arising from the mucosa or metastases from other primary tumors.
3. Fallopian tube cancers are usually asymptomatic and are rarely diagnosed preoperatively.
4. The classic triad of pain, profuse watery discharge, and menorrhagia—known as hydrops tubae profens—is rare but considered pathognomonic for fallopian tube carcinoma.
5. These are treated with TAHBSO and adjunctive chemotherapy.
6. Prognosis is similar to that of ovarian cancer.

Gestational Trophoblastic Disease

Gestational trophoblastic disease (GTD) is a diverse group of interrelated disease processes resulting in the abnormal proliferation of trophoblastic (placental) tissue. GTD represents a spectrum of neoplasms that can be grouped into four major classifications (Table 31-1): molar pregnancies (80%), invasive moles (10% to 15%), choriocarcinomas (2% to 5%), and very rare placental site trophoblastic tumors (PSTTs). These neoplasms share the ability to produce human chorionic gonadotropin (hCG) that serves both as a tumor marker for diagnosing the disease and as a tool for measuring the effects of treatment. GTD is also extremely sensitive to chemotherapy and is therefore the most curable gynecologic malignancy.

■ BENIGN GESTATIONAL TROPHOBLASTIC DISEASE

Benign GTD is composed of molar pregnancies, also known as **hydatidiform moles**. These account for 80% of all GTD. Ninety percent of molar pregnancies are classified as "**classic**" or **complete moles** and are the result of molar degeneration but have no associated fetus. Ten percent of molar pregnancies are classified as **partial** or **incomplete moles** and are the result of molar degeneration in association with an abnormal fetus. The characteristics of complete and incomplete molar pregnancies are compared in Table 31-2.

Ninety percent of molar pregnancies are benign. The remainder may present as malignant disease in the form of invasive moles, choriocarcinoma, or PSTTs.

■ COMPLETE MOLAR PREGNANCIES

Pathogenesis

Although the cause of molar pregnancy is unknown, it is believed that most **complete moles** result from the fertilization of an enucleate ovum or "**empty egg**," one whose nucleus is missing or nonfunctional, by one normal sperm (Figure 31-1). All chromosomes are therefore **paternally derived**. The most common chromosomal pattern for complete moles is **46,XX**. Rarely, a complete mole may be formed by the fertilization of an empty egg by two normal sperm. In this case as well, all chromosomes are parentally derived.

The placental abnormality in a complete mole is characterized by trophoblastic proliferation and hydropic degeneration in the absence of fetal parts. Although most molar pregnancies are benign, complete moles have a **higher malignant potential** than do incomplete moles (see Table 31-2).

Epidemiology

The incidence of molar pregnancy is about 1 : 1000 pregnancies among white women in the United States. The global rate is highest among Asian women in the Far East where molar pregnancies occur in 1 : 200 pregnancies. There is a decreased rate of GTD in black women in the United States.

Risk Factors

GTD occurs most commonly in women under age 20 or over age 40. Higher incidences have also been found in geographic areas where the diet is low in beta-carotene and folic acid. There is also an

Classification of GTD

Benign GTD
Molar pregnancy (80% of GTD)
 Complete mole (classic mole)
 Incomplete mole (partial mole)
*Malignant GTD**
Invasive mole (10% to 15% of GTD)
Choriocarcinoma (2% to 5% of GTD)
Placental site trophoblastic tumors (PSTTs)

Note: *Malignant GTD is divided into nonmetaplastic and metastatic with good prognosis or poor prognosis.
Source: Adapted from Hacker N, Moore JG. Essentials of Obstetrics and Gynecology. Philadelphia: WB Saunders, 1998:485.

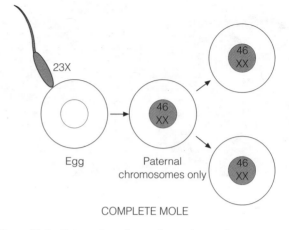

COMPLETE MOLE

Figure 31-1 • Cytogenic makeup of complete molar pregnancy. A complete mole arises from the fertilization of an empty enucleate ovum by a normal sperm. The sperm duplicates its own chromosomes, resulting in a 46XX diploid karyotype; all of the chromosomes are of paternal origin.

increased incidence among women who have had prior miscarriages or a prior history of GTD.

Clinical Manifestations

History

The most common presenting symptom of molar pregnancy is irregular or heavy **vaginal bleeding** during early pregnancy (97%). The bleeding is typically painless but may be associated with uterine contractions. Table 31-3 lists other conditions associated with complete molar pregnancy, in descending order of frequency. Due to earlier diagnosis and treatment

of molar pregnancy, these conditions are seen less often.

These conditions may contribute to medical complications associated with high beta-hCG levels including severe nausea and vomiting (from **hyperemesis gravidarum**); irritability, dizziness, and photophobia (from **preeclampsia**); or nervousness, anorexia, and tremors (from **hyperthyroidism**). In fact, preeclampsia occuring prior to 22 weeks gestation is pathoneumonic for molar pregnancy.

Comparison of Characteristics of Complete versus Incomplete Molar Pregnancies

Features	Complete/Classic Mole	Incomplete/Partial Mole
Genetics		
Most common karyotype	46,XX	69,XXY
Chromosomal origin	All paternally derived	Extra paternal set
Pathology		
Coexistent fetus	Absent	Present
Chrorionic villi	Hydropic (swollen)	Focal, viable edema
Trophoblastic hyperplasia	Diffuse, severe	Focal, minimal
Clinical presentation		
Symptoms/signs	Abnormal vaginal bleeding	Missed abortion
Uterine size	50% large for dates	Appropriate for dates
	30% small for dates	
Persistent (malignant) GTD		
Nonmetastatic	15% to 25%	3% to 4%
Metastatic	4%	0

TABLE 31-3

Symptoms Associated with Molar Pregnancy

Symptoms	Percent
Vaginal bleeding	90–97
Passage of molar vesicles	80
Discrepancy between uterine size and dates	30–50
Bilateral theca lutein cysts	15–50
Hyperemesis gravidarum	10–25
Preeclampsia before 24 weeks gestation	10–15
Hyperthyroidism	10
Trophoblastic pulmonary emboli	2

Source: Adapted from Frederickson H, Wilkins-Haug L, OB/GYN Secrets. 2nd ed. Philadelphia: Hanley and Belfus, 1997:141.

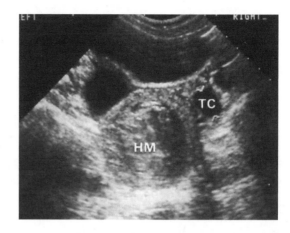

Figure 31-2 • Ultrasound scan of a hydatidiform mole (HM) with a theca lutein cyst (TC) in the ovary.
(Reproduced with permission from Chamberlain G. Lecture Notes on Obstetrics, 7th ed. Oxford: Blackwell Science, 1996.)

Physical Examination

In a complete molar pregnancy, the pelvic examination may reveal the expulsion of **grapelike molar clusters** into the vagina or blood in the cervical os. Occasionally, the physician may find large bilateral **theca lutein cysts** that result from high levels of β-hCG. The abdominal examination in molar pregnancy may be remarkable for the absence of fetal heart sounds and size/date discrepancies. Similarly, the physical examination may show sequelae of preeclampsia or hyperthyroidism, including tachycardia, tachypnea, and hypertension.

Diagnostic Evaluation

In the presence of a molar pregnancy, quantitative serum **β-hCG** levels can be extremely high (>100,000 mIU/mL), relative to values for normal pregnancy. Confirmation of GTD is usually made using pelvic ultrasound (US) that reveals a **"snowstorm" pattern** (due to swelling of chorionic villi). In the case of a complete mole, no fetus is present in the uterus (Figure 31-2).

Differential Diagnosis

The differential diagnosis for gestational trophoblastic neoplasia includes conditions that can result in abnormally high β-hCG levels and/or enlarged placentas such as multiple gestation pregnancy, erythroblastosis fetalis, intrauterine infection, fibroids, threatened abortion, ectopic pregnancy, or normal intrauterine pregnancy.

Treatment

The treatment for molar pregnancy, regardless of the duration of pregnancy, is **immediate removal of the uterine contents**. If fertility preservation is important to the patient, treatment includes dilation and suction evacuation (D&E) followed by gentle scraping with a sharp curet. After the uterine contents have been removed, intravenous oxytocin can be administered to stimulate uterine contraction and minimize blood loss. If the patient with a molar pregnancy has completed childbearing, **hysterectomy** is an alternate therapy. The risk of recurrent disease remains 3% to 5%—even after hysterectomy.

Follow-Up

The prognosis for molar pregnancy is excellent, with 95% to 100% cure rates. Persistent disease will develop in 15% to 25% of patients with complete moles and in 4% of patients with incomplete moles. For this reason, close follow-up is essential.

After evacuation of a molar pregnancy, **serial β-hCG titers** should be monitored using radioimmunoassay weekly until three consecutive negative results. The levels should then be followed monthly until normal for at least 1 year. Figure 31-3 demonstrates the normal regression of β-hCG titers after molar evacuation. Because accurate monitoring depends on the ability to accurately follow β-hCG levels, it is essential to **prevent pregnancy** during the follow-up period.

Patients who are cured of the disease can have normal pregnancies after treatment with no increase in the rate of spontaneous abortion, complications, or congenital malformations. The risk of developing GTD in subsequent pregnancies is less than 5% for women with a history of GTD.

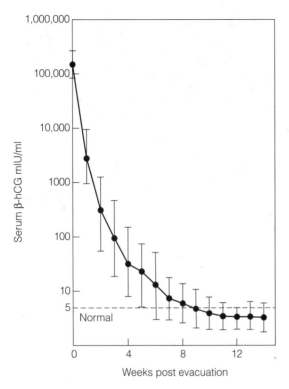

Figure 31-3 • Normal regression of β-hCG levels after molar evacuation.

KEY POINTS

1. Ninety percent of molar pregnancies are complete moles and are the result of the fertilization of an empty ovum by one sperm.
2. The most common karyotype is 46,XX.
3. There is no associated fetus and patients usually present with irregular vaginal bleeding or passage of vesicles.
4. Complete molar pregnancy can also include symptoms resulting from hyperemesis gravidarum, preeclampsia, or hyperthyroidism.
5. Complete molar pregnancy is diagnosed by β-hCG levels and pelvic ultrasound showing a "snowstorm" pattern.
6. It is treated with immediate suction evacuation of the uterus and gentle curettage.
7. Complete molar pregnancy requires close follow-up with weekly and then monthly β-hCG levels for 1 year with concurrent reliable contraception to prevent pregnancy.
8. Complete molar pregnancy results in persistent malignant disease in 15% to 25% of cases and has a risk of recurrence of <5%.

■ INCOMPLETE MOLAR PREGNANCY

Pathogenesis

An **incomplete** or **partial mole** is formed when a normal ovum is fertilized by two sperm simultaneously (Figure 31-4). This results in a triploid karyotype with 69 chromosomes, of which two sets are paternally derived. The most common karyotype is **69,XXY** (80%). The placental abnormality in an incomplete mole is characterized by focal hydropic villi and trophoblastic hyperplasia of the syncytial layer.

Incomplete moles often appear with a **coexistent fetus** with a triploid genotype and multiple anomalies. Most fetuses associated with incomplete moles only survive several weeks **in utero** before being spontaneously aborted in the late first or early second trimester. Incomplete moles are almost always benign and have a much **lower malignancy potential** than complete moles.

Clinical Manifestations

History

Incomplete molar pregnancy often presents with **delayed menses** and a **pregnancy diagnosis**. Ninety percent of patients with incomplete moles present with **miscarriage** or missed abortions. As a result, incomplete moles may be diagnosed somewhat later than complete molar pregnancies. Diagnosis is often made on pathologic examination of the products of conception. Patients with incomplete moles may have similar but **much less severe symptoms** than those with complete molar pregnancy.

Physical Examination

In incomplete molar pregnancy, the physical examination is typically normal except for the absence of fetal heart sounds.

Treatment

Treatment is **immediate removal of the uterine contents**. Less than 4% of patients with incomplete moles will develop persistent malignant disease.

Follow-Up

Meticulous follow-up with serial β-hCG levels as described in the previous section on complete molar pregnancy is critical to treatment of this disease. Reliable contraception is also important to prevent

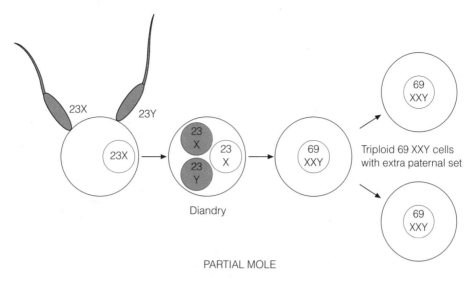

Figure 31-4 • Cytogenetic makeup of incomplete molar pregnancy. An incomplete mole arises from the simultaneous fertilization of a normal ovum by two sperm (diandry). The resulting triploid karyotype is most commonly 69, XXY.

PARTIAL MOLE

Diandry

Triploid 69 XXY cells with extra paternal set

pregnancy and allow accurate β-hCG levels of measurement.

KEY POINTS

1. Incomplete moles account for 10% of molar pregnancies and result from the simultaneous fertilization of a normal ovum by two sperm.
2. These most commonly have a 69,XXY karyotype.
3. Incomplete moles are composed of molar degeneration and have a coexistent abnormal fetus.
4. Patients usually present with spontaneous or missed abortions.
5. Incomplete moles are diagnosed by β-hCG levels and pelvic ultrasound.
6. These moles are treated with immediate suction evacuation of the uterus and gentle curettage.
7. Persistent malignant disease develops in only 4% of cases.
8. Incomplete moles require close follow-up with weekly and then monthly β-hCG levels for 1 year with concurrent reliable contraception to prevent pregnancy.

■ MALIGNANT GESTATIONAL TROPHOBLASTIC DISEASE (GTD)

Pathogenesis

Molar pregnancies are typically benign and make up 90% of all gestational trophoblastic disease; however, 10% of patients with GTD are diagnosed with a persistant (malignant) form of the disease. Malignant GTD is divided into three histologic types: **invasive moles**, **choriocarcinoma** and **PSTT**. In 50% of cases, malignant GTD occurs months to years after a molar pregnancy. Another 25% occur after an antecedent normal pregnancy, and 25% after a miscarriage, ectopic pregnancy, or abortion.

For the purpose of treatment and prognosis, malignant GTD (invasive moles, choriocarcinoma, PSTT) can be classified as **nonmetastatic** if there is no disease spread beyond the uterus or **metastatic** if the disease has progressed beyond the uterus. Metastatic disease can further be classified as **good prognosis** or **poor prognosis** depending on factors such as length of time since antecedent pregnancy, β-hCG level, presence of brain or liver metastases, the type of antecedent pregnancy, and the result of prior chemotherapy trials (Figure 31-5).

The staging for gestational trophoblastic neoplasia is shown in Table 31-4. This system has not been found to be clinically useful because it does not account for important prognostic factors such as degree of metastasis, type of antecedent pregnancy,

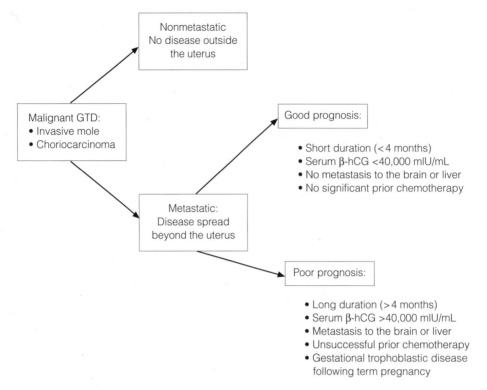

Figure 31-5 • Classification of malignant GTD.

TABLE 31-4

Staging of Gestational Trophoblastic Tumors

Stage	Extent of Disease*
I	Confined to the uterine corpus
II	Metastases to the pelvis or vagina
III	Metastases to the lung
IV	Distant metastases

Note: *Metastasis sites in order of frequency are lung, vagina, pelvis, brain, and liver.
Source: Adapted from Frederickson H, Wilkins-Haug L. OB/GYN Secrets. 2nd ed. Philadelphia: Hanley & Belfus, 1997:143.

or duration of disease. In the United States, the World Health Organization (WHO) and National Institutes of Health (NIH) have devised systems that incorporate these prognostic factors and better reflect disease outcome. Table 31-5 shows the WHO system.

Clinical Manifestations

Although the three forms of malignant GTD are histologically different, **clinical presentation** has shown to have more prognostic value than histology. GTD occurring after a molar pregnancy is typically diagnosed by plateauing or rising beta-hCG levels during monitoring following the evacuation of the molar pregnancy. Unlike other forms of malignant GTD, PSTTs more characteristically have chronically low levels of β-hCG. Women with β-hCG levels >100,000 mIU/ml, excessive uterine size for dates, and prominent theca lutein cysts are at the highest risk of malignant GTD.

Women with malignant GTD that follows other types of antecedent pregnancies (normal, miscarriage, ectopic, or abortion) can have a variety of subtle presenting symptoms making diagnosis very difficult. The one exception is choriocarcinoma, which tends to present with signs or symptoms of metastatic disease. Even in that case, the symptoms may mimic any number of disease processes and diagnosis is often delayed.

Treatment

One distinguishing feature of malignant GTD is its **extreme sensitivity to chemotherapy**. The treatment

TABLE 31-5

WHO Scoring System Based on Prognostic Factor for GTD*

Risk Factor	Score			
	0	1	2	4
Age (y)	≤39	≥39		
Antecedent pregnancy	Hydatidiform mole		Abortion	Term
Pregnancy event to treatment interval (mo)	<4	4–6	7–12	>12
Human chorionic gonadotropin (IU/L)	<10³	10³–10⁴	10⁴–10⁵	>10⁵
ABO blood groups (female × male)		O × A	B	
			A × O	AB
No. of metastases		1–4	4–8	>8
Site metastases		Spleen	Gastrointestinal tract	Brain
		Kidney	Liver	
Largest tumor mass, including uterine (cm)		3–5	>5	
Prior chemotherapy drugs			Single drug	Two or more

Note: *The total score for a patient is obtained by adding the individual scores for each prognostic factor.
Total score: ≤4 = low risk; 5–7 = middle risk; ≥8 = high risk.
Source: World Health Organization Scientific Group. Gestational Trophoblastic Disease. Technical Report Series 692. Geneva: WHO, 1983.

for nonmetastatic disease is single-agent chemotherapy, usually **methotrexate** or **actinomycin-D**. Good prognosis metastatic GTD is typically treated with single-agent chemotherapy, whereas poor prognosis malignant GTD is treated with a multiagent regimen (MAC: methotrexate, actinomycin-D, chlorambucil). With chemotherapy, the cure rate for metastatic malignant disease is 95% to 100% for good prognosis disease, and 50% to 70% for poor prognosis disease.

Surgery does not generally play a role in the treatment of malignant GTD except for PSTT, which is not sensitive to chemotherapy and is treated with hysterectomy. Radiation is usually reserved for treating brain and liver metastases.

Follow-Up

As with other forms of GTD, careful follow-up with serial β-hCG levels as described is critical to the management of malignant GTD. Likewise, reliable contraception is critical in order to maintain accurate measurement of β-hCG levels.

■ INVASIVE MOLES

Pathogenesis

Invasive moles may result from a **malignant transformation** of a persistence of benign disease (75%), or **recurrence** of GTD (25%). With invasive moles, the molar villi and trophoblasts penetrate locally into the myometrium, sometimes reaching through to the peritoneal cavity. Despite this, invasive moles **rarely metastasize**.

Epidemiology

Invasive moles have an overall incidence of 1 : 15,000 pregnancies.

Clinical Manifestations

History

Most patients with invasive moles are identified as a result of plateauing or rising β-hCG after treatment for a molar pregnancy.

Physical Examination

The physical examination in patients with invasive moles is similar to that for molar pregnancy.

Diagnostic Evaluation

The work-up for invasive moles is similar to that for benign disease including serial quantitative β-hCG levels and pelvic ultrasound.

Treatment

Invasive moles are typically nonmetastatic and respond well to single-agent chemotherapy with methotrexate (with or without folinic acid rescue) or actinomycin-D.

Follow-Up

As with other forms of GTD, careful follow-up with serial β-hCG levels as described is critical to the management of invasive molar pregnancies. Likewise, reliable contraception is critical in order to maintain accurate measurement of β-hCG levels.

KEY POINTS

1. Invasive moles can result from persistent molar pregnancy (75%) or from recurrent GTD (25%).
2. Diagnosis of invasive mole is usually made by detecting plateauing or rising β-hCG levels after molar evacuation.
3. These moles have an overall incidence of 1:15,000 normal pregnancies.
4. Invasive moles contain molar villi and trophoblasts that can penetrate into and through the myometrium.
5. These moles are generally not metastatic and respond well to single-agent chemotherapy (95% to 100% cure rate).

■ CHORIOCARCINOMA

Pathogenesis

Choriocarcinoma is a **malignant necrotizing tumor** that can arise from trophoblastic tissue weeks to years after **any type of gestation**. Although 50% of patients who develop choriocarcinoma have had a preceding molar pregnancy, 25% develop the disease after a normal-term pregnancy and 25% after miscarriage, abortion, or ectopic pregnancy.

Choriocarcinoma invades the uterine wall and venous channels with trophoblastic cells, causing destruction of uterine tissue, necrosis, and hemorrhage. The characteristic histologic pattern of gestational choriocarcinoma includes sheets of anaplastic cytotrophoblasts and syncytiotrophoblasts in the absence of chorionic villi. This tumor is **often metastatic** and usually **spreads hematogenously** to the lungs, vagina, pelvis, brain, liver, intestines, and kidneys.

Epidemiology

Choriocarcinoma is very rare in the United States where its incidence is only 1:40,000 pregnancies, but may be as high as 1:114 in parts of Asia.

Clinical Manifestations

History

Patients with choriocarcinoma, unlike those with invasive moles, often present with symptoms of **metastatic disease**. Vaginal metastases may cause vaginal bleeding, whereas metastases to the lungs may cause hemoptysis, cough, or dyspnea. Central nervous system (CNS) lesions may cause headaches, dizziness, blackouts, or other symptoms common to space-occupying lesions.

Physical Examination

Patients with choriocarcinoma often have signs of metastatic disease, including uterine enlargement, vaginal mass, and neurologic signs from CNS involvement.

Diagnostic Evaluation

As with other forms of GTD, the primary work-up for choriocarcinoma includes measurement of quantitative β-hCG levels and pelvic ultrasound. However, given the likelihood of metastasis, diagnostic assessment for choriocarcinoma should include a thorough evaluation of metastatic disease in the lungs, liver, kidneys, spleen, and brain.

Differential Diagnosis

Choriocarcinoma has been found to metastasize to virtually every tissue in the body. It is known as **the** great imitator because its signs and symptoms are similar to those of many disease entities. Also, given that choriocarcinoma can occur from weeks to years after any type of gestation and is relatively rare, the diagnosis is often delayed when the disease occurs outside the context of a prior molar pregnancy.

Treatment

Treatment of choriocarcinoma mirrors that of invasive moles. Nonmetastatic and good prognosis metastatic disease are treated with single-agent chemotherapy, whereas poor prognosis metastatic choriocarcinoma is treated with multiagent chemotherapy. The cure rate for good prognosis disease is 95% to 100%, and for poor prognosis disease cure rate is 50% to 70%.

Follow-Up

Again, as with all other forms of GTD, choriocarcinoma requires close monitoring of β-hCG levels over time in conjunction with reliable contraception.

> ### KEY POINTS
>
> 1. Choriocarcinoma is a rare form of GTD with an overall incidence of 1:40,000 pregnancies.
> 2. It is a malignant, necrotizing tumor that can occur weeks to years after any type of gestation.
> 3. Patients present with signs and symptoms of metastases to the lungs, vagina, liver, brain, or kidneys.
> 4. Choriocarcinoma is diagnosed by pelvic ultrasound, serial b-hCG levels, and a thorough workup for metastatic disease.
> 5. It is treated with single- or multiagent chemotherapy depending on the presence of disease outside the uterus and on the disease prognosis category.
> 6. The cure rate for good prognosis disease is 95% to 100%; the cure rate for poor prognosis disease is 50% to 70%.

■ PLACENTAL SITE TROPHOBLASTIC TUMORS (PSTTs)

PSTTs are extremely rare tumors that arise from the placental implantation site. The cells from placental site tumors infiltrate through the myometrium and grow between its smooth muscle cells and then invade the myometrium and blood vessels. Histologically, these tumors are characterized by the absence of villi and the proliferation of cytotrophoblasts.

Bleeding is the most common symptom of PSTT and may occur weeks to years after an antecedent pregnancy. Unlike other forms of GTD, these tumors produce chronic low levels of β-hCG and human placental lactogen. They are also generally not sensitive to chemotherapy but, fortunately, they rarely metastasize beyond the uterus. Therefore, hysterectomy is the treatment of choice for PSTT.

> ### KEY POINTS
>
> 1. PSTTs are extremely rare and arise from the placental implantation site.
> 2. These tumors are characterized by the absence of villi and the proliferation of cytotrophoblasts.
> 3. PSTTs spread by invasion into the myometrium and blood vessels.
> 4. Patients most commonly present with vaginal bleeding and persistently low levels of β-hCG.
> 5. PSTTs are not sensitive to chemotherapy, so they are treated by hysterectomy.

Breast cancer is the most common malignancy in women in the United States, representing approximately 32% of female cancers. It is also the second most common cause of cancer deaths in women (after lung cancer deaths), accounting for some 44,000 deaths per year. A woman has a 1:8 chance of having breast cancer in her lifetime. Yet, despite its incidence, the cause of breast cancer still remains unknown.

In addition to breast cancer, as many as 50% of women will have benign breast lesions over their lifetime. Therefore, understanding the range of benign and malignant breast lesions and their symptoms is enormously important. Obstetrician-gynecologists, primary care physicians, and surgeons perform the evaluation of breast masses, discharge, or pain as well as screen for breast cancer. The anatomy and physiology of the breast as well as how to diagnose and treat these lesions should be understood by all physicians involved in the care of women.

ANATOMY

Breast tissue extends from the second to the sixth rib vertically. Medically, it extends to the lateral margin of the sternum, and to the mid-axillary line as the lateral border. The axillary tail of Spence extends into the axilla. Breast parenchyma is divided into segments containing **mammary glands** that consist of 20 to 40 lobules drained by **lactiferous ducts** that open individually into the nipple. Fibrous bands spanning between two fascia layers—called **Cooper's suspensory ligaments**—support the breast. The breast is divided into four quadrants for ease of description: upper outer quadrant (UOQ), lower outer quadrant (LOQ), upper inner quadrant (UIQ), and lower inner quadrant (LIQ) (Figure 32-1). The major blood supply to the breast are the **internal mammary** and the **lateral thoracic arteries**. The medial and central aspects are supplied by the anterior perforators of the internal mammary artery and the UOQ is supplied by the lateral thoracic.

The **axillary lymph nodes** drain up to 97% of the ipsilateral breast, and secondarily drain the supraclavicular and jugular nodes. These nodes are subdivided into three levels for the purposes of specifying disease progression. Level I lymph nodes lie lateral to the pectoralis minor; level II lymph nodes lie deep to the pectoralis minor muscle; level III lymph nodes lie medial to the pectoralis minor. The internal mammary nodes are responsible for 3% of drainage, mainly of the UIQ and LIQ. The interpectoral nodes (Rotter's) lie between the pectoralis major and pectoralis minor muscles.

The **innervation** of the breast requires careful attention during surgical dissection. Nerves at risk include the intercostobrachial nerve that transverses the axilla to supply sensation to the upper medial arm; the long thoracic nerve (of Bell) of C5, C6, and C7 that innervates the serratus anterior muscle, injury of which can lead to the "winged" scapula; the thoracodorsal nerve that innervates the latissimus dorsi muscle; and the lateral pectoral nerve that innervates the pectoralis major and minor muscles.

PHYSIOLOGY

Breast development is classified into **Tanner stages 1–5** (see Chapter 20). The breast responds to cyclic hormones, as well as to changes during pregnancy and menopause. **Estrogen** promotes ductal development and fat deposition. **Progesterones** promote the lobular-alveolar development that makes lactation possible. **Prolactin** is involved in milk production,

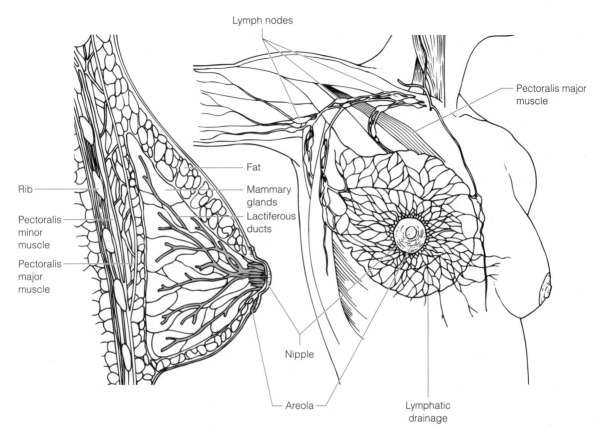

Figure 32-1 • Anatomy of the female breast.

whereas **oxytocin** from the posterior pituitary causes milk letdown. In postmenopausal women, the decreased estrogenic state is associated with tissue atrophy, loss of stroma, and replacement of atrophied lobules with fatty tissue.

■ EVALUATION OF THE BREAST

Routine Evaluation

Routine **monthly self-examination** and **yearly physician evaluation** are recommended for all women over age 20. Self-examination should be performed approximately 5 days after menses when the breast is least engorged and tender. Physical examination involves careful inspection of the skin for contour or color changes with the patient in upright and supine positions. This is followed by palpation for lymphadenopathy, masses, nipple discharge, or pain. The self-breast exam should be reviewed at each annual gynecology visit. Patients are often motivated by the fact that the majority of breast masses are found by patients or their partners.

In addition to physician and self-breast exams, the third part of routine breast care is the **screening mammography**. Current mammography screening guidelines by the American Cancer Society include a mammogram every 1 to 2 years between the age 40 to 50 and a mammogram annually after age 50. Women with a strong family history of breast cancer should begin mammogram screen five years earlier than the age at which the youngest family member was when diagnosed with breast cancer.

Evaluation of the Breast Masses

If a patient is found to have a **breast mass** on the physician's exam or her own self-exam, a thorough history and exam are crucial. When evaluating a breast mass, important information includes the timing, the manner in which it was discovered, associated tenderness, and the relationship of changes to the menstrual cycle.

If a mass is identified, its location, size, shape, consistency, and mobility should be noted, as well as any associated tenderness or skin change. Worrisome lumps are dominant, discrete, and dense. Carcinomatous lumps are usually firm, nontender, poorly circumscribed, and immobile. Lymph nodes are worrisome if larger than 1 cm, fixed, irregular, firm, or multiple.

Abnormal breast masses should be evaluated radiographically. **Mammogram findings** that may indicate malignancy include a spiculated mass; architectural distortion with retraction; asymmetric localized fibrosis; microcalcifications with linear, branched patterns; increased vascularity; or altered subareolar duct pattern. **Ultrasound** is useful to assess whether a mass greater than 0.5 cm is solid or cystic.

If a concerning breast mass is seen on radiologic study or palpated, it should be biopsied for **pathologic diagnosis**. One method of obtaining cells for diagnosis is **needle aspiration** for palpable cystic lesions. The fluid is sent for cytology if it is turbid or bloody. **Fine-needle aspiration** (FNA) biopsy is used to sample a palpable solid mass. This is performed by making multiple passes through the mass from different angles while aspirating the syringe on a 20 to 22-gauge needle. Diagnostic accuracy approaches 80% to 90%.

Excisional biopsy is performed if the FNA does not obtain fluid or tissue or if the mass turns out to be solid. The mass should also be excised if the fluid is bloody, the mass persists after fluid is removed, the mass is persistent after two aspirations, or fluid reaccumulates within 2 weeks. Excisional biopsy is also performed if cytology is nondiagnostic. Excisional biopsy can also performed under needle or wire guidance when a nonpalpable lesion is found by mammography. The mass should be excised with 1 cm rim of normal tissue to qualify for "lumpectomy," thus avoiding the need for repeat surgery if the mass is malignant.

Evaluation of Nipple Discharge

When a patient presents with **nipple discharge**, it is important to find out the nature of any nipple discharge: whether it is bilateral, the number of duct openings involved, and how the discharge is related to stimulation or masses. The vast majority of discharge has a benign etiology; however, any concerning discharge should be sent to cytology. **Bloody discharge** is associated with intraductal papilloma or invasive papillary cancer. **Galactorrhea** is associated

with pregnancy, pituitary adenoma, acromegaly, hypothyroidism, stress, and medications such as oral contraceptive pills (OCPs), antihypertensives, and psychotropic drugs. **Serous discharge** is associated with normal menses, OCPs, fibrocystic change, or early pregnancy. **Yellow-tinged discharge** is associated with fibrocystic change or galactocele. **Green, sticky discharge** is associated with duct ectasia. **Purulent discharge** indicates superficial or central breast abscess.

Evaluation of Breast Pain

Breast pain (mastodynia, mastalgia) is a common complaint that is rarely a symptom of breast cancer. It can be a component of premenstrual syndrome (PMS), associated with hormone replacement therapy (HRT), or caused by menstrual irregularities or fibrocystic change. The patient's medical history, including benign or malignant diseases of the breast, is relevant. Any history of radiation or surgery to the breast, oophorectomy, adrenalectomy, family history of breast disease, and constitutional symptoms such as weight loss or gain, chest wall pain, or amenorrhea are relevant.

KEY POINTS

1. Breast cancer is the most common neoplasm in women, occurring in 1:8 women in the United States.
2. Routine monthly self-examination and annual physician evaluation are recommended for all women over age 20.
3. Current routine mammogram recommendations include a mammogram every 1 to 2 years from age 40 to 50, and yearly after age 50.
3. Evaluation of breast masses include careful physical exam, evaluation with mammography and ultrasound of any abnormal findings, and biopsy of suspicious findings to rule out malignancy.
4. Knowledge of anatomy of the breast is crucial for surgical treatment.

■ BENIGN BREAST DISEASE

Benign breast symptoms and findings are common and occur in approximately 50% of women, with a higher incidence in younger women. The decision to biopsy any abnormal breast findings for definitive diagnosis is influenced by the patient's risk factors for malignant disease. Two-thirds of tumors in reproductive-age women are benign, whereas half of palpable masses in perimenopausal women and the majority of lesions in postmenopausal women are malignant.

Fibrocystic Disease

Epidemiology

Fibrocystic change of the breast includes a spectrum of clinical findings due to exaggerated stromal response to hormones and growth factors. It can include cystic change, nodularity, stromal proliferation, and epithelial hyperplasia. In the absence of atypical hyperplasia, **fibrocystic change is not associated with increased cancer risk**. Peak incidence is between age 32 to 40, but changes can persist throughout a woman's entire life.

Diagnosis

Patients with fibrocystic disease present with breast swelling, pain, and tenderness. Fibrocystic disease may have more focal symptomatic areas, involve both breasts, and vary throughout the menstrual cycle. Evaluation with mammogram and/or ultrasound should be performed for suspicious lesions.

Treatment

Often, symptoms of fibrocystic breast disease are ameliorated with **reduction of nicotine** and **caffeine**. High doses of **vitamin E** (600 IU per day for 8 weeks) and the use of Primrose oil have been found to improve symptoms in many patients. **Progestins** such as norethynodrel and norethindrone acetate have also had some success in relieving symptoms. If symptoms persist and are severe, the androgen **danazol**, 200–400 mg a day for 4 to 6 months, can be used. Side effects include amenorrhea, weight gain, hirsutism, voice deepening, acne, and liver dysfunction. Another possible treatment for severe symptoms is **tamoxifen**, 10–20 mg once a day on cycle days 5 through 25 for 4 months. Its anti-estrogenic affect is mediated through binding estrogen receptors. The use of **bromocriptine** is currently being studied.

Fibroadenoma

Epidemiology

Breast fibroadenomas are benign tumors with epithelial and stromal components. They are the most common breast lesions found in women under age 32.

Diagnosis

Fibroadenomas are often palpated on physical examination as round, well-circumscribed, mobile firm lesions that are rubbery and nontender. Most masses are 1–5 cm in diameter at the time of detection. Lesions larger than 5 cm are termed giant fibroadenomas and need to be ruled out as cystosarcoma phyllodes. These are usually solitary but can be multiple, and occur bilaterally up to 25% of the time. These lesions often change during the menstrual cycle, pregnancy, and with OCP use.

Treatment

A young patient with classic presentation of a fibroadenoma and no family history of breast cancer can be followed clinically if stable. Otherwise, FNA for cytology is highly sensitive for detecting cancer or phyllodes tumors. If the fibroadenoma is large or worrisome, excisional biopsy is recommended to remove the tumor and establish pathologic diagnosis.

Cystosarcoma Phyllodes

Epidemiology

Phyllodes tumors are a rare variant of fibroadenoma and involve epithelial and stromal proliferation. It is diagnosed most commonly in premenopausal women, although it can occur at any age.

Diagnosis

This lesion appears as a large, bulky, mobile mass. The overlying skin is warm, erythematous, shiny, and engorged. The mass is **large** (4–5 cm), smooth, and well-circumscribed, and is characterized by **rapid growth**. Most lesions are benign; however, some physicians consider cystosarcoma phyllodes a low-grade malignancy and a few tumors do develop true sarcomatous potential. These tumors are worrisome for aggressive malignancies; pathologic diagnosis must therefore be made.

Treatment

The clinical course of these tumors is unpredictable as most appear benign, but 10% do contain malignant cells. There is also a high rate of local recurrence after simple excision. Recommended therapy is therefore **wide local excision** with a 1-cm margin for small tumors and simple mastectomy for large lesions.

Intraductal Papilloma

Epidemiology

Intraductal papilloma is a benign solitary lesion that involves the epithelial lining of lactiferous ducts. It is the most common cause of **bloody nipple discharge** in the absence of a concurrent mass.

Diagnosis

Intraductal papilloma usually appears with bloody nipple discharge in premenopausal women. The serosanguinous discharge is sent for cytology to rule out invasive papillary carcinoma, which has similar symptoms 20% to 32% of the time. To identify the papilloma, the physician can open the involved duct to visualize the tumor.

Treatment

Definitive diagnosis and treatment is by excision of the involved ducts after localization by physical examination. Intraductal papillomas rarely undergo malignant transformation.

Mammary Duct Ectasia (Plasma Cell Mastitis)

Epidemiology

This subacute inflammation of the ductal system causes dilated mammary ducts. There is infiltration of plasma cells and significant periductal inflammation. This lesion most commonly occurs **at** or **after menopause**.

Diagnosis

Patients present with nipple discharge, noncyclic breast pain, nipple retraction, or subareolar masses. The discharge is multicolored, sticky, originating from multiple ducts, and often bilateral. The patient should have a mammogram, and excisional biopsy is indicated to rule out carcinoma.

Treatment

Definitive treatment is local excision of the inflamed area, occasionally requiring extensive subareolar duct excision.

KEY POINTS

1. Benign breast symptoms and findings are common and occur in approximately 50% of women, with a higher incidence in younger women.
2. Two-thirds of tumors in reproductive-age women are benign, whereas half of palpable masses in perimenopausal and the majority of lesions in postmenopausal women are malignant.
3. The decision to biopsy any abnormal breast findings for definitive diagnosis is influenced by the woman's risk factors for malignant disease.
4. The most common benign breast diseases are fibrocystic disease and fibroadenomas.

■ MALIGNANT BREAST DISEASE

Epidemiology

Breast cancer is the most common nonskin malignancy affecting women in the United States. One in every eight American women will develop this disease during her lifetime and will have a 3.5% chance of dying from it. It accounts for 28% of all cancers in women and 18% of women's cancer deaths.

The risk of getting breast cancer increases with age. Four out of every five women with breast cancer are over age 50. While the incidence of diagnosis is increasing, the death rate is decreasing, likely due to earlier detection and improved therapies. Currently, breast cancer is the leading cause of death in U.S. women age 40 to 55.

Risk Factors

Numerous risk factors are associated with breast cancer (Table 32-1). One major risk factor is **increasing age**. For example, an American woman's annual risk increases from 1:5900 at age 32 to 1:290 by age 80. A **personal history of breast cancer** increases the risk of disease in the contralateral breast by a factor of 5. Exposure to **ionizing radiation** before age 32 and alcohol abuse can significantly increase the risk of breast cancer. Diagnosis of atypical **ductal** or **lobular hyperplasia** on biopsy increases risk by a factor of 5. The presence of ductal or lobular carcinoma in situ, noninvasive carcinomas, also increases cancer risk.

■ TABLE 32-1

Breast Cancer Risk Factors

Breast Cancer Risk Factors	Relative Risk
Sex	99% in women
Age	85% over age 40
Proliferative fibrocystic change	2–5:1
Previous breast cancer, 1 breast	5:1
Nulliparous versus parous	3:1
First birth after age 34	4:1
Menarche before age 12	1.3:1
Menopause after age 50	1.5:1
Affluent versus poor	2:1
Jewish versus non-Jewish	2:1
Western hemisphere	1.5:1
Cold climate versus warm climate	1.5:1
Chronic psychologic stress	2:1
Obesity	2:1
Obesity, hypertension, diabetes	3:1
High dietary fat	3:1
White versus Asian	5:1
Second-degree relative	1.5:1
First-degree relative	
Unilateral premenopausal	1.8:1
Bilateral premenopausal	8.8:1
Unilateral postmenopausal	1.2:1
Bilateral postmenopausal	4.0:1

Source: Adapted from DiSaia PJ, Creasman WT. Clinical Gynecologic Oncology, 5th ed. St Louis: Mosby-Yearbook, 1997:403.

A **family history** of gynecologic malignancies also significantly increases the risk. Having a first-degree relative with breast cancer increases a woman's risk greatly depending on the number of affected relatives, their age at diagnosis, and the bilaterality of their disease. A strong family history is suspicious for a **genetic predisposition**, which contributes to an estimated **5% of breast cancers**. Six familial syndromes have been identified with an increased risk of breast cancer. The best known of these are the BRCA1 and BRCA2 genes are associated with bilateral premenopausal breast cancer and breast cancer associated with ovarian cancer.

Between 0.5% and 4.0% of breast cancer is diagnosed surrounding pregnancy or lactation. Compared to nonpregnant women with breast cancer at similar stage and age, **survival rates seem equivalent** for women with breast cancer.

The question of whether or not **postmenopausal HRT** changes the risk of breast cancer is still debated. Some physicians suggest that estrogen replacement given with progesterone may actually decrease a woman's risk of breast cancer, just as it does the risk of endometrial cancer. The theory is that unopposed endogenous estrogens provide a favorable environment for breast cancer development. This is consistent with the epidemiologic finding that nulligravida, polycystic ovarian disease, early menarche (before age 12), and late menopause (after age 55) patients are also at higher risk. On the other hand, evidence from meta-analyses suggests that patients who use HRT for more than 5 years may be at *increased* relative risk of developing breast cancer. Interestingly, in these studies, HRT users diagnosed with cancer had earlier stage disease at diagnosis and much better prognoses. Studies of **OCP exposure reveal no increased risk** of breast cancer.

Prevention

Early pregnancy, prolonged lactation, chemical or surgical sterilization, exercise, abstinence from alcohol, and a low-fat diet may help prevent breast cancer. Increasing evidence suggests that tamoxifen may be effective in suppressing the development of breast cancer. By binding to the estrogen receptor, **tamoxifen competively inhibits estrogen binding** and maintains inhibition of breast cancer cells. Tamoxifen is currently used widely in patients with early stage, surgically treated breast cancer and has been shown to decrease contralateral breast cancer by 40%.

Diagnosis

The trifeca of routine breast care is the monthly **self-breast exam**, the annual **clinician breast exam**, and annual **mammography** for women over age 40 or those who are at high risk for breast cancer.

Patients may present clinically with **breast masses**, **skin change**, **nipple discharge**, or symptoms of metastatic disease. Skin dimpling can occur due to tethering of Cooper ligaments from the mass underneath. The skin can appear erythematous and warm, with nipple retraction or inversion. Tissue edema or a **"peau d'orange"** appearance may occur due to dermal lymphatic invasion and blockage. The superficial epidermis of the nipple may appear eczematous or ulcerated, as in Paget's disease.

Bloody discharge needs to be evaluated to rule out invasive papillary carcinoma. Palpable masses are often detected by the patient or partner on self-exam and are usually nontender, irregular, firm, and immobile. **Fifty percent of tumors occur in the UOQ** (Figure 32-2). These tumors can be multifocal, multicentric, or bilateral. Mammography is the best tool to detect early lesions, reducing mortality by 32% to 50%. Recent studies have shown that mammography is less effective in women with dense breast tissue; for example, in African American women.

A nonpalpable suspicious lesion found on mammogram requires **localized needle biopsy** or **stereotactic FNA** for pathologic diagnosis.

The evaluation for metastatic disease with a thorough history, physical, and imaging is also an important part of breast disease management. Breast cancer tends to metastasize to the **bone, liver, lung, pleura, brain,** and **lymph nodes.** Patients may present with constitutional symptoms of weight loss, anorexia, and fatigue. They may have symptoms of dyspnea, cough, and bony pains.

Noninvasive Disease

Ductal Carcinoma In Situ (DCIS)

Epidemiology
DCIS—also called intraductal carcinoma—involves proliferation of malignant epithelial cells contained within mammary ducts (Figure 32-3). It is more common than lobular carcinoma in situ, and is considered a **premalignant lesion**. Average age at diagnosis is mid 50s.

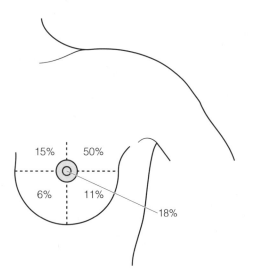

Figure 32-2 • Relative location of malignant lesions of the breast.

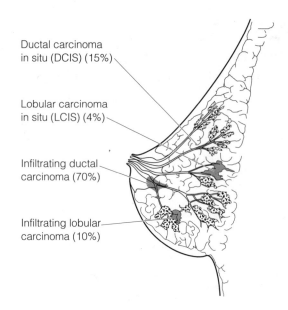

Figure 32-3 • Subtypes of breast cancer. DCIS is believed to be a precursor to invasive ductal carcinoma; LCIS is, in contrast, more akin to atypical hyperplasia and carries a risk of future ductal or invasive lobular carcinoma anywhere in the breast.

Diagnosis
Eighty percent of DCIS are detected by screening mammography revealing clustered microcalcifications. It can occasionally be palpated. Diagnosis can be established by needle localization biopsy or excisional biopsy of a palpable lesion. Thirty-five percent of lesions are multicentric; bilateral disease is rare.

Treatment
The risk of subsequent invasive ductal carcinoma or local recurrence of intraductal carcinoma is approximately 5% per year. Of recurrent disease, 50% will be DCIS; the other 50% will be invasive carcinoma. Current treatment is therefore conservative surgical **excision of all microcalcifications with wide margins.** Simple mastectomy is occasionally necessary for extensive lesions.

Lobular Carcinoma In Situ (LCIS)

Epidemiology
LCIS is the proliferation of malignant epithelial cells contained within breast lobules (Figure 32-3). The average age at diagnosis is the mid 40s and patients tend to be premenopausal.

Diagnosis
LCIS is usually diagnosed incidentally on biopsy for another finding as it is **not palpable** and **not seen on**

mammograms. It is usually multicentric and is bilateral 50% to 90% of the time. There is a 20% risk of subsequent invasive ipsilateral and contralateral breast carcinoma.

Treatment

Therapy is usually by local excision. There is a 1% risk of recurrent disease, which may be intraductal, invasive ductal, or lobular carcinoma.

Invasive Breast Diseases

Infiltrating Ductal Carcinoma

This is the **most common breast malignancy**, accounting for 70% of all breast cancers. The tumor arises from the ductal epithelium and infiltrates the supporting stroma (Figure 32-3). Less common but more favorable subtypes include medullary carcinoma, colloid carcinoma, tubular carcinoma, and papillary carcinoma.

Invasive Lobular Carcinoma

Lobular carcinoma arises from the lobular epithelium and infiltrates the breast stroma (Figure 32-3). It accounts for 8% to 10% of all breast cancers and tends to be bilateral.

Paget's Disease of the Nipple

Paget's disease accounts for 1% to 3% of all breast malignancies. It is often concomitant with DCIS or invasive carcinoma in the subareolar area. The malignant cells enter the epidermis of the nipple, causing the classic eczematous changes of the nipple. Examination reveals crusting, scaling, erosion, discharge, and possibly a breast mass.

Inflammatory Breast Carcinoma

This is an extremely aggressive malignancy, accounting for 1% to 4% of all breast cancers. It is a poorly differentiated tumor characterized by dermal lymphatic invasion. Symptoms include edema, erythema, warmth, and diffuse induration of the skin described as "**peau d'orange.**" It is usually accompanied by axillary lymphadenopathy, and has distant metastases on presentation 17% to 36% of the time.

Strategies for the Treatment of Invasive Breast Cancer

1. **Determine Primary Treatment Strategy.** Radical mastectomy was once the standard of care for invasive breast cancer. However, we now know that, in most cases, conservative treatment with

lumpectomy and radiation therapy results in identical survival as modified radical mastectomy. Once a plan for the primary treatment is made, lymph node and hormone receptor status can be determined so that strategies for adjuvant therapy can be made.

2. **Determine Lymph Node Status. Lymph node status** is a major prognostic factor for recurrence and morbidity with invasive breast cancer. It is therefore generally accepted that **all women should undergo ipsilateral axillary lymph node dissection** whether treated with lumpectomy and radiation or with mastectomy.

3. **Determine Hormone Receptor Status.** In addition to establishing lymph node status, the **hormone receptor status** is also determined. In general, hormone receptor positive tumors are well differentiated and exhibit a less aggressive clinical behavior, including lower recurrence rate and lower capacity to proliferate. Moreover, receptor positive tumors are more likely to respond to hormonal manipulation. Estrogen and progesterone positive status therefore carries a more favorable prognosis than negative hormone receptor status.

4. **Determine Type of Adjuvant Therapy.** Once lymph node and hormone receptor status are determined, a strategy for adjuvant therapy can be employed. The goal of adjuvant therapy is to **control micrometastases** after local disease is controlled with lumpectomy and radiation or with mastectomy. Adjuvant treatment is usually given as follows.

- **Lymph node negative patients**: Low-risk women in this group (nonpalpable tumors or tumors <1 cm) have a low recurrence risk rate and generally do not require adjuvant treatment. Higher-risk patients (large, aneuploid or estrogen receptor negative tumors) are treated with adjuvant chemotherapy if premenopausal and adjuvant tamoxifen if postmenopausal and estrogen-receptor positive.

- **Lymph node positive premenopausal patients**: These patients have a higher recurrence risk so **adjuvant chemotherapy** is used regardless of hormone receptor status. Most typically, a combination of cyclophosphamide [C], methotraxate [M], and 5-fluorouricil [F] is used. Adjuvant chemotherapy results in significantly decreased risk of recurrence and decreased mobidity. **Tamoxifen** is added in those premenopausal women whose tumors are estrogen-receptor positive.

- **Lymph node positive and hormone receptor posi-**

tive postmenopausal patients: This group can have significantly decreased recurrence and morbidity when primary treatment is followed with hormone therapy containing **tamoxifen**. Tamoxifen competively binds to estrogen receptors thus inhibiting the effect of estrogen on breast tissue.

- **Lymph node positive and hormone receptor negative postmenopausal patients**: This group is also treated with combination chemotherapy given that their tumors are not hormone-receptor nega-

tive and therefore not responsive to hormone therapy.

5. **Treat Metastatic or Recurrent Disease.**

- **Estrogen-receptor negative patients**: This group is best treated with combination chemotherapy that may include doxorubicin (Adriamycin) [A], and vincristine [V], in addition to CMF. There is a 75% response to chemotherapy but this is only temporary (6 to 8 months) with the average additional

---

■ TABLE 32-2

TNM Staging of Breast Cancer

Cancer Stage	Primary Tumor Size	Lymph Node Involvement	Distant Metastases
0	T_{is}	N_0	M_0
I	T_1	N_0	M_0
IIa	T_0	N_1	M_0
	T_1	N_1	M_0
	T_2	N_0	M_0
	T_2	N_0	M_0
IIb	T_2	N_1	M_0
	T_3	N_0	M_0
IIIa	T_0	N_2	M_0
	T_1	N_2	M_0
	T_2	N_2	M_0
	T_3	N_1, N_2	M_0
IIIb	T_4	Any N	M_0
	Any T	N_3	M_0
IV	Any T	Any N	M_1

Key: TNM Classification
T: Primary Tumor
  T_x Primary tumor unassessable
  T_0 No evidence of primary tumor
  T_{is} Carcinoma in situ; intraductal carcinoma, lobular carcinoma in situ, or Paget's disease of the nipple with no tumor
  T_1 Tumor <2 cm in largest dimension
      T_{1a} Tumor <0.5 cm
      T_{1b} Tumor <1 cm but >0.5 cm
      T_{1c} Tumor <2 cm but >1 cm
  T_2 Tumor <5 cm but >2 cm
  T_3 Tumor >5 cm
  T_4 Tumor any size extending to chest wall or skin
      T_{4a} Extension to chest wall
      T_{4b} Edema or ulceration of skin of breast or satellite skin nodules on ipsilateral breast
      T_{4c} Both T_{4a} and T_{4b}
N: Regional Lymph Nodes
  N_x Regional lymph nodes cannot be assessed
  N_0 No regional lymph node metastases
  N_1 Metastasis to mobile ipsilateral axillary lymph node
  N_2 Metastasis to the ipsilateral axillary lymph node, fixed
  N_3 Metastatis to ipsilateral internal mammary lymph node
M: Distant Metastasis
  M_x Presence of distant metastasis cannot be assessed
  M_0 No evidence of distant metastasis
  M_1 Distant metastasis, include metastasis to ipsilateral supraclavicular lymph nodes
Source: Adapted from American Joint Committee on Cancer. Manual for Staging of Cancer, 4th ed. Philadelphia: J.B. Lippincott, 1992:147.

survival being 1½–2 years from the time of recurrence.

- **Estrogen receptor positive patients**: In the face of metastatic disease, these patients benefit most from hormonal therapy rather than chemotherapy. Premenopausal women may be treated with oophorectomy or gonadotropin-releasing hormone (GnRH) antagonists, whereas postmenopausal women are treated with tamoxifen. The one exception to this are those estrogen-receptor positive women who have visceral involvement requiring immediate therapy. In these cases, chemotherapy is used given its relatively quicker responsive compared to hormone therapy.

Prognosis

The most reliable predictor for survival is the stage of breast cancer at the time of diagnosis. The 5-year disease-free survival rate in patients with breast cancer is 80% for stage I, 60% for stage II, 20% for stage III, and minimal for stage IV disease (Table 32-2). The current overall 5-year survival rate has increased to 94%. **Positive estrogen and progesterone receptor status carries a more favorable prognosis.** Premenopausal women tend to have more aggressive disease, with a 26% 5-year mortality rate when diagnosed in their 20s versus 15% when diagnosed in their 40s. Stage of cancer is the most important prognostic factor for breast cancer. Other prognostic indicators include lymph node status, hormone receptor status, tumor size, nuclear grade, histologic type, proliferative rate, and oncogene expression.

Follow-Up

Follow-up after breast cancer treatment should include a **physical exam** every 3 months in the first year, every 4 months in the second year, and every 6 months thereafter. The first **follow-up mammogram** is usually performed 6 months after treatment. Routine chest x-ray and bone scans have now been replaced with **clinical monitoring** for **metastatic disease** (dry cough, exertional dyspnea, bone and body pains, pleuritic chest pain, etc.). Blood **tests for bone disease (alkaline phosphatase)** and **liver function tests** (LFTs) are obtained every 6 months. Women taking tamoxifen should be followed for irregular bleeding given the possibility of increased endometrial cancer with tamoxifen use. **Endometrial biopsy** should be performed where indicated.

Hormone Use after Breast Cancer Treatment

Some premenopausal patients may wish to become pregnant after breast cancer treatment. Traditionally, this has been discouraged for fear that pregnancy-related estrogens may stimulate dormant cancer cells. Studies now suggest that **there is no difference in survival rates in women who become pregnant after breast cancer treatment**. For women who wish to avoid fertility after cancer treatment, there has been **no adverse effect shown with the use of oral contraceptives** containing estrogen.

The use of postmenopausal HRT in breast cancer survivors has been widely debated. To date, studies suggest that **HRT use does not influence the survival outcomes** of patients after breast cancer treatment. Conversely, the benefits of short-term HRT for symptom relief and osteoporosis prevention have been demonstrated. Patients and providers must be aware, however, that the possibility of developing a new lesion or recurrence during posttreatment HRT use does exist.

KEY POINTS

1. Numerous risk factors have been identified for breast cancer (increasing age, family history, high-fat diet, ionizing radiation, late child bearing, atypical hyperplasia); however, most patients have no known risk factors.
2. Only 5% to 10% of breast cancer is related to genetic predisposition.
3. Women who use HRT for more than 5 years are potentially at increased risk of developing breast cancer.
4. Studies of OCP exposure reveal no increased risk of breast cancer.
5. DCIS (15%) is a preinvasive disease and is treated with lumpectomy and radiation therapy. LCIS (4%) is treated with local resection.
6. Invasive breast disease—including infiltrating ductal carcinoma (70%) and infiltrating lobular carcinoma (10%)—is treated with lumpectomy and radiation or with modified mastectomy with equal risk of recurrence and survival.
7. All women with invasive breast disease should have ispilateral axillary lymph node dissection and determination of estrogen-receptor status.
8. The standard adjuvant treatment for premenopausal women with positive nodes, regardless of hormone-receptor status, includes 6 months of cyclophosphamide, methotrexate, and fluorouracil combination chemotherapy.

9. The standard adjuvant treatment for post-menopausal women with positive nodes, and positive estrogen-receptor status is tamoxifen.

10. Follow-up for patients with breast cancer includes mammography, frequent physical exam, serum and clinical monitoring for metastatic disease.

11. While there is debate over the use of estrogens in breast cancer survivors, pregnancy, OCP use, and HRT use after breast cancer treatment have been found to influence breast cancer survival.

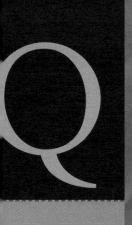

Questions

1. A 23-year-old woman presents with multiple lesions on her labia and perineum. These tender ulcers have been causing discomfort for 36 hours. The patient also complains of dysuria and fatigue. A Tzanck prep of one of the lesions reveals multinucleated giant cells. The woman is concerned that this was transmitted sexually and would like to be tested for other sexually transmitted diseases.

   Which of the following tests should be ordered?
   a. rapid plasma reagin (RPR)
   b. HIV
   c. Chlamydiazyme DNA probe
   d. Gonorrhea culture or DNA probe
   e. All of the above

2. Which of the following regimens can be used to cure the patient described in question 1?
   a. Acyclovir 400 mg PO TID
   b. Ceftriaxone 250 mg IM × 1
   c. Azithromycin 1 g PO × 1
   d. Metronidazole 500 mg PO BID
   e. None of the above

3. You are caring for a young couple whose chief complaint is 2 years of primary infertility. As part of an initial evaluation, the hysterosalpingogram shows bilateral occlusion of the fallopian tubes. As part of your counseling, you offer them a referral to a reproductive endocrinologist for treatment. You explain that their treatment will most likely involve ovulation induction coupled with in vitro fertilization. They are concerned about the possible side effects of "fertility drugs."

   You inform them that the two most common major side effects of gonadotropin ovulation induction are
   a. ovarian cancer and ovarian hyperstimulation syndrome.
   b. multiple gestation pregnancy and polycystic ovarian syndrome.
   c. multiple gestation pregnancy and ovarian hyperstimulation syndrome.

   d. polycystic ovarian syndrome and ovarian cancer.
   e. None of the above; fertility drugs have no major side effects.

4. A 61-year-old woman whose last menstrual period was 3 years ago presents with a complaint of vaginal bleeding that has occurred over the past 3 days. She weighs 210 pounds and has a history of obesity, hypertension, and non-insulin dependent diabetes (NIDDM). Although she had irregular periods most of her life, she did conceive and deliver one child. The patient has some mild symptoms associated with menopause but has never been on hormone replacement therapy. Initial tests reveal endometrial hyperplasia. When you meet with the patient to give her the results she is very concerned regarding the implications of your diagnosis.

   You inform her that
   a. endometrial hyperplasia does not place her at increased risk of endometrial cancer.
   b. endometrial hyperplasia is her only risk factor for endometrial cancer.
   c. the likelihood of developing cancer depends largely on the degree of cytologic atypia.
   d. the likelihood of developing cancer depends largely on the degree of histologic atypia.
   e. endometrial hyperplasia is a noninvasive, superficial cancer of the endometrium.

5. A 22-year-old gravida 2 para 0 at 33 weeks gestation is found to have a BP of 166/114 on a routine office visit. Her BP at her first prenatal visit at 7 weeks was 124/72. Her urine dip at this most recent visit shows 3+ protein although it previously had 0 to trace protein. The patient is also complaining of a persistent headache although she has no history of migraines. Her ALT and AST are elevated at 92 and 105, respectively.

   After starting an antihypertensive agent and magnesium sulfate, what do you do next?

a. Order bed rest for the remainder of the pregnancy
b. Order bed rest until week 37, then amniocentesis for fetal lung maturity, then deliver
c. Immediate induction of labor for anticipated vaginal delivery
d. Immediate delivery via cesarean section
e. Continue expectant management

6. A 29-year-old gravida 3 para 2 at 38 weeks gestation presents to labor and delivery complaining of the sudden onset of abdominal pain and bright-red vaginal bleeding. On examination, her uterus is firm and tender to palpation and the tocodynamometer reveals regular contractions every 1 to 2 minutes. The fetal heart monitor shows no evidence of fetal distress. The patient had a normal ultrasound at week 34 that showed the infant in the vertex presentation.
   Which of the following is the *most likely* diagnosis in this patient?
   a. Labor
   b. Premature rupture of membranes
   c. Placenta accreta
   d. Placenta previa
   e. Placental abruption

7. A 67-year-old woman presents with vulvar pruritus for the prior year that has been increasing over the past few months. She went through menopause at age 49 and has been on estrogen and progesterone since that time. On physical examination, there are velvety-red lesions bilaterally on the vulva. There is also some white placque.
   The first step in the management of this patient is
   a. to treat with antifungals.
   b. to treat with topical steroids.
   c. wide local excision of the lesions.
   d. to perform a punch biopsy of the vulvar lesion.
   e. cryotherapy.

8. A 27-year-old African American woman presents at 16 weeks gestation for a prenatal visit.
   Which of the following genetic tests would *only be offered* if one of the others was positive?
   a. Screening for thalassemia
   b. Screening for sickle-cell anemia
   c. Amniocentesis
   d. Expanded maternal serum α-fetoprotein
   e. Screen for cystic fibrosis

9. A 36-year-old gravida 3 para 2 comes to you concerned because she typically had very regular menses but has not had a period in 8 weeks. She didn't worry initially because she had a Paragard IUD placed 3 years ago after the birth of her last child. However, a serum pregnancy test confirms that she is pregnant. On physical exam, the strings are visible in the cervical os. Pelvic ultrasound confirms an 8.2-week intrauterine pregnancy.
   How do you proceed?
   a. Expectant management
   b. Gentle traction on the strings to attempt removal of the IUD
   c. Dilation and evacuation of uterus to prevent septic abortion
   d. Prophylactic antibiotics to prevent septic abortion
   e. Kidney, ureters, bladder, and upright radiographs to delineate the relationship of the IUD to the fetus

10. During your pediatric gynecology rotation, you see a 13-year-old girl who is brought in by her mother. The mother is concerned that her daughter has not yet begun to menstruate. After a thorough history you perform a physical examination that reveals age-appropriate pubic and axillary hair and breast buds, which the mother says developed in the past year. To reassure the patient and her mother, you explain the typical chronological order of pubertal development.
    Which of the following is the *most common* chronological order of these developmental stages?
    a. Gonadarche, thelarche, pubarche, menarche
    b. Gonadarche, menarche, thelarche, pubarche
    c. Thelarche, gonadarche, pubarche, menarche
    d. Thelarche, gonadarche, menarche, pubarche
    e. Thelarche, pubarche, gonadarche, menarche

11. A 23-year-old woman presents with a single papule on her right labia. It is nontender and approximately 1 cm in diameter. The rest of her physical exam is negative except for palpable inguinal adenopathy. She last had intercourse 2.5 weeks ago and wants to be tested for sexually transmitted diseases.
    Which of the following would *only be ordered* if additional history was present?
    a. Gonorrhea culture or DNA probe
    b. Chlamydiazyme DNA probe
    c. Rapid plasma reagin
    d. HIV
    e. HSV Ab titer

12. Dark field microscopy is performed on the above patient, revealing motile spirochetes. You treat the patient with which of the following?
    a. 1 g azithromycin PO
    b. Acyclovir 400 mg PO TID
    c. Acyclovir 400 mg IV TID
    d. Benzathine penicillin G 2.4 M units × 1
    e. Penicillin G 2.4 M units IV Q 4 h

13. A 19-year-old woman presents with complaints of no periods for the past 7 months. During this time she

started college and feels her stress level has increased. The patient has also changed her eating habits, which has led to a weight decrease from 120 to 105 pounds. She has noted no other changes in her health.

Which of the following tests should be ordered initially?

a. Thyroid stimulating hormone (TSH), Prolactin
b. β-hCG, Prolactin, TSH
c. Follicle stimulating hormone, β-hCG
d. Prolactin, β-hCG, DHEAS
e. Testosterone, β-hCG

14. The labs ordered for the patient discussed above were all normal.

Which of the following would be the *best way* to assess this patient's estrogenization?

a. Progesterone challenge test
b. ACTH stim test
c. LH/FSH ratio
d. Estradiol levels
e. Endometrial biopsy

15. You are working in the emergency room when you are asked to see a patient with vaginal bleeding. She is a 27-year-old gravida 2 para 0 at 8 weeks gestation who has had 3 days of heavy vaginal bleeding. The woman's pregnancy test is positive, her hematocrit is stable at 37.6, and her blood type is A negative. On pelvic exam you note tissue being extruded from the cervical os. You remove the tissue manually and find an open cervical os. Pelvic ultrasound confirms an intrauterine pregnancy. You explain to the patient that she is in the midst of a miscarriage and obtain her consent for a dilation and curettage of the uterus, which is uneventful. You then give the patient a RhoGAM injection (RhIgG) and refer her for follow-up with her gynecologist. Two weeks later you receive a copy of the pathology report stating the tissue was consistent with an incomplete molar pregnancy. You phone the patient's gynecologist to relay the information and to ask some questions about the molar pregnancies because you've never treated a patient with this diagnosis.

Which of the following would the gynecologist identify as characteristic of incomplete molar pregnancy?

a. Incomplete moles result from the fertilization of an empty ovum with one sperm and therefore typically have a karyotype of 46,XX.
b. Incomplete moles do not have an associated fetus.
c. Patients with incomplete moles typically present with signs of hyperthyroidism, preeclampsia, and/or hyperemesis gravidarum.
d. Incomplete moles have a lower rate of persistent disease and low malignant potential compared to complete molar pregnancies.

e. Incomplete moles are treated with methotrexate and serial β-hCGs to a level of zero.

16. A 27-year-old woman presents complaining of foul-smelling vaginal discharge. On exam she has a gray–green discharge and the cervix has punctate epithelial papillae, giving it a "strawberry" appearance. On wet prep a unicellular organism with flagella can be seen.

This organism is *most likely*

a. *Candida albicans.*
b. *Trichomonas vaginalis.*
c. *Gardnerella vaginalis.*
d. *Bacteroides fragiles.*
e. *Haemophilus ducreyi.*

17. A 27-year-old woman comes to the emergency department complaining of a vaginal discharge. On speculum exam, you observe that she has a mucousy yellow discharge and that her cervix appears erythematous. On bimanual exam, the patient has cervical motion tenderness, no uterine tenderness, and no adnexal tenderness. Her temperature is 36.7°C, white blood cell count of 8.4, and the rest of the vital signs and laboratory results are within normal limits.

The treatment of choice for this patient is

a. azithromycin 1 g PO for 7 days.
b. doxycycline 100 mg PO BID for 7 days.
c. ceftriaxone 250 mg IM times 1 and doxycycline 100 mg PO BID for 7 days.
d. cefoxitin 2 g IV Q 6h and doxycycline PO as an inpatient.
e. ampicillin, gentamicin, and clindamycin IV as an inpatient.

18. A 51-year-old woman comes to your office complaining of hot flashes and trouble sleeping at night. Her last menstrual period was 6 months ago and her periods were irregular for 1 year prior to that.

Elevation in which of the following tests confirms your diagnosis?

a. hCG
b. TSH
c. FSH
d. PRL
e. LH

19. Of the following, which classic triad characterizes preeclampsia?

a. Visual changes, proteinuria, pitting pedal edema
b. Headache, visual changes, right upper quadrant pain
c. Hypertension, visual changes, right upper quadrant pain
d. Hypertension, proteinuria, and nondependent edema
e. Hypertension, proteinuria, and pitting pedal edema

20. A 24-year-old woman found a firm, rubbery 1.5 cm mass on breast self-exam. On examination in your office there is no skin change, nipple discharge, enlarged lymph nodes, or tenderness. She has no known family history of breast cancer. Ultrasound reveals a solid 2 cm mass.

    Recommended patient management at this point should be
    a. diagnosis is fibroadenoma; no further follow-up necessary.
    b. mammography.
    c. wide local excision.
    d. observation or fine-needle aspiration.

21. A 40-year-old patient presents with 2.0 cm breast mass. On examination in your office there is no skin change, nipple discharge, enlarged lymph nodes, or tenderness. She has no known family history of breast cancer. A mammogram is read as normal, a fine-needle aspiration is nondiagnostic, and the mass persists.

    What is the next management step for this patient?
    a. Follow clinical exams
    b. Repeat fine-needle aspiration
    c. Excisional biopsy
    d. Ultrasound

22. A 23-year-old G1 P0 at week 38 is being managed with magnesium sulfate while she undergoes induction of labor for severe preeclampsia. She received a 4 gram bolus followed by a constant infusion of 2.0 grams per hour. However, the nurse found the patient to have absent patellar reflexes and a respiratory rate of 6 breaths/minute. The patient is can be aroused but is very drowsy.

    In addition to discontinuing the magnesium, what should your next management step be?
    a. Administer terbutaline
    b. Intubate immediately
    c. Administer calcium gluconate
    d. Give betamethasone
    e. Do nothing further

23. A 19-year-old woman presents with a complaint of 6 months of amenorrhea. She notes that she has not had a period since starting college last fall. The patient notes no weight loss during that time and has, in fact, gone from 173 to 181 pounds over the past few months but believes the weight gain is secondary to change in diet during college. She denies nipple discharge, frequent headaches, and vaginal discharge. She notes no other symptoms.

    Which of the following tests is *most likely* to be abnormal indicating her diagnosis?
    a. Thyroid-stimulating hormone
    b. Follicle-stimulating hormone
    c. Prolactin

d. Luteinizing hormone
e. β-hCG

24. A 63-year-old woman comes to you with 6 weeks of postmenopausal bleeding. Review of her history reveals menarche at age 10 and a lifetime history of oligomenorrhea. She reports being overweight most of her life and currently weighs 225 pounds. She is 5'4" tall. The patient experienced menopause at age 56 and has never been on hormone replacement therapy. She is basically healthy except for borderline hypertension and adult onset diabetes mellitus, for which she takes oral hyperglycemic agents.

    Which of the following would be the *most important* thing to do next for this patient?
    a. A TSH and PRL level
    b. An FSH level
    c. A Pap smear
    d. An endometrial biopsy
    e. Dilation and curettage of the uterus
    f. Pelvic ultrasound
    g. Hysteroscopy
    h. Hysterectomy
    i. Total abdominal hysterectomy and bilateral salpingo-oophorectomy
    j. Begin hormone replacement therapy

25. A 29-year-old G0 has been a type 1 diabetic for 17 years and now presents for pregestational counseling. In addition to the standard pregestational advice such as checking a rubella titer, and to take folic acid, you counsel her regarding tight blood sugar control prior to becoming pregnant.

    Assuming that the patient lowers her HgbA1c prior to pregnancy, the risk of which of the following complications will be unchanged?
    a. Caudal regression syndrome
    b. Cardiac anomalies
    c. Fetal macrosomia
    d. Neural tube defects
    e. All of the above

26. A 28-year-old class A2 diabetic at 34 weeks of gestation presents for a prenatal appointment. In addition to managing her insulin and performing routine counseling, you also discuss plans for delivery.

    In general, in the well-controlled, insulin-requiring gestational diabetic woman, which mode and timing of delivery is usually employed?
    a. Expectant management; await the natural onset of labor
    b. Offer cesarean section in labor
    c. Offer expectant management until week 42, and vaginal delivery in labor

d. Offer induction of labor between weeks 39 to 40 gestation

e. Offer cesarean section if expected weight is >4000 grams

27. A 25-year-old G1 P0 at 9 weeks gestation presents for her initial prenatal visit. She has no medical or surgical history, and has a certain LMP that is consistent with her examination. The patient has donated blood in the past and knows that she is Rh negative.

   In which of the following situations would the patient be cared for *without being treated* with RhoGAM?
   a. First-trimester bleeding
   b. Second-trimester bleeding
   c. Routinely at the beginning of the third trimester
   d. Contractions at 34 weeks gestation
   e. At the time of an amniocentesis

28. A 27-year-old woman presents to the emergency department complaining of vaginal discharge and abdominal pain. On physical examination she has a temperature of 38.1°C and on abdominal exam has tenderness in the right upper quadrant and lower abdomen with minimal peritoneal signs. On speculum exam, the patient has a mucousy yellow discharge. On bimanual exam, she has cervical motion tenderness and bilateral adnexal tenderness. Her white blood cell count is 14.3 and a pelvic ultrasound shows a normal uterus and normal ovaries bilaterally.

   The *most likely* diagnosis for this patient is which of the following?
   a. Cervicitis
   b. Endomyometritis
   c. Pelvic inflammatory disease
   d. Tubo-ovarian abscess
   e. Appendicitis

29. A 73-year-old woman presents complaining of vulvar pruritus. She has had these symptoms for about 3 months and self-treatment with an over-the-counter antifungal medication has failed. On physical examination the patient has an atrophic vulva with fusion of the labia majora and minora. A biopsy is performed and the result shows lichen sclerosus.

   Which of the following treatments would be recommended first?
   a. Topical estrogen
   b. Topical testosterone
   c. Topical ketoconazole
   d. Topical corticosteroid
   e. Oral estrogen supplementation
   f. Oral ketoconazole
   g. Surgical repair of fused labia
   h. Expectant management

30. A 29-year-old woman presents complaining of vulvar pain that increases with ambulation and intercourse. She also notes a lump on her right labia that has increased in size over the past 48 hours and is quite painful. The patient has had these same symptoms in the past but it never became red or painful. On examination she has a 5 cm tender cyst on the medial aspect of her right labia, with a surrounding erythema of the labia that extends 1–2 cm away.

   How would you manage this patient?
   a. Expectant management
   b. Sitz baths only
   c. Incision and drainage
   d. Insertion of Word catheter
   e. Needle aspiration drainage
   f. Antibiotics
   g. Biopsy of the cyst
   h. Marsupialization of the cyst
   i. Excision of the cyst

31. Of the following, which can cause both primary and secondary amenorrhea?
   a. Asherman's syndrome
   b. Gonadal agenesis
   c. Anorexia nervosa
   d. Sheehan's syndrome
   e. Kallmann's syndrome

32. Your see a 23-year-old G0 P0 who is interested in obtaining more information on available contraceptive methods. She is a nonsmoker who has had chlamydia once in the past. She has had four male sexual partners in the past and used condoms intermittently. Her family history is notable for her mother who is currently being treated for postmenopausal breast cancer and doing well. The patient wants to know if she is a candidate for oral contraceptive pills.

   You tell her that the absolute *contraindications* for the use of estrogen-containing oral contraceptives include
   a. a history of pulmonary embolism.
   b. a smoker over age 35.
   c. a history of depression.
   d. diabetes mellitus.
   e. fibroid uterus.
   f. hyperlipidemia.
   g. breastfeeding.
   h. hypertension.
   i. migraine headaches.

33. A 29-year-old G2 P1 comes for prenatal care. She has a history of delivery of a 4250 g baby. She herself had been a big baby at birth. The patient is concerned because her prepregnancy weight was 162 pounds and she gained 70 pounds during this pregnancy. At 26 weeks gestation the

patient had a glucose loading test of 50 g glucose. When her blood glucose level was measured 1 hour later, it was 164.

As her obstetrician, what would you do next?

a. Check a hemaglobin A1C
b. Start her on an appropriate insulin regimen
c. Check a 3-hour glucose tolerance test
d. Start her on an oral hyperglycemia agent
e. Start her on a diabetic diet

34. A 17-year-old gymnast presents in generally good health except for the absence of menses. She states that she developed breasts later than her friends and never began menstruation. On physical examination, she has Tanner stage 5 development of breasts and pubic hair. On speculum exam, her cervix appears normal and she has a normal bimanual exam.

The *most likely* etiology of this patient's primary amenorrhea is

a. anorexia nervosa.
b. gonadal agenesis.
c. transverse vaginal septum.
d. testicular feminization.
e. hypogonadotropic hypogonadism.

35. A 29-year-old G3 P1 presents complaining of no menses for 4 months after stopping her birth control pills. She is concerned that the use of the oral birth control pills (OCPs) has left her with amenorrhea. The patient has had no recent changes in weight, exercises two to three times a week, and notes no particular changes in either her work or home life. Her obstetric history includes a therapeutic abortion at age 21, a normal spontaneous delivery at age 25, and a miscarriage at age 27. After the dilation and curettage at the time of the miscarriage, the patient was hospitalized with an infection of her uterus. Since that time she has taken OCPs.

Given this history, which of the following is the *most likely* etiology of this patient's amenorrhea?

a. Vaginal agenesis
b. Asherman's syndrome
c. Mayer-Rokitansky-Küster-Hauser syndrome
d. Testicular feminization
e. Hypogonadotropic hypogonadism

36. Ultrasound can be useful in diagnosing potential causes of third-trimester bleeding.

Ultrasound is the primary diagnostic tool for which cause of third-trimester bleeding?

a. Uterine rupture
b. Placental abruption
c. Placenta previa
d. Cervical neoplasm
e. Vaginal laceration

37. A 19-year-old woman presents complaining of 7 months of amenorrhea. She notes that she has not had a period since 2 to 3 months after starting college. She notes weight loss during that time from 131 to 114 pounds over the past few months but believes the weight loss is secondary to a change in diet during college. She also has insomnia, heat intolerance, and occasionally hot flashes.

Which of the following tests would *most likely* indicate her diagnosis?

a. Thyroid stimulating hormone
b. Luteinizing hormone
c. Prolactin
d. β-hCG
e. ACTH stim test

38. You performed an annual gynocologic exam on your next patient 3 weeks ago. She is returning at this time because she is interested in changing from an oral contraceptive pill to another form of birth control. She is a 38-year-old G4 P3 whose only current sexual partner is her husband of 6 years. The patient has had a total lifetime history of 7 male partners and a remote history of *Chlamydia cervicitis* in college years ago. She is a healthy, one-half a pack per day smoker who has had three uncomplicated vaginal deliveries and one ectopic pregnancy at 8 weeks gestation, which was treated with methotrexate. She has had regular monthly periods with a moderate amount of dysmenorrhea all of her life. The woman did not mention it at her annual visit, but over the past 3 months she has had menometorrhagia (heavy irregular menses). She denies any postcoital spotting and had a normal Pap smear with negative cervical cultures 3 weeks ago. Neither she nor her husband is ready to commit to permanent sterilization. The patient was doing some research over the Internet about intrauterine devices (IUDs) and she wants to know if this would be an option for her and her husband.

You explain that, at this time, you do not recommend an IUD because of her

a. age.
b. smoking history.
c. history of multiple sexual partners.
d. history of pelvic inflammatory disease.
e. prior ectopic pregnancy.
f. undiagnosed vaginal bleeding.
g. desire for future fertility.

39. Risk factors for placental abruption include all of the following *except*

a. hypertension.
b. advanced maternal age.
c. cocaine use.
d. preterm premature rupture of membranes.
e. heroin abuse.

40. A 19-year-old G3 P1 patient with a history of a miscarriage in her last pregnancy presents to the emergency department with some vaginal spotting. She reports that her last menstrual period occurred 7 weeks earlier. She has had no vaginal discharge other than the spotting, no cramping, and no abdominal pain. Her physical examination reveals a slightly enlarged uterus, no tenderness, and a closed cervical os. A serum β-hCG-level is sent off and returns 1146. A pelvic ultrasound shows no intrauterine pregnancy, a 2 cm left ovarian simple cyst, and no free fluid.

Your diagnosis of this patient is which of the following?
a. Threatened abortion/rule out ectopic pregnancy
b. Ectopic pregnancy
c. Inevitable abortion
d. Missed abortion
e. Normal pregnancy

41. In the patient described above, when should a repeat β-hCG be drawn?
a. 24 hours
b. 48 hours
c. 72 hours
d. 1 week
e. It does not need to be drawn again

42. A 30-year-old G0 P0 comes to you for a second opinion after being diagnosed by her primary gynecologist with a bicornuate uterus. She and her husband are planning to start a family and want to know how this diagnosis would affect a future pregnancy.

You explain that the most likely complication associated with the presence of bicornuate uterus is which of the following?
a. Infertility requiring medical or surgical intervention
b. Recurrent miscarriage
c. Preterm rupture of membranes
d. Premature labor and delivery
e. Bicornuate uterus should have no effect on the pregnancy, labor, or delivery.

43. A 71-year-old woman presents with light vaginal bleeding. She has no other complaints. The bleeding began 30 days ago and she has bled three or four times since then. She has no other medical history. On physical exam she is a thin woman with no obvious findings. Her uterus is small and postmenopausal and her ovaries are not palpable. Her vagina and introitus are slightly atrophic with no lesions and she has no obvious hemorrhoids. The patient had a normal Pap smear 8 months ago and no history of abnormal Pap smears. On pelvic ultrasound, there is a 1 cm × 1.2 cm lesion in her intrauterine cavity.

Which of the following is the most likely cause of this patient's bleeding?

a. Atrophy
b. Cervical cancer
c. Endometrial polyp
d. Endometrial cancer
e. Excess hormones

44. A 19-year-old G3 P1 at 31 weeks gestation presents with contractions every 3 to 4 minutes. On examination, her cervix is found to be dilated 2 cm and 50% effaced. The patient's history is remarkable for a delivery at 33 weeks gestation in her last pregnancy of a 5 lb 3 oz infant 3 years ago, and a miscarriage 2 years ago. She has a history of a half pack per day smoking for 6 years.

Which of the following is the most predictive risk factor for recurrent preterm labor?
a. History of spontaneous abortion
b. Prior preterm delivery
c. Large fetus
d. Cigarette smoking
e. Teenage pregnancy

45. A 32-year-old woman comes to your office for an annual exam. She complains of a dull, achy pain in her right lower abdomen. She reports having the pain three to four times throughout the year. The pain is not associated with her menses. She has occasionally had a late period that was very heavy but in general, her periods are otherwise regular. She denies intermenstrual bleeding or postcoital spotting. You examine her and send off labs for thyroid-stimulating hormone and prolactin, both of which are normal, and a β-hCG, which is negative. A pelvic ultrasound reveals a 3.5 cm right ovarian cyst that is thin-walled, fluid-filled, and without septations.

How would you treat this patient?
a. Take her to the OR for an ovarian cystectomy.
b. Start her on an oral contraceptive pill to suppress cyst formation and reevaluate her at her next annual visit.
c. Reassure her and repeat the pelvic ultrasound in 6 to 8 weeks.
d. Reassure her that all is well and prescribe a non-steroidal anti-inflammatory drug for her discomfort.
e. Take her to the OR for a right oophorectomy.

46. A 19-year-old G1 P0 at 38 weeks gestation presents to labor and delivery. On arrival, she is having contractions every 2 to 3 minutes and claims that her "water broke" 2 days earlier but that she didn't come in because she hadn't reached her due date. She has a temperature of 101.2°F, heart rate of 110, blood pressure of 116/72, and uterine tenderness on palpation. The fetal heart rate is in the 170s with small accelerations and no decelerations.

Which of the following is your diagnosis of this patient?

a. Labor
b. Preterm labor
c. Chorioamnionitis
d. Maternal fever
e. Preterm rupture of membranes

47. A 37-year-old G2 P0 at 42 weeks gestation with diet-controlled, Class A1, gestational diabetes presents in labor. The fetal heart rate tracing is reassuring, and the patient is contracting well every 2 to 3 minutes. She progresses slowly over the course of the day until she is fully dilated. She begins the second stage of labor and pushes for 1.5 hours. Finally the head delivers, but once it does there is a shoulder dystocia.

Which of the following actions is likely to *worsen* the shoulder dystocia?
a. Suprapubic pressure
b. Fundal pressure
c. Increased flexion of the hips
d. Delivery of the posterior arm
e. Episiotomy

48. A 27-year-old G1 P0 at 40 weeks gestation presents to labor and delivery with contractions every 6 to 8 minutes.

Of the following findings, which is the *most worrisome* on the fetal heart tracing?
a. Repetitive early decelerations, minimal variability
b. No heart rate decelerations, minimal variability
c. Repetitive late decelerations, absent variability
d. No heart rate decelerations, moderate variability
e. Repetitive variable decelerations, moderate variability

49. A 56-year-old G0 P0 Caucasian female weighing 250 pounds is concerned about her risks of breast cancer. Her history includes prior oral contraceptive pill (OCP) use for 5 years in her 20s and hormone replacement therapy (HRT) used for 3 years since she reached menopause. Her mother was diagnosed with unilateral breast cancer at age 37.

Which of the following is the correct decreasing order of relative risk factors?
a. OCP + HRT use > obesity > nulliparous > late menopause > family history
b. Nulliparous > obesity > family history > late menopause > OCP + HRT use
c. Family history > nulliparous > late menopause > OCP + HRT use > obesity
d. Family history > OCP + HRT use > obesity > nulliparous > late menopause

50. A 36-year-old woman was diagnosed with metastatic breast cancer. She underwent mastectomy and axillary node dissection. Estrogen and progesterone receptor status were both positive.

What would be your next step in treatment?
a. Tamoxifen alone
b. Chemotherapy followed by tamoxifen
c. No further therapy
d. Chemotherapy alone

51. A 52-year-old woman presents for a routine examination after 18 months of amenorrhea. Her medical history is otherwise without complications. Her physical examination is within normal limits.

Because of this patient's menopausal state, you counsel her that combination hormone replacement therapy can
a. worsen her menopausal symptoms.
b. decrease her risk of osteoporosis.
c. decrease her risk of breast cancer.
d. increase her risk of liver cancer.
e. increase her risk of uterine cancer.

52. A 24-year-old G2 P1 at 24 weeks gestation presents with left lower quadrant pain that has increased over the past 3 weeks. On exam she has local abdominal tenderness, low-grade fever, and moderate leukocytosis. A pelvic ultrasound reveals a normal intrauterine pregnancy at 24 weeks, a 6 cm left anterior fibroid, and normal ovaries.

How would this patient be best managed?
a. Observation and analgesics
b. Immediate dilation and evacuation followed by removal of the fibroid
c. Immediate induction of labor followed by removal of the fibroid
d. Laparoscopic myomectomy
e. Abdominal myomectomy

53. A 19-year-old primigravid patient presents for an initial prenatal visit at 7 weeks gestation. She is concerned because she used both cocaine and heroin in the month before she discovered she was pregnant. In a long discussion with her about the risks of substance abuse during pregnancy, you tell her that use of which of the following has the highest correlation with congenital abnormalities?
a. Alcohol
b. Caffeine
c. Cocaine
d. Opiates
e. Smoking tobacco

54. A 37-year-old G2 P2 black female presents with a history of regular menses complicated by heavy vaginal bleeding and heavy cramping. She has no intermenstrual bleeding or postcoital spotting. The woman is a very healthy and fit person and has declined therapy for her pain and bleeding in the past. She has become used to these symptoms but is concerned because her last period lasted 10 days and she was changing her menstrual pad nearly every 2 to 3 hours. The patient also complains of more dull achy pain and abdominal pressure than with previous menstrual periods. Her hematocrit at the visit is 33.9 and a pelvic ultrasound reveals multiple large fibroids, the largest measuring 4–5 cm. Most appear to be intramural, but the cavity appears to contain some submucosal fibroids as well. Her ovaries are normal and there is no hydronephrosis. The patient is now interested in treating her fibroids but would like to preserve her future fertility if possible.

In this situation, the patient's symptoms would best be treated with

a. expectant management.
b. oral contraceptive pills.
c. Depo-Lupron.
d. hysteroscopic myomectomy.
e. abdominal myomectomy.
f. total abdominal hysterectomy.
g. vaginal hysterectomy.
h. total abdominal hysterectomy and bilateral salpingo-oophorectomy.

55. While on call in the hospital, you are paged to the emergency department to see a 25-year-old G2 P0 patient from your clinic. She is a law student who had a condom failure 50 hours before the visit. She was using no other form of contraception. The woman has a history of a first-trimester termination of pregnancy in the past and is not ready to start a family. She heard from a classmate that there is a pill that can be taken to prevent pregnancy after intercourse.

What do you tell this patient?

a. You have nothing to offer her because RU-486 was never approved for use in the United States.
b. You have nothing to offer her because, although there is a "morning after" pill, it must be given within the first 48 hours after unprotected intercourse.
c. It is very unlikely that she is pregnant and she should come back if she doesn't get a period within 6 weeks.
d. Take one 35 µg birth control pill now, and another 12 hours from now.
e. Take two 50 µg birth control pills now, and two more 12 hours from now.

56. A 32-year-old woman presents for her first prenatal visit. She has a history of two singleton births, at 39 and 40 weeks; a twin birth at 28 weeks; and two miscarriages. All four of her children are alive and well.

Which of the following is her designation of gravity (G) and parity (P)?

a. G5P3024
b. G5P2224

c. G6P3024
d. G6P2124
e. G6P2224

57. The patient described above has a last menstrual period of May 4, 2004.

What is estimated date of confinement using Nägele's rule?

a. January 11, 2005
b. January 12, 2005
c. February 4, 2005
d. February 11, 2005
e. February 12, 2005

58. If this same patient did not know when her last menstrual period was, which of the following would be the most useful to determine her estimated date of confinement?

a. Physical examination
b. Maternal perception of fetal movement
c. Abdominal ultrasound at 16 weeks gestation
d. Transvaginal ultrasound at 8 weeks gestation
e. Doppler ultrasound

59. Your next patient in clinic is a young woman who recently underwent a dilation and evacuation of the uterus for a complete molar pregnancy. She is now being followed with weekly β-hCG levels to monitor for recurrent disease. Initially, her β-hCG levels declined. Unfortunately, the levels then plateaued and, 8 weeks after evacuation, began to rise and have continued to rise over the past 2 weeks. The patient has not been sexually active since the evacuation and has been reliably taking oral contraceptive pills. You inform her of the rising levels and your suspicion of an invasive molar pregnancy. The evaluation for metastatic disease is negative. Together you make a plan for her follow-up care.

Which of the following is *true* regarding this patient's diagnosis?

a. She is at lower risk for persistent disease because she had a complete molar pregnancy than she would have been had she had an incomplete molar pregnancy.
b. She will likely require multi-agent chemotherapy treatments.
c. Invasive moles rarely metastasize.
d. The patient will most likely need radiation therapy in addition to multi-agent chemotherapy.
e. She should avoid contraceptive methods that contain estrogen after treatment of her invasive mole.

60. A 37-year-old G7 P6 with a dichorionic/diamnionic, vertex/vertex twin gestation at 38 weeks presents to labor and delivery for induction of labor. She is started on oxytocin and begins having contractions after several

hours. The patient progresses slowly over the next 16 hours until she is 5 cm dilated and, at this point, develops a fever and fetal tachycardia. The woman is diagnosed with chorioamnionitis and antibiotic therapy is started. She delivers the babies vaginally 6 hours later. Right after delivery of the second infant, there is a large, continuous hemorrhage from the vagina.

The *most likely* cause of this is

a. vaginal laceration.
b. cervical laceration.
c. uterine atony.
d. uterine rupture.
e. placenta accreta.

61. You have just completed a total abdominal hysterectomy and bilateral salpingo-oophorectomy on a 64-year-old postmenopausal woman with endometrial cancer. You send the specimen to the pathologist for review.

Which of the following is the *most likely* cell type for endometrial cancer?

a. Squamous carcinoma
b. Clear-cell carcinoma
c. Endometrioid adenocarcinoma
d. Papillary serous carcinoma
e. Adenosquamous carcinoma

62. Your patient, a 59-year-old woman, is being followed for endometrial cancer. She underwent a total abdominal hysterectomy and bilateral salpingo-oophorectomy and had no evidence of disease in her lymph nodes. She is diagnosed with grade II endometrioid adenocarcinoma with invasion of over one-half of the myometrium.

In discussing the results with your patient you explain that, in general, the most important prognostic factor in endometrial cancer is the

a. histologic grade.
b. depth of myometrial invasion.
c. histologic type.
d. volume of original tumor.
e. presence of lymph node metastases.

63. A 21-year-old G1 P0 at 42 weeks gestation presents with mild contractions every 4 to 5 minutes and a cervical examination of 1 cm dilation, 50% effaced at −2 station. The fetal heart rate tracing reveals a baseline in the 140s with repetitive variable decelerations. The patient has had routine prenatal care and a normal fetal survey at 18 weeks gestation.

Which of the following is the *most likely* cause of these decelerations?

a. Uteroplacental insufficiency
b. Maternal hypotension
c. Oligohydramnios
d. Fetal acidemia
e. Fetal head compression

64. A 32-year-old G2 P2 patient is 7 days postpartum after repeat cesarean section. She presents to labor and delivery complaining of fever and chills. She is breast-feeding and her breasts are sore and tender.

In your differential diagnosis of fever in this patient, which of the following is *ruled out* because of the timing of the presentation?

a. Endomyometritis
b. Wound infection
c. Mastitis
d. Pyelonephritis
e. Onset of lactation, or milk "let-down"

65. A 30-year-old G0 P0 comes to you for a second opinion after being diagnosed with a uterine septum by her primary gynecologist. She and her husband are planning to start a family and want to know how this diagnosis would affect a future pregnancy.

You explain that the *most likely* complication associated with the presence of a uterine septum is which of the following?

a. Infertility requiring medical or surgical intervention
b. Recurrent miscarriage
c. Preterm labor and delivery
d. Breech or other malpresentation at term
e. A uterine septum should have no effects on the pregnancy, labor, or delivery

66. A 19-year-old woman presents for a routine examination. Her physical examination is entirely normal; however, her Pap smear shows a low-grade squamous intraepithelial lesion (LSIL). Subsequent colposcopy reveals a few lesions on the anterior aspect of the cervix, entirely visualized. The lesions turn white after treatment with acetic acid and have atypical vascularity. A biopsy returns CIN II or high grade squamous intraepithelial lesion (HSIL).

Which of the following is the standard of care for management of this patient?

a. Imiquimod (Aldara) treatment
b. Loop electrosurgical excision procedure
c. Cold knife cone biopsy
d. Cryotherapy
e. Simple hysterectomy
f. Radical hysterectomy
g. Radiation therapy

67. A 27-year-old G1 P0 at 40 weeks gestation presents to labor and delivery in active labor. Over the course of several hours, she progresses from 3 cm to 8 cm dilation. At this point, she is in

a. stage I of labor, latent phase.
b. stage I of labor, active phase.
c. stage II of labor, latent phase.
d. stage II of labor, active phase.
e. stage III of labor.

68. A couple comes in to see you because they have been unsuccessfully trying to conceive for the past 14 months. After a thorough history, you learn that the woman has never been pregnant and that the man has fathered no children to his knowledge. You also learn that the timing of their intercourse has been appropriate for conception.

As an initial work-up, what do you do next?

a. Do nothing because this couple is not "technically" infertile until they have been trying to conceive for 18 months
b. Semen analysis for the husband and menstrual tracking, ovulation tracking, and thyroid-stimulating hormone, follicle-stimulating hormone, and prolactin levels for the wife
c. Semen analysis and testicular biopsy for the husband and ovulation tracking, hysterosalpingogram, and laparoscopy for the wife
d. Offer the couple clomiphene citrate (Clomid) because it has few side effects and the best success rate in couples with unexplained infertility
e. Refer the couple to an infertility specialist capable of performing in vitro fertilization

69. A healthy 34-year-old G0 has been trying to conceive for the past 2 years. She has a history of regular menses each month, which are notable for severe cyclic pain cramping before and during menstruation. She also reports a history of dysmenorrhea and dyspareunia. On exam, her uterus is retroverted and not easily mobile. There is nodularity noted on the uterosacral ligaments. A pelvic ultrasound reveals a normal uterus and normal bilateral adnexa. Laparoscopy reveals stage I endometriosis.

Given that she is trying to conceive, the most appropriate management is which of the following?

a. Expectant management
b. Oral contraceptive pills
c. Lupron
d. Danazol
e. Resection and/or ablation of endometriosis implants

70. You are asked to give a lecture to medical students on the subject of ovarian and fallopian tube cancers.

When discussing the pathogenesis of ovarian cancer, you explain that most ovarian cancers are derived from

a. epithelial tissue.
b. germ cells.
c. sex cord tissue.
d. stromal tissue.
e. metastasis from other sites.

71. A 23-year-old G1 P0 at 35 weeks gestation presents with a vaginal gush of fluid. On sterile speculum examination, the patient has a pool of clear fluid in the vagina that is nitrazine and fern positive. She is contracting every 3 to

4 minutes, and her cervix on visualization appears to be dilated 2–3 cm.

Which of the following is the best course of action?

a. Tocolysis with magnesium or terbutaline
b. Betamethasone and tocolysis
c. Betamethasone and no tocolysis
d. Expectant management
e. Amnio/dye test

72. You are assisting in a gynecologic oncology clinic when you see a 57-year-old G3 P3 female who is a former nurse. She presents with 6 months of pelvic discomfort, increasing abdominal girth, and early satiety. Physical exam reveals a large abdomino/pelvic mass. A pelvic ultrasound and CT scan show a 10 cm right ovarian mass, ascites, and studding of the peritoneum. In your discussion with the patient you predict that this most likely represents a malignant ovarian neoplasm. She asks about the primary method of treatment for ovarian carcinoma.

You explain that the mainstay of treatment for epithelial ovarian neoplasms is

a. radiation alone.
b. right salpingo-oophorectomy.
c. total abdominal hysterectomy.
d. surgery plus platinum-based chemotherapy.
e. surgery followed by radiation therapy.
f. platin-based chemotherapy alone.

73. During your internship you are contacted by a family friend who was diagnosed with fallopian tube carcinoma while undergoing a hysterectomy for fibroids. She is concerned that she may have missed symptoms of her disease and wants to know which symptoms are associated with fallopian tube cancer.

You inform your patient that most women with fallopian tube carcinoma have no symptoms at all; however, the one symptom that is pathognomonic for fallopian tube cancer is

a. increasing abdominal girth.
b. watery vaginal discharge.
c. vague abdominal pain.
d. postmenopausal bleeding.
e. early satiety.

74. A 57-year-old Caucasian female on screening mammography is found to have a cluster of microcalcifications with a spiculated mass in the outer upper quadrant. The mass is not palpable on physical examination, and there are no skin changes or nipple discharge.

The next step in this patient's management should be which of the following?

a. Follow with clinical exams for development of palpable mass or skin changes
b. Stereotactic fine-needle aspiration

c. Ultrasound to localize tumor
d. Mastectomy for probable malignancy

75. A 41-year-old G2 P1 at 16 weeks gestation is concerned about her risk of fetal problems given her advanced maternal age. She undergoes evaluation with a triple screen test, survey ultrasound, and amniocentesis. Unfortunately, these tests are abnormal and the fetus is found to have multiple congenital abnormalities incompatible with life. After much discussion, the couple opts to terminate the pregnancy at 16 weeks gestation.

You tell them the safest option for termination would be

a. single-dose RU-486 (mifepristone) followed by vaginal prostaglandin administration.
b. suction curettage.
c. sharp curettage.
d. dilation of the cervix with laminaria, followed by evacuation of the uterus using forceps and suction curettage.
e. intra-amniotic instillation of hypertonic saline.
f. induction of labor with vaginal prostaglandins.
g. induction of labor with high-dose oxytocin.

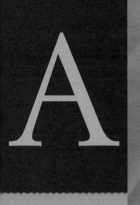

Answers

1. e (Chapter 16)

This patient's history is most consistent with genital herpes. In this setting, other sexually transmitted diseases should be screened for including gonorrhea, chlamydia, syphilis, hepatitis B, hepatitis C, and HIV. In addition, if there is any question about whether this is a primary or secondary outbreak, IgG and IgM titers to HSV can be sent.

2. e (Chapter 16)

There is no cure for a herpes simplex virus infection. Therefore, patients with oral and genital herpes may experience recurrent lesions. Acyclovir and several other antiviral medications can be used to decrease symptom outbreak by several days. In patients who get recurrent lesions, these medications can be used prophylactically to prevent outbreaks. Ceftriaxone is used to treat gonococcus, azithromycin to treat chlamydia, and metronidazole to treat bacterial vaginosis.

3. c (Chapter 26)

Two of the most common major side effects of gonadotropin ovulation induction are multiple gestation pregnancy and ovarian hyperstimulation syndrome. In more recent studies on the possible association between the use of ovulation induction agents and ovarian cancer have yet to prove an association. Polycystic ovarian syndrome can be a cause of infertility that can be treated with ovulation induction. It is not a side effect of ovulation induction.

4. c (Chapter 14)

Endometrial hyperplasia is the abnormal proliferation of glandular and stromal elements of the endometrium. It is a premalignant condition, not a preinvasive cancer. Like endometrial cancer, risk factors include conditions that predispose the patient to prolonged exposure to unopposed endogenous or exogenous estrogen such as obesity, early menarche, late menopause, chronic anovulation, and unopposed exogenous estrogen administration. Both hypertension and diabetes also increase the risk of endometrial hyperplasia and endometrial cancer. Endometrial hyperpla-

sia, if left untreated, could develop into endometrial cancer, depending on the degree of cytologic atypia. The risk of progression to endometrial cancer is 1% with simple hyperplasia, 3% with complex hyperplasia, 8% with atypical simple hyperplasia, and 29% with atypical complex hyperplasia.

5. c (Chapter 8)

Severe preeclampsia is defined as having any of the following: blood pressure greater than 160/110; >5000 mg of proteinuria in 24 hours; symptoms such as severe headache or epigastric pain, oliguria, pulmonary edema; or any of the elements of hemolytic anemia, elevated liver enzymes, low platelets (HELLP) syndrome. This patient meets several of these criteria. The ultimate treatment for severe preeclampsia is delivery of the fetus. Steps should be taken to stabilize the mother with antihypertensives and magnesium sulfate. Prior to 32 weeks gestation, it is common to use expectant management in order to gain fetal maturity and administer betamethasone. However, delivery should not be delayed in the setting of a headache and liver function test elevations. Immediate induction of labor for an anticipated vaginal delivery is therefore the management plan of choice. As part of this treatment, cervical ripening with prostaglandins, amniotomy, and pitocin may be used.

6. e (Chapter 5)

The classic signs of placental abruption include the sudden onset of painful contraction and vaginal bleeding. The uterus is typically firm and tender and the irritation of the separation will often initiate regular contractions. Even though the patient is having regular contractions, no cervical change is described; therefore, a diagnosis of labor cannot be made. Given the normal ultrasound, a placenta previa is unlikely. While placenta accreta can occur outside of the setting of a placenta previa, bleeding associated with this form of abnormal placentation occurs after delivery when the placenta does not separate from the uterine wall. The most common presentation of rupture of membranes is a gush of fluid rather than blood.

7. d (Chapter 27)

When a postmenopausal patient presents with vulvodynia or vulvar pruritus, cancer must be ruled out with biopsy of any visualized lesions. If there are no obvious lesions, colposcopy can be performed with acetic acid and any aceto-white lesions can be biopsied. Even in this patient, where Paget's syndrome may be suspected, a diagnosis should be made before more aggressive surgical therapy is attempted.

8. c (Chapter 3)

How patients are managed with genetic screens depends on their risk factors. African Americans are at an increased risk to carry the sickle-cell disease and thalassemias. They are not at increased risk for cystic fibrosis (CF); however, CF testing is now offered to all women during their prenatal care. The expanded maternal serum α-fetoprotein (MSAFP) that is used to screen for neural tube defects and Down syndrome is also offered to all women. Invasive prenatal diagnosis with amniocentesis or chorionic villus sampling (CVS) are only offered to those women of advanced maternal age or who are known to be at high risk for chromosomal or other genetic anomalies (e.g., balanced translocations). If the patient and her partner are known to be carriers of thalassemia, sickle-cell anemia, or cystic fibrosis, an amniocentesis should be performed to diagnose the fetus. Further, if the MSAFP was positive for a risk of either chromosomal abnormality or neural tube defect, an amniocentesis can be performed to confirm or rule out these diagnoses.

9. b (Chapter 24)

The failure rate of an intrauterine device (IUD) is extremely low—less than 2%. Of those who do conceive with the IUD in place, the spontaneous miscarriage rate is 40% to 50%. When an intrauterine pregnancy occurs with an IUD in place, the physician should attempt to remove the IUD by using gentle traction on the strings. If the device cannot be removed in this manner, it should be left in place for the duration of the pregnancy.

10. a (Chapter 20)

The four stages of puberty include gonadarche—the initiation of luteinizing hormone and follicle-stimulating hormone release, thelarche—the onset of breast development, pubarche—the development of pubic and axillary hair, and menarche—the onset of menstruation. The mean ages of the stages of puberty are as follows: gonadarche at age 8, thelarche at around age 9.8, pubarche at age 10.5, menarche at age 12.8. A normal variant of the order is gonadarche, pubarche, thelarche, menarche.

11. e (Chapter 16)

This patient's history is most consistent with syphilis, and is least consistent with genital herpes. Because of concern for other sexually transmitted diseases (STDs) with the transmission of syphilis, the battery of tests sent would include those for gonorrhea, chlamydia, HIV, hepatitis B, and hepatitis C. Syphilis would be screened for with an RPR or VDRL and confirmed with an FTA-ABS or MHA-TP. There would be no reason to send for antibody titers of HSV because even if the patient were exposed, it would not change the management of the situation. If the patient did develop lesions more consistent with HSV, it would be reasonable to send IgG and IgM titers if there is any question about whether this is a primary or secondary outbreak. These antibody titres are not sent routinely in patients requesting STD screens.

12. d (Chapter 16)

The history is now confirmed with the identification of the causative organism of syphilis, *Treponema pallidum*, which is seen as a motile spirochete on dark field microscopic inspection of a slide made from the contents of the chancre. Because this patient clearly has primary syphilis of only several weeks duration, she can be treated with a single dose of IM benzathine penicillin G. A positive screen for syphilis without any symptoms would be considered of unknown duration and the patient would be treated with three weekly doses of penicillin G. Tertiary syphilis and neurosyphilis both require treatment with IV penicillin.

13. b (Chapter 21)

This patient has secondary amenorrhea. While it is possible that her weight loss and stress have led to the secondary amenorrhea, it is still important to rule out other causes. The most common cause of secondary amenorrhea is pregnancy, thus the β-hCG should be ordered. Thyroid dysfunction and elevated prolactin levels can both lead to amenorrhea and should be ordered. An elevated follicle-stimulating hormone level would be seen in someone with early menopause; however, this 19-year-old patient with no other complaints is unlikely to have premature ovarian failure. Secondary amenorrhea can also be seen in patients with polycystic ovarian syndrome and, if these patients are showing signs of masculinization, a testosterone or dehydroepiandrosterone sulfate (DHEAS) level is reasonable; however, in this patient, without any particular symptoms, it is unnecessary.

14. a (Chapter 21)

The progesterone challenge test involves giving 7 to 14 days of progesterone, usually 10 mg of medroxyprogesterone acetate (Provera). Within a few days after the last dose of progesterone, the patient should undergo a menstrual period that may be lighter than usual, indicating that the uterus is receiving some estrogen stimulation. Estradiol levels are a poor way to measure estrogenization, particularly when the day of the cycle is unknown. An endometrial biopsy can show that the endometrial lining has had estrogen stimulation and can be done in the luteal phase. However, in this patient, it is unclear where in the cycle she is, so this test is not useful in this setting. The adrenocoricotropic hormone stim test for Addison's and CAH disease and the LH:FSH ratio once used in polycystic ovarian disease have little bearing on this clinical situation.

15. d (Chapter 31)

Molar pregnancies account for 80% of all gestational trophoblastic disease and 10% of molar pregnancies are incomplete. Incomplete moles result from the simultaneous fertilization of an ovum with two sperm and therefore typically have a triploid karyotype of 69,XXY. Unlike complete moles, incomplete molar pregnancies have an associated fetus with a triploid genotype and multiple anomalies. Incomplete moles most often result in miscarriages or missed abortions. Patients may have signs of hyperthyroidism, preeclampsia, and/or hyperemesis gravidarum, but these symptoms occur more infrequently in incomplete moles and are generally less pronounced than when they occur in complete moles. Incomplete moles are treated with immediate evacuation of the uterine contents and monitoring of serial β-hCGs to a level of zero. Methotrexate is not indicated at this point in treatment. Compared to complete moles, incomplete moles have a low rate of persistent disease and a low malignant potential.

16. b (Chapter 16)

This history and exam are most consistent with *Trichomonas vaginalis* infection. The finding of a "strawberry cervix" is considered pathognomonic for *Trichomonas*, but is only present about 10% of the time. Diagnosis is most often confirmed by visualizing the motile organism on wet prep. Overgrowth with *Gardnerella vaginalis* can lead to bacterial vaginosis. Diagnosis is made by a positive "whiff" test and identification of clue cells on the wet prep. This patient's history is not consistent with candidiasis, which is diagnosed by symptoms and identification of yeast on potassium hydroxide prep.

17. c (Chapter 16)

Cervical motion tenderness with no other findings on exam is most consistent with cervicitis. The two most common organisms that cause cervicitis are *N. gonorrhoeae* and *C. trachomatis*. The treatment for cervicitis should cover both gonococcus and chlamydia. The most common way to treat this is with a single IM dose of ceftriaxone and a week of PO doxycycline. Because of concern for patient compliance, a single dose of azithromycin is often used to treat chlamydia rather than the week course of doxycycline.

18. c (Chapter 20)

An elevated level of follicle-stimulating hormone (FSH) is used to confirm menopause when the diagnosis is uncertain. In a patient such as the one described, diagnosis would usually be made on a clinical basis. A human chorionic gonadotropic (hCG) would be sent in a younger woman to rule out pregnancy with secondary amenorrhea of 6 months. Thyroid-stimulating hormone (TSH) and prolactin would also be sent to rule out sources of secondary amenorrhea in a patient with an unknown etiology.

19. d (Chapter 8)

The classic triad of preeclampsia includes hypertension, proteinuria, and nondependent edema in the face and hand. Because edema can be nonspecific, clinicians decreasingly use it as a part of diagnosis. The generalized vasoconstriction seen in preeclampsia can result in visual changes, headaches, strokes, seizures, oliguria, renal failure, or liver capsule pain or rupture. These symptoms, along with worsening blood pressure, or changes in liver function tests, platelets, and creatinine are used to monitor the severity of the disease.

20. d (Chapter 32)

In a low-risk patient without worrisome family history or signs of malignancy on physical exam, breast masses can be followed clinically with frequent follow-up exams. Mammography is not recommended in young patients because of dense breast parenchyma leading to poor sensitivity. Definitive diagnosis can be made with a fine-needle aspiration (FNA) for cytology, which has a greater than 90% sensitivity for breast disease. A lumpectomy or wide local excision is unnecessary if the FNA is diagnostic. In this patient the most likely diagnosis is fibroadenoma; however, many patients will request a biopsy to make sure they do not have cancer.

21. c (Chapter 32)

A mammogram is used to assess breast masses in women older than 25. The needle aspiration can be diagnostic, so it should be used as the first step in achieving pathologic diagnosis. If this is nondiagnostic, an excisional biopsy should be performed for histologic diagnosis. An ultrasound is not helpful in this case because a fine-needle aspiration would have already revealed whether the mass was a cyst. Regardless, a pathologic specimen is still needed.

22. c (Chapter 8)

Magnesium sulfate is often used in obstetrics for tocolysis in the management of preterm labor and for seizure prophylaxis in the management of preeclampsia. The therapeutic range is between 4 and 8 meq/mL. Patellar reflexes are generally lost at 10 and respiratory depression occurs at 12. Levels of 20 or greater are associated with respiratory and cardiac arrest. This patient is at risk for respiratory and cardiac arrest. She should be given calcium gluconate to reverse the effects of magnesium sulfate. Because the patient is breathing on her own, intubation is not necessary at this point, although constant assessment is necessary in case the patient's condition should deteriorate. Terbutaline is a tolcolytic used to treat preterm labor and betamethasone is a steroid used antenatally to encourage fetal lung development when preterm delivery is anticipated between 28 and 34 weeks of gestation.

23. e (Chapter 21)

The most common cause of secondary amenorrhea is pregnancy, which is the most likely diagnosis that can be made from the tests being ordered. You would expect her to have an elevated β-hCG level confirming a pregnancy diagnosis. She doesn't have symptoms of either hypo- or hyperthyroidism or of elevated prolactin, but these tests are usually ordered as well. LH and FSH would not be ordered and would offer no helpful information in making a diagnosis. Many women who become pregnant may not realize they are until quite late into the pregnancy particularly if they are obese and/or have a history of oligomenorrhea.

24. d (Chapter 29)

The most common presenting symptom in endometrial cancer is abnormal vaginal bleeding. The diagnostic evaluation of postmenopausal bleeding requires an endometrial biopsy to evaluate the endometrial tissue. Modern endometrial biopsy is as accurate as a D&C, which was formally the gold standard in evaluation of postmenopausal bleeding. D&C only becomes necessary if an office endometrial biopsy cannot be obtained (e.g., cervical stenosis). While other diagnostic tools are helpful in evaluation of postmenopausal bleeding, sampling of the endometrial biopsy is required. A pelvic ultrasound is helpful in evaluating the endometrial stripe thickness (5 mm or less is normal in menopause), and in looking for endometrial polyps or fibroids and ovarian neoplasms as a source of bleeding. If not done within the past year, a Pap smear should be performed to evaluate the cervix for dysplasia and cancer. In rare instances, endometrial cancer can also be picked up on Pap smear. Checking thyroid-stimulating hormone and prolactin can be helpful in evaluating the patient for thyroid disease and hyperprolactinemia as sources of bleeding. An elevated follicle-stimulating hormone (FSH) level would confirm the postmenopausal state but this is already clinically evident. No surgical management should be pursued until a tissue diagnosis has been made. Hormone replacement therapy may be used to treat endometrial atrophy and postmenopausal symptoms, but only after a tissue diagnosis is made.

25. c (Chapter 9)

The fetal complications of diabetes vary widely, including abnormalities in growth ranging from intrauterine growth restricted and small-for-dates infants to fetal macrosomia with delayed organ maturity. Congenital anomalies are increased two- to threefold over pregnancies without diabetes. These range from cardiovascular abnormalities to neural tube defects and the rare caudal regression syndrome.

These infants are also at increased risk for sudden intrauterine fetal demise (IUFD). HgbA1c is predictive of the risk of congenital anomalies, but is not well associated with fetal macrosomia.

26. d (Chapter 9)

Offer induction of labor at 39 to 40 weeks gestation. This is done given the increased risk of intrauterine fetal demise (IUFD) after 40 weeks in diabetic pregnancies. Alternatively, in patients who are poorly controlled or are interested in earlier induction, induction is offered from 37 to 39 weeks gestation. However, before electively inducing labor prior to 39 weeks in these patients, fetal lung maturity should be verified. Cesarean section is offered if the estimated fetal weight is >4500 grams to avoid the increased incidence of shoulder dystocia and Erb's palsy.

27. d (Chapter 7)

Management of Rh-negative patients with RhoGAM has led to a marked reduction in women who have been sensitized to the Rh antigen. The recommendations for treatment with RhoGAM include use anytime in the first two trimesters with vaginal bleeding or amniocentesis, at the beginning of the third trimester at approximately 28 weeks gestation, during the third trimester if there are signs of a fetal-maternal hemorrhage that is greater than can be negated by the 28-week dose of RhoGAM, and postpartum if the infant is Rh positive. RhoGAM is not routinely given during preterm labor unless the patient has not yet received a dose in the pregnancy.

28. c (Chapter 17)

This patient's constellation of findings is most consistent with pelvic inflammatory disease (PID), likely complicated by Fitzhugh-Curtis syndrome with a perihepatitis leading to the right upper quadrant tenderness. Tubo-ovarian abscess should be on the differential diagnosis, but is unlikely with a normal pelvic ultrasound. Appendicitis should also be considered and, if the appendix is not visualized on ultrasound, a CT would more definitively rule this out.

29. d (Chapter 13)

Postmenopausal women presenting with vulvar pruritius or vulvodynia should usually have a biopsy to rule out vulvar dysplasia or cancer. If vulvar candidiasis seems to be the etiology of the symptoms, topical antifungals such as ketoconazole may be used first. If the diagnosis is lichen sclerosus, a medium to high potency topical steroid is the first line treatment. A topical 2% testosterone cream can also be used for lichen sclerosis only if there is evidence of atrophy secondarily. Surgical treatment of the effects of lichen sclerosis is rarely indicated. If the etiology of a vulvar biopsy is vulvar eczema, a topical hydrocortisone should be used. If it is secondary to atrophy, topical estrogen is the treatment of choice. Further, in a patient with vulvar atrophy who is not on hormone replacement therapy, oral supplementation should be offered as well.

30. d (Chapter 13)

This patient has a Bartholin's abscess. In this setting, the patient should undergo I&D with placement of a Word catheter. The patient should do sitz baths three to four times a day as well. If there is surrounding cellulitis as in this case, antibiotics to cover skin flora are used as well. If the patient merely had an enlarged Bartholin's cyst, sitz baths alone could be considered. With an abscess or cyst of this size, needle drainage would not be used because the cavity of the cyst would continue to be or become infected. If the Word catheter failed to treat the Bartholin's cyst, marsulialization could then be attempted. If this patient had been over age 40 when she first developed her Bartholin's cyst, then biopsy would be indicated. In the rare case of Bartholin's cyst malignancy, total excision is indicated.

31. c (Chapter 21)

Anorexia nervosa, exercise, weight loss, and stress can all lead to primary or secondary amenorrhea depending on their timing in a woman's life. Kallmann's syndrome, which is the congenital absence of GnRH and gonadal agenesis, causes only primary amenorrhea. Sheehan's syndrome, which is pituitary infarction, usually postpartum, and Asherman's syndrome are primarily associated with secondary amenorrhea.

32. a (Chapter 24)

Absolute contraindications for oral contraceptives (OCPs) include deep venolus thrombosis (DVT), pulmonary embolism, cardiovascular disease, stroke, breast or endometrial cancers, melanoma, hepatic tumor, or abnormal liver function (impacts clearance of hormones). Smoking over age 35 is a relative contraindication given their increased risk of DVT, stroke, heart disease, pulmonary embolism, and so on if they take OCPs. Other relative contraindications include migraines, diabetes mellitus, sickle-cell disease, hypertension, depression, and hyperlipidemia. Smokers over age 35 and lactating women are generally encouraged to use progesterone-only contraception such as the progesterone only pill or Depo-Provera. Lactation itself is only a relative contraindication to combined OCP use.

33. c (Chapter 8)

Check a glucose tolerance test by administering 100 mg of oral glucose and measuring a fasting blood glucose level immediately before the dose, then measuring levels at 1, 2, and 3 hours after the dose. This is the test used to confirm diabetes in pregnancy. Once the diagnosis is made, you can proceed to the next stage in management by diet, exercise, and/or insulin administration. Recently oral hyperglycemic agents have begun being used in pregnancy both alone and to decrease amounts of insulin required. They are still not used postpartum in breast-feeding women. Hemoglobin A_{IC} levels measure the concentration of glycosylated hemoglobin and are best used in patients with overt previously existing diabetes mellitus to correlate with glucose control over 6 to 8 weeks, not for the initial diagnosis of diabetes mellitus. Hemoglobin levels of <8.5% at conception are associated with a 3% incidence of congenital anomalies, whereas levels >8.5% at conception are associated with a 22% incidence of congenital anomalies.

34. e (Chapter 21)

This patient likely has primary amenorrhea due to a lack of GnRH pulsatility, which is secondary to the exercise and stress from her competitive athletics. Anorexia nervosa should also be considered in all women with primary and secondary amenorrhea, but there is no other evidence in this patient to support that diagnosis. The anatomic causes were each ruled out on physical exam. A transverse vaginal septum was ruled out by visualization of the cervix. In testicular feminization, the patient would have breast development, but no uterus—a normal bimanual exam of the pelvic organs and a visualized cervix rules this out. Patients with gonadal agenesis with either 46,XY or 46,XX karyotypes will not have breast development, although those with 46,XX will have a uterus.

35. b (Chapter 21)

When considering the differential diagnosis of amenorrhea, it should be classified as primary or secondary. Primary amenorrhea is the absence of menses prior to age 16. Anatomic etiologies include vaginal agenesis, transverse vaginal septum, Mayer-Rokitansky-Küster-Hauser syndrome and other müllerian anomalies that lead to no development of either the vagina or the uterus. Secondary amenorrhea is the absence of menses for three menstrual cycles or a minimum of 3 months. Hormonal etiologies are related to the lack of either release or response to GnRH, FSH, or LH. Noninherited etiologies of hypogonadotropic hypogonadism include anorexia, stress, and athletics. Asherman's syndrome, which is intrauterine scarring, is usually secondary to infection or instrumentation.

36. c (Chapter 4)

Ultrasound can be very useful in diagnosing potential causes of third-trimester bleeding. Placenta previa can be diagnosed with 90% accuracy on ultrasound. Most placental abruptions, however, are not seen on ultrasound. Diagnosis of placental abruption is made based on a detailed history of risk factors and the clinical picture of bleeding associated with abdominal pain. About 30% of abruptions are small and asymptomatic and are diagnosed after delivery. The presentation of uterine rupture can also be quite variable and requires a detailed history and physical. Uterine rupture can cause sudden abdominal pain, vaginal bleeding, fetal distress, abnormal abdominal contouring, cessation of uterine contractions, and regression of the presenting part. Cervical neoplasm is usually best diagnosed with Pap smear, colposcopy, biopsy, and CT. Vaginal laceration diagnosis requires a careful speculum exam.

37. a (Chapter 21)

This patient has signs and symptoms of hyperthyroidism with the weight loss, insomnia, and heat intolerance. These could also be put together as a constellation of stress or even anorexia; however, there is no specific test to diagnose either of these.

38. f (Chapter 24)

Absolute contraindications of the IUD include current pregnancy; undiagnosed abnormal bleeding; suspected gynecologic malignancy; acute cervical, uterine, or salpingeal infection; and history of pelvic inflammatory disease. Relative contraindications include nulliparity or desire for future childbearing, prior ectopic pregnancy, history of STDs, multiple sexual partners, moderate or severe dysmenorrhea, and congenital malformations of the uterus. Age and smoking history should not impact the decision to use an IUD in a multiparous woman. This patient should not, however, continue on combination OCPs given that her age and smoking history put her at increased risk for stroke and heart attack. This woman should have her vaginal bleeding thoroughly evaluated with a pregnancy test, TSH, PRL, endometrial biopsy, and pelvic ultrasound as indicated. If her work-up is reassuring and her period returns to normal, she could then be offered an IUD.

39. e (Chapter 5)

The primary cause of placental abruption is unknown but there are many associated precipitating and predisposing factors for abruption. Maternal hypertension is the most common risk factor for placental abruption accounting for 50% of cases, half of which are due to chronic hypertension and half of which are due to pregnancy-induced hypertension. Other risk factors for abruption include prior history of abruption, advanced maternal age, multiparity, cocaine abuse, and vascular disease. Some precipitating factors include trauma (external fetal version, motor vehicle accidents, abdominal trauma), sudden uterine volume loss (delivery of first twin, rupture of membranes with polyhydramnios), preterm premature rupture of membranes, and short umbilical cord. While abuse of most illicit drugs are associated with fetal complications, heroin abuse is *not* associated with placental abruption.

40. a (Chapter 2)

This patient has the diagnosis of a threatened abortion. If the physical exam shows a closed cervical os in the setting of

vaginal bleeding and either a viable intrauterine pregnancy (IUP) or a pelvic ultrasound and β-hCG that are too early to show a viable IUP, the diagnosis is threatened abortion. If the IUP cannot be seen, but there is not enough evidence to confirm an ectopic pregnancy, the patient is also considered to have a diagnosis of rule-out ectopic pregnancy. A patient in early pregnancy who presents with abdominal or pelvic pain and vaginal bleeding is at risk for ectopic pregnancy. The diagnostic work-up includes a history, physical examination, β-hCG, CBC, type and screen (T&S), and pelvic ultrasound. The definitions of ectopic pregnancy and the different types of abortions are described in Chapter 2.

41. b (Chapter 2)

In patients who have the diagnosis of rule-out ectopic pregnancy because their β-hCG is still too low for an intrauterine pregnancy (IUP) to be seen on pelvic ultrasound, the β-hCG should be checked every 48 hours. In a normally developing IUP, the β-hCG should double every 48 hours or at least increase by a minimum of 66%.

42. d (Chapter 14)

Typically, women with a bicornuate uterus should not have difficulty conceiving or carrying a pregnancy throughout the first trimester. Recurrent first-trimester miscarriages are more commonly associated with a uterine septum due to limited blood supply if the embryo implants on the septum. However, the primary problem in women with bicornuate uteri is one of small endometrial cavity size of either horn of the uterus. These women are therefore at increased risk of preterm labor and delivery. They may also experience second-trimester miscarriages as well as breech presentation and other malpresentations that predispose to cesarean section.

43. c (Chapter 22)

In patients with postmenopausal bleeding, it is imperative to make a diagnosis, because they are considered to have cancer until proved otherwise. The lesion in this woman's uterus is most likely an endometrial polyp; endometrial cancer would rarely present this way. This patient has none of the risk factors for endometrial cancer such as obesity, hypertension, or diabetes. Cervical cancer would be unlikely to present this way and would not be likely to occur so soon after a normal Pap smear. Excess endogenous or exogenous hormones could cause irregular postmenopausal bleeding; however, this patient is unlikely to be on hormones given that she has mild atrophy. Finally, the atrophy itself can cause postmenopausal bleeding, but the eroded site of the bleeding would usually be visualized and this would be rare with mild atrophy.

44. b (Chapter 6)

Preterm labor is described as contractions leading to cervical change before 37 weeks gestation. Risk factors include prior preterm delivery, prior preterm labor, PPROM, uterine abnormalities, polyhydramnios, bacterial vaginosis, placental abruption, preeclampsia, chorioamnionitis, and pregestational weight less than 50 kg. Multiple prior dilations of the cervix in a therapeutic or spontaneous abortion—particularly in the second trimester—has been associated with cervical incompetence; this would be unlikely in this patient, who has reached 31 weeks gestation. A large fetus can be correlated with polyhydramnios, which is correlated with preterm labor, but this association is weaker than prior preterm delivery. Teenage pregnancy is correlated with lower socioeconomic status, which is correlated with many complications of pregnancy, including preterm delivery, but again this is weaker than prior preterm delivery. Smoking is correlated more with lower birth weight than with preterm delivery.

45. c (Chapter 14)

Management of ovarian cysts varies with the age of the patient and the size and characteristics of the cyst. Cysts of any size in a premenarchal or postmenopausal female should be evaluated via laparotomy. In reproductive age women, cysts larger than 6 cm generally require surgical exploration and management given the risk of torsion and neoplasm. In this patient population, cysts smaller than 6 cm are typically physiologic cysts and will generally resolve on their own. Discomfort can be managed with NSAIDs and suppression of future cyst formation can be achieved with oral contraceptive pills. It is critical, however, that a repeat pelvic ultrasound be performed to assure regression of the cyst.

46. c (Chapter 6)

Chorioamnionitis is an infection of the fluid around the fetus that usually involves the uterus and the fetus as well. The five diagnostic signs include elevated maternal white blood count and temperature, fetal tachycardia, uterine tenderness, and vaginal discharge. If diagnosis is uncertain, amniocentesis can be performed and tested for Gram stain, glucose, white blood count, and culture. Neither the sensitivity nor the specificity of the first three tests is over 80% and, although culture is the gold standard, it can take several days to obtain results. Recently, it has been suggested that IL-6 in the amniotic fluid is more sensitive. This patient is likely in labor, but this cannot be confirmed without a cervical exam. She does not have either preterm labor or preterm rupture of membranes because she is not preterm (<37 weeks). The patient does have a fever, but that is not a diagnosis.

47. b (Chapter 6)

The management of shoulder dystocia, as with any emergency situation, should be discussed and considered frequently so that clinicians can react quickly and efficiently to its occurrence. A common algorithm would be to begin with suprapubic pressure to dislodge the anterior shoulder and the McRobert maneuver to increase the pelvic diameter. An episiotomy is commonly performed if these maneuvers fail. This is usually followed with the Wood screw maneuver, delivery of the posterior arm, or the Rubin maneuver. If none of these maneuvers works after several attempts, more aggressive interventions include fracturing the fetal clavicle. A final maneuver that has been described, the Zavanelli maneuver, is to place the fetal head back into the maternal pelvis and perform a cesarean delivery. Fundal pressure, which would further impact the anterior fetal shoulder behind the maternal pubic symphysis, is *not* recommended.

48. c (Chapter 4)

Fetal heart rates are evaluated, paying attention to baseline rate, variability, accelerations, and decelerations. The baseline rate should be between 110 and 160 bpm. Minimal and absent variability are worrisome for hypoxia and acidemia of the fetus, with absent variability being worse than minimal. Three types of decelerations have been described—early, variable, and late. Early decelerations begin and end with contractions and are thought to be a result of fetal head compression. Variable decelerations are sharp drops in the fetal heart rate with quick return to baseline and can be either isolated or correlated with contractions; these are believed to result from compression of the umbilical cord. Late decelerations begin after the contraction has begun and end after it has ended. These are usually shallow and can be quite subtle and difficult to detect. Late decelerations are correlated with decreased placental perfusion that can be secondary to inadequate blood flow to the uterus or increased vascular resistance of the placenta.

49. b (Chapter 32)

Nulliparous women are at a 3:1 relative risk versus parous women. Obesity is her next risk factor, putting her at 2 times the risk. Having a first-degree relative who developed unilateral breast cancer premenopausally leads to a 1.8 relative risk. Women who reach menopause after age 50 are at 1.5 times the risk, whereas OCP use and short-term HRT show no evidence of increasing breast cancer risk.

50. d (Chapter 32)

In advanced stage breast cancer in premenopausal women, chemotherapy has been shown to significantly improve survival regardless of hormone receptor status. The current chemotherapy regimen is 6 cycles of some combination of Adriamycin, cytoxan, fluorouracil, and methotrexate. Chemotherapy offers a response rate of 15% to 40%. Node-positive postmenopausal women are treated with tamoxifen for 2 to 5 years if estrogen receptor (ER) status is positive, and not used if ER negative.

ANSWERS

51. b (Chapter 20)

It is generally accepted that the indications for hormone replacement therapy (HRT) include symptomatic relief of postmenopausal symptoms and protection from osteoporosis. Estrogen replacement in a postmenopausal patient has been shown to decrease the risk of osteoporosis, and urogenital atrophy. Because isolated estrogen can increase the risk of endometrial cancer, this is given in conjunction with either continuous or cyclic progesterone to protect the uterus. There is no long-term evidence that combination HRT increases the risk of uterine, breast, or colon cancer. HRT has no known effect of liver cancer.

52. a (Chapter 14)

Fibroids may grow in size during pregnancy due to the stimulatory effects of high levels of estrogen, progesterone, and growth factors. Although growth of fibroids during pregnancy cannot be predicted, studies estimate that about half of fibroids will significantly increase in size during pregnancy, particularly during the first trimester. Rapid growth can result in decreased blood supply to the fibroid and necrosis known as "red" or "hemorrhagic" degeneration and pain. Fibroids during pregnancy may cause local abdominal tenderness, low-grade fever, and moderate leukocytosis. This can usually be treated with analgesics and observation. Myomas that are symptomatic and pedunculated may be clamped and ligated. Other possible complications of fibroids greater than 3 cm include increased rates of preterm labor, placental abruption, fetal malpresentation, pelvic pain, and cesarean section. Fibroids located in the cervix or in the lower uterine segment may obstruct the birth canal during vaginal delivery. Fibroids should otherwise not be removed during pregnancy or delivery given their risk of bleeding, which may necessitate a hysterectomy.

53. a (Chapter 11)

Although none of the substances are recommended in pregnancy, only alcohol, which is associated with fetal alcohol syndrome and with cardiac defects in particular, is associated with congenital anomalies. Cocaine use during pregnancy has been correlated with central nervous system effects and developmental delay in the exposed child. Tobacco use has been correlated with small for gestational age fetuses and increased respiratory disease in childhood. Caffeine and opiates don't have particularly noted fetal effects, although fetuses exposed to opiates throughout pregnancy will need to be weaned off the drug postpartum.

54. d (Chapters 14, 25)

Most women with fibroids are asymptomatic. However, when fibroids cause symptoms such as pelvic pain, bleeding, or infertility, treatment can be considered. Oral contraceptive pills are contraindicated in patients with fibroids because they result in increased estrogen levels, which can stimulate fibroid growth (similar to growth from increased estrogen levels during pregnancy). Medical treatment of fibroids can range from use of NSAIDs, Provera (medroxyprogesterone), Danazol (danocrine), and Depo-Lupron (leuprolide acetate). All of these work to decrease circulating estrogen levels and thereby shrink fibroids. Unfortunately, leiomyoma often recur after discontinuation of these medicines. Surgical treatment will vary depending on the location of the fibroids and desire for future fertility. Submucosal fibroids, which can cause bleeding and result in fertility difficulties, can be resected via hysteroscopy. This patient's symptoms—heavy bleeding and mild anemia—are most likely due to submucosal fibroids. Given this and her desire for future fertility, hysteroscopic myomectomy would be the best therapeutic approach. Intramural and subserosal fibroids, which are often the cause of pelvic pressure, pain, and urinary symptoms, can be removed via laparoscopic or abdominal myomectomy if future fertility is desired. For the patient with severe symptoms who no longer desires childbearing, vaginal or abdominal hysterectomy can be offered depending on the size of the uterus.

55. e (Chapter 25)

Emergency contraception can be offered to a patient if unprotected intercourse has occurred no more than 72 hours prior to treatment. The "morning after pill" or postcoital pill is a two-dose regimen of 100 µg of ethinyl estradiol combined with levonorgestrel, given 12 hours apart. The high-dose hormones in this regimen can cause nausea, therefore an antiemetic should be given to the patient prior to each OCP dose. To complete the patient's evaluation, a pregnancy test should be performed prior to administering the morning after pill and again if the patient does not have a menstrual period within 6 weeks. The patient should be offered an STD screen as well. Recently, emergency contraception, which is progesterone only, has been used to decrease side effects. It is unclear whether its efficacy is markedly different.

56. d (Chapter 1)

The gravity and parity designation is as follows: gravity is the number of pregnancies that patient has had and parity is the number of deliveries that a patient has had, in which a twin delivery counts as one delivery. Parity is further broken down into the four-digit designation of term, preterm, aborted, and living (TPAL). A term pregnancy is any gestation past 37 weeks. A preterm pregnancy is any gestation that is longer than 20 weeks but less than 37 weeks or results in a fetus that weighs more than 500 grams. Aborted pregnancies include both spontaneous abortions and elective terminations of pregnancy. Living refers to the total number of living children. This patient has had 5 previous pregnancies and is currently pregnant, so her gravity is 6. She has had 2 term deliveries, 1 preterm pregnancy (remember, a twin delivery is one delivery), 2 miscarriages, and 4 living children. Thus, her parity would be 2-1-2-4.

57. d (Chapter 1)

Nägele's rule of dating a pregnancy stems from the fact that the estimated date of confinement (EDC) is 280 days from the last menstrual period (LMP). On average, that will be 9 months and 1 week from the LMP. Thus, Nägele's rule is to subtract 3 months and add 7 days (and 1 year).

58. d (Chapter 1)

Dating of a pregnancy is important to establish as soon as possible. Usually, 280 days from the LMP is used as the EDD, which is then confirmed by physical examination and eventually a second-trimester ultrasound. However, physical examination is not a particularly accurate way to date a pregnancy, and ultrasound becomes less accurate as a pregnancy continues. Ultrasound is considered to have a 7% to 10% range of accuracy, and a rule of thumb is that it can be off by up to 1 week in the first trimester, 2 weeks during the second trimester, and 3 weeks during the third trimester. Thus, in a patient who had no clear LMP to date the pregnancy, a transvaginal ultrasound performed as early as possible would be the best way to date this pregnancy.

59. c (Chapter 31)

This patient most likely has an invasive molar pregnancy that may be the result of persistent molar disease (75%) or recurrent disease (25%). Most patients with invasive moles are diagnosed as a result of plateauing or rising β-hCG levels following molar evacuation. Invasive moles typically penetrate locally into the myometrium and into the peritoneal cavity. Despite this, invasive moles rarely metastasize, but it is still important that the patient be evaluated for possible metastatic disease. The mainstay of treatment for invasive molar pregnancies is chemotherapy; single agent for nonmetastatic disease as this patient has or multiagent chemotherapy for metastatic disease. Radiation therapy is only indicated for treatment of brain and liver metastases. As with all forms of gestational trophoblastic disease, close follow-up with serial β-hCG levels and reliable birth control during the surveillance period is imperative to successful treatment. There is no contraindication to contraceptives containing estrogen or progesterone.

60. c (Chapter 12)

Postpartum hemorrhage is defined as blood loss greater than 500 cc after vaginal delivery or greater than 1000 cc after cesarean delivery. It can be caused by any of the answers mentioned here, including abnormal placentation; uterine atony; maternal trauma of the perineum, vagina, cervix, or uterus; and coagulation defects. Of all the etiologies mentioned, this patient's hemorrhage is most consistent with uterine atony. This patient has multiple risk factors for uterine atony, including a multiple gestation, chorioamnionitis, prolonged labor, exposure to oxytocin, and multiparity.

61. c (Chapter 29)

Nearly 75% of endometrial cancers are endometrioid adenocarcinomas.

62. a (Chapter 29)

The histologic grade is the most important prognostic factor in endometrial cancer. The tumor grade tells what percent of the tumor shows characteristics of solid growth patterns. Grade 1 is less than 5% solid growth, grade 2 is 6% to 50% solid growth, and grade 3 is greater than 50% solid growth. Other important prognostic factors include depth of myometrial invasion, histologic type (adenocarcinoma versus clear cell versus papillary serous, etc.), pelvic lymph node metastases, original tumor volume, adnexal metastases, and positive peritoneal washings.

63. c (Chapter 7)

Repetitive decelerations are never reassuring and indicate that close attention needs to be paid to the fetal heart tracing until their resolution. The most worrisome repetitive decelerations are late ones that can be a result of uteroplacental insufficiency or maternal hypotension. Repetitive early decelerations can result from descent of the fetal head that leads to head compression with contractions. Variable decelerations result from cord compression. In the postdate patient, spontaneous or repetitive variable decelerations most likely result from oligohydramnios, which leads to more frequent cord compression. Fetal acidemia usually leads to decreased fetal heart rate variability rather than decelerations.

64. e (Chapter 12)

Although the onset of lactation can commonly cause a fever in the first 24 to 72 hours postpartum, it is unlikely to do so 7 days postpartum. However, mastitis, a wound infection, or endomyometritis are all quite likely to result in fever. Patients who deliver by cesarean section, as well as many patients who deliver vaginally, may have had an indwelling catheter for 24 hours, which can predispose them to urinary infections. Thus, while pyelonephritis isn't the most likely diagnosis, it should be in the differential diagnosis and ruled out with urinalysis and culture and physical examination.

65. b (Chapter 14)

The most likely complication is an increased rate of miscarriage due to implantation on a largely avascular septum. Later in pregnancy, uterine septum is associated with increased risk of preterm labor, abnormal fetal life, and cesarean section.

66. b (Chapter 28)

Although this patient had a LSIL Pap smear, her biopsy showed HSIL. Thus, in this patient with HSIL, the standard of care is to perform a cervical conization also known as a LEEP, LLETZ, or loop using electrocautery. There is debate about whether the margins of the LEEP are too distorted by the electrocautery; however, this is currently the most common management of these lesions. A cold knife cone biopsy could also be performed, but is likely to cost more as it must be done in the OR and is not absolutely necessary. Cryotherapy and laser could also be used, but it is difficult to tell how clean the margins are since there is no tissue to send to pathology when these techniques are utilized. Simple hysterectomy is usually reserved for patients with early or preinvasive cervical cancer and for those who have completed childbearing. Radiation therapy and radical hysterectomy are commonly used to treat advanced cervical cancer, but the associated morbidity should be avoided in this young patient with precancerous disease. Although cervical dysplasia and condyloma are both associated with exposure to the human papilloma virus, imiquimod or Aldara is a topical therapy for vulvar condyloma and is not indicated in the direct treatment of cervical dysplasia.

67. b (Chapter 4)

Labor is described as having three stages. Stage I is from the onset of labor until complete dilation of the cervix, stage II is from the end of stage I until delivery of the infant, and stage III is from the end of stage II until delivery of the placenta. Stage I of labor is divided into the latent and active phases. The latent phase is from the onset of labor until the rate of change of cervical dilation reaches its maximum; this usually occurs between 3–5 cm. The active phase is from the point of maximum rate of change until almost full dilation, where some patients will go through a transition or deceleration phase as they dilate the remaining 0.5 to 1.0 cm.

68. b (Chapter 26)

Infertility is the inability to conceive after 12 months of unprotected intercourse. At this point, it is reasonable to begin an initial diagnostic evaluation. Care should be taken to evaluate both the female and the male partner since 40% of infertility is due to female factors and 40% is due to male factors. For the female partner, the initial investigation should include a thorough history and physical, demonstration of ovulation (tracking the menstrual cycle, measuring the basal body temperature, monitoring the cervical mucus, measuring the midluteal progesterone, and documenting any premenstrual or ovulatory symptoms), and some baseline lab values (TSH, FSH, and prolactin). For the male partner, the initial investigation should include a thorough history and physical and a semen analysis to evaluate the sperm volume, motility, and morphology. This basic work-up can be done easily and without the assistance of a reproductive endocrinologist.

69. e (Chapter 15)

Endometriosis is the presence of endometrial cells outside the uterine cavity. The treatment options vary widely. For a patient in whom endometriosis is suspected but symptoms do not severely affect quality of life, symptoms can be managed with NSAIDs, oral contraceptive pills, or Depo-Provera, all of which induce a state of pseudopregnancy by suppressing ovulation and menstruation. Danazol, an androgen derivative, and Lupron, a GnRH agonist, can be used to induce a reversible state of pseudomenopause by suppressing FSH and LH and consequently decreasing the level of estrogen. These are all temporizing measures. For a patient who is trying to conceive, fulguration of endometrial implants has been found to increase the rate of fertility depending on the stage of the disease.

70. a (Chapter 30)

There are a variety of benign (80%) and malignant (20%) ovarian tumors. Over 65% of ovarian tumors and 95% of ovarian cancers arise from the coelomic epithelium on the ovary. Germ cell tumors account for 15% to 20% of ovarian neoplasms. Sex cord–stromal tumors account for 5% to 10% and Krukenberg or metastatic tumors from other primary cancers account for 5% of ovarian tumors.

71. d (Chapter 6)

The management of PPROM is widely debated. Before 32 to 34 weeks gestation, most institutions use betamethasone to help induce fetal lung maturity; however, it is rarely used beyond 34 weeks gestation. The use of tocolysis varies greatly, ranging from no use whatsoever to tocolysis at less than 26 to 28 weeks gestation to tocolysis until 34 weeks, as in preterm labor. Many patients with PPROM go into labor within 48 to 72 hours; for those who don't, the risks of prolonged ROM include chorioamnionitis, abruption, and cord prolapse. With these risks weighed against the risks of prematurity, induction of labor has been considered between 32 and 36 weeks gestation. Some institutions send the amniotic fluid for fetal lung maturity testing and induce labor if it is mature. Tocolysis at 35 weeks gestation would not be used in this patient, thus the most appropriate plan presented would be expectant management. If the patient stopped contracting, many practitioners would induce or augment labor at that point.

72. c (Chapter 30)

The mainstay of treatment for ovarian cancer is surgery with complete surgical staging, including total abdominal hysterectomy, bilateral salpingo-oophorectomy (TAHBSO), omentectomy, and cytoreduction of any visible tumor. The patient then undergoes chemotherapy, typically with cisplatin and taxol.

73. a (Chapter 30)

Most fallopian tube cancers are asymptomatic and diagnosed only incidentally during an abdominal procedure. Watery vaginal discharge is the hallmark of fallopian tube carcinomas. Other symptoms include vague low abdominal pain and discomfort; symptoms that can be mistaken for many common illnesses.

74. b (Chapter 32)

Identification of nonpalpable lesions by mammography is critical for earlier diagnosis. Although these microcalcifications can be due to a benign condition, 25% to 30% of such characteristics on mammography are associated with an invasive breast cancer. If the cluster of microcalcifications is associated with a well-demarcated mass, it is more likely to be benign. The chance of benign diagnosis is much lower when associated with an irregular spiculated mass. Ultrasound is not useful because the mass is not palpable, so a stereotactic fine-needle aspiration would be necessary for sampling. Tissue diagnosis is recommended prior to major surgical treatments.

75. d (Chapter 25)

RU-486 has a 90% success rate but is only an option for first-trimester terminations and is best when used before 7 weeks. Dilation and suction evacuation, and induction of labor via intraamniotic instillation of hypertonic saline, or induction of labor with vaginal prostaglandins and/or Pitocin are valid options. Dilation and evacuation of the uterus is the method of choice as it has been shown to be safer than other techniques for patients between 13 and 16 weeks gestation. This differs from suction curettage in that the cervix is typically dilated for several hours using laminaria osmotic dilators. Also, special forceps are used to assist in evacuation of the uterus. Lastly, identification of the main fetal parts should be performed to ensure complete removal. Prior to termination of pregnancy, the patient should have her Rh status checked and should be given RhoGAM (Rh IgG) if indicated.

ANSWERS

References

American College of Obstetricians and Gynecologists. 2002 Compendium of Selected Publications. Washington DC: American College of Obstetricians and Gynecologists, 2002.

American College of Obstetricians and Gynecologists. Precis: An Update in Obstetrics and Gynecology. Washington DC: 1998.

American College of Obstetricians and Gynecologists. Prolog: Gynecologic Oncology and Surgery. 3rd ed. Washington DC: 1996.

American Joint Committee on Cancer. Manual for Staging of Cancer, 4th ed. Philadelphia: J.B. Lippincott; 1992:147.

Beckman CC, Ling F. Obstetrics and Gynecology for Medical Students. Baltimore: Williams and Wilkins, 1998.

Berek JS, Adashi EY, Hillard PA. Novak's Gynecology. 13th ed. Baltimore: Williams and Wilkins, 2002.

Blackwell RE. Women's Medicine. Boston: Blackwell Science, 1996.

Braunwald E, et al. Harrison's Principles of Internal Medicine. 15th ed. New York: McGraw-Hill, 2001.

Burnett AF. Clinical Obstetrics and Gynecology: A Problem-Based Approach. Malden, MA: Blackwell Science, 2001.

Carlson K, Eisenstat S, Frigoletto F, Schiff I. Primary Care of Women. St. Louis, MO: Mosby–Yearbook, 1995.

Chamberlain G, Malvern J. Lecture Notes on Gynaecology. Oxford: Blackwell Science, 1996.

Champion RH. Textbook of Dermatology. 5th ed. Oxford: Blackwell Science, 1992:2852.

Champion RH, Burton JL, Ebling FJG, eds. Textbook of Dermatology. 6th ed. Malden: Blackwell Science, 1998.

Clark SL, et al. Critical Care Obstetrics. 3rd ed. Malden: Blackwell Science, 1997.

Cotran R, Robbins S, Kumar V. Robbins Pathologic Basis of Disease. Philadelphia: WB Saunders, 1999.

Cox FEG, ed. Modern Parasitology: A Textbook of Parasitology. 2nd ed. Oxford: Blackwell Science, 1993.

Creasy RK. Management of Labor and Delivery. Malden: Blackwell Science, 1997.

Crissey JT, Lang H, Parish LC. Manual of Medical Mycology. Cambridge: Blackwell Science, 1995.

Cunningham FG, et al. Williams Obstetrics. 21st ed. New York: McGraw-Hill, 2001.

DeCherney A, Pernoll M. Current Obstetric and Gynecologic Diagnosis and Treatment. 9th ed. New York: McGraw-Hill, 2003.

DiSaia PH, Creasman WT. Clinical Gynecologic Oncology. 6th ed. St. Louis, MO: Mosby-Yearbook, 1998.

Emans SJ, Laufer MR, Goldstein DP. Pediatric and Adolescent Gynecology. 4th edition. Philadelphia, PA: Lippincott–Raven, 1998.

Fitzpatrick TB, et al. Color Atlas and Synopsis of Clinical Dermatology. 2nd ed. New York: McGraw-Hill, 1994.

Frederickson G, Wilkins-Haug L. OB/GYN Secrets. Philadelphia: Hanley & Belfus, 1998.

Gabbe SG, Niebyl RJ, Simpson JL. Obstetrics: Normal and Problem Pregnancies. 4th ed. New York: Churchill Livingston, 2002.

Hacker N, Moore JG. Essentials of Obstetrics and Gynecology. Philadelphia: WB Saunders, 1997.

Heffner, Linda. Human Reproduction at a Glance. Oxford: Blackwell Science, 2002.

Hunter JAA, Savin JA, Dahl MV. Clinical Dermatology. 2nd ed. Oxford: Blackwell Science, 1995.

Katzung B. Basic and Clinical Pharmacology. 8th ed. New York: Lange Medical Books/McGraw-Hill, 2001.

Kurman RJ. Blaustein's Pathology of the Female Genital Tract. 5th edition. New York: Springer-Verlag, 2002.

Mead PB, Hagar DW, Sebastian F. Infection Protocols for Obstetrics and Gynecology. 2nd ed. Montvale: Medical Economics Publishing, 2000.

Meyer MB, Tonascia JA. Maternal smoking, pregnancy complications, and perinatal mortality. Am J Obstet Gynecol 1977;128:494.

Norwitz E, Schorge J. Obstetrics & Gynecology at a Glance. Malden, MA: Blackwell Science, 2001.

Parker SL, Tong T, Bolden S, Wingo PA. Cancer Statistics, CA Cancer J Clin 1996;46:5–27.

Pernoll ML. Obstetrics and gynecology. In: Rypins' Clinical Sciences Review. 16th ed. Philadelphia: Lippincott, 2001.

Repke, JT. Intrapartum Obstetrics. New York: Churchill Livingston, 1996.

Retzky SS, Rogers RM. Clinical Symposia: Urinary Incontinence in Women. Vol. 47. Summit: Ciba Geigy, 1995.

Robbins S, Cotran R, Kumar V. Robbins Pathologic Basis of Disease. Philadelphia: WB Saunders, 1991:1158–1159.

Rock J, Thompson JD. TeLinde's Operative Gynecology. 8th edition. Philadelphia, PA: Lippincott-Raven: 1997.

Sadler TW. Langman's Medical Embryology. 6th ed. Baltimore: Williams & Wilkins, 2000.

Scott JR, et al. Danforth's Obstetrics and Gynecology. 8th edition. Baltimore: Lippincott-Williams & Wilkins, 1998.

Singer A, et al. Lower Genital Tract Precancer: Colposcopy, Pathology and Treatment. 2nd ed. Oxford: Blackwell Science, 2000.

Speroff L, Darney P. A Clinical Guide for Contraception. 2nd ed. Baltimore: Williams and Wilkins, 1996.

Speroff L, Glass RH, Kase NG. Clinical Gynecologic Endocrinology and Infertility. 6th ed. Baltimore: Williams & Wilkins, 1996.

Stenchever M, et al. Comprehensive Gynecology. 4th ed. St. Louis, MO: Mosby Yearbook, 2001.

Stenchever MA, Goff B. Atlas of Clinical Gynecology. Vol. II: Gynecologic Pathology. Philadelphia, PA: Appleton & Lange, 1998.

Weinberger SE. Principles of Pulmonary Medicine. 3rd ed. Philadelphia: WB Saunders, 1998.

World Health Organization Scientific Group. Gestational Trophoblastic Disease. Technical Report Series 692. Geneva: WHO, 1983.

Index